Life Saving Sleep

New Horizons in Mental Health Treatment

Better sleep heals: stress, anxiety, depression,
posttraumatic stress, suicidal thoughts, suicidal behaviors,
sedative dependency, sleeping pill use, headaches,
brain fog, and nightly trips to the bathroom.

Barry Krakow, MD

ADVANCE PRAISE

"Barry Krakow is one of the godfathers of sleep medicine. His ideas and publications have influenced the field as much as any provider within the past 30 years. This book illustrates a number of his principles and teachings and is a must-read for anyone seeking to improve their sleep quality. Beyond publishing more than 100 research papers with over 5000 citations, I personally find Barry's books truly shine in communicating directly to patients and the public, and *Life Saving Sleep* is his best work yet."

> Matthew Rodgers, MD
> Sleep and Family Medicine
> Medical Director Virtual Health Europe

"An impassioned clarion call! Both the general public and healthcare professionals alike will benefit from Dr. Krakow's experience, knowledge, and insights regarding the foundation of vibrant health and wellbeing: restorative sleep. This book will empower patients and professionals to find real solutions for vexing sleep problems."

> Robert J. Vanecek, PhD, ABPP, BCB, BCB-HRV
> Clinical Health Psychologist

"No one understands the nexus of sleep disorders and mental health better than Dr. Krakow. *Life Saving Sleep* should be included in every medical school's curriculum. This holistic guide is a must-read for every healthcare practitioner and highly recommended for everyone who sleeps."

> A. Joseph Borelli, Jr., MD
> Medical Director/Board of Directors of bleepsleep.com

"Sleeping pills will not improve your sleep quality, but this book will, and so much of physical and mental health depends on quality sleep."

> Chris Aiken, MD
> Editor of the *Carlat Psychiatry Report;* Mood disorders section editor, *Psychiatric Times*; Instructor in Clinical Psychiatry Wake Forest University, Author of *The Depression and Bipolar Workbook*

"Dr. Barry Krakow's latest book, *Life Saving Sleep*, is designed as a 'sleeper's manual' offering practical techniques for dealing with sleep disorders from the common to the complex. But it is far more than that. The book provides a radical paradigm shift in the way sleep disorders are understood in psychiatry. Where the disorders of sleep have long been treated as a result of psychiatric disturbances, Dr. Krakow's insight is to see them as a cause, rather than a result, of mental afflictions. This profound change promises new, more effective approaches to the problems of both mind and sleep."

> Forouz Jowkar, MS, PhD
> Advanced Fellow, American Academy of Anti-Aging and
> Functional Medicine

"Dr. Krakow has written a powerful manual for optimal sleep and mental wellness by masterly integrating a number of holistic concepts. He is one of the few sleep doctors in the world who not only understands breathing-related sleep disorders, but is able to properly diagnose and treat many patients that don't benefit from conventional treatment by the sleep community. This is a must-read book for anyone who breathes or sleeps."

> Steven Y. Park, MD
> Author of Amazon best-selling book, *Sleep Interrupted: A physician reveals the #1 reason why so many of us are sick and tired.*

"Dr. Krakow's *Life Saving Sleep* is a wake-up call! The connection between sleep quality and our mental and physical health is too often under-estimated or completely overlooked. This book explains why sleep matters so much as well as what can go wrong. Even more importantly, it shares in plain language the most effective devices, techniques and therapies that can ensure we get a good night's sleep. From my own experience, Dr Krakow introduced me to the ASV device, and it is no exaggeration to say that it has changed my life!"

> Frits Dirk van Paasschen,
> Author of the *Disruptors' Feast* and Former CEO of Coors Brewing
> Company and Starwood Hotels and Resorts

"Many psychiatric conditions occur with obvious sleep symptoms, yet mental health professionals may overlook these co-occurring sleep disorders. Dr. Krakow's astute and unique approach bridges this gap in healthcare. Like no other book in this field, *Life Saving Sleep*, is an eye-opener that will change the way you think, feel, and sleep for the rest of your life."

    Stephen B. Safer, LCSW

    Clinical Psychotherapist and Author of *UniverseSoul* and

    The Infinity Frequency

"Well written, entertaining; complex information explained succinctly in easily understandable ways. Greatly broadened the scope of my knowledge on the mental health-sleep interface. And I found immediate and accessible knowledge to enhance clinical efficacy in my patients."

    Jerald M. Gottlieb, PhD, PC

    Clinical Psychologist

"In his excellent and clearly written book, Dr. Krakow describes sleep problems with feeling and provides an empathetic reaction to the many symptoms. He describes comprehensive treatment approaches with realistic methods including pros and cons. I believe his book will be of great help to many people struggling with poor sleep."

    Gerold Yonas, PhD

    Physicist, engineer, and former Chief Scientist of President Reagan's

    Strategic Defense Initiative and Author of *Death Rays and Delusions*, a

    firsthand account of the creation of the "Star Wars" beam weapon program

"I have followed Dr. Krakow's brilliant research career for many years. His knowledge of sleep and insomnia have enlightened me and allowed for improved patient care. You will find his approach much different. The book not only describes sleep disorders beautifully, he gives you the "how" to help you regain restful sleep. I highly recommend a careful read to initiate the self-healing, which is possible with the information."

    James E. Metz, DDS, Diplomat ABDSM

    Founder of The Metz Center, Columbus, Ohio, and

    The Metz Appliance for control of obstructive sleep apnea

"As a patient of Dr. Krakow, I finally learned how to get a good night's sleep. His new book is an outstanding how-to guide to teach chronic insomniacs and others with complex sleep disorders the most effective ways to gain restful and quality sleep."

Zack Schuler

Founder and CEO, NINJIO, LLC

"Dr. Krakow's research and clinical practice have made a huge difference to my own health and happiness. Friends have been coming to me with their sleep problems for a decade now—sometimes desperately, often hopelessly—and always overwhelmed by uncertainty. While most sleep advice covers only narrow or outdated models, this book turns the good doctor's wealth of experience into a practical, up-to-date guide for the hopeless, desperate and overwhelmed."

Patri Friedman, Coauthor of *Seasteading: How Floating Nations Will Restore the Environment, Enrich the Poor, Cure the Sick, and Liberate Humanity from Politicians,*

Founder, Seasteading Institute, Ephemerisle Festival, GP, Pronomos Capital

"Dr. Krakow has clearly elucidated the unfortunate stumbling blocks that prevent practitioners in both primary and psychiatric care from fully grasping the detrimental effects of sleep dysfunction. As a physician using CPAP, I found myself coming to grips with my own lack of knowledge in an area I felt I knew well. Reading Dr. Krakow's book as he connected the dots between sleep dysfunction and mental health, as well as the brain, heart, and vascular damage, allowed me to look into my own mirror of medical blind spots and commit to reevaluating the real importance of this medical stepchild: sleep dysfunction. Thank you, Dr. Krakow for this long overdue examination of such a quiet but pervasive shadow that untreated can be lethal. A must-read for all of us treating patients."

Jeff Stuart Sollins, MD

Internal and Wholistic Medicine

Founder, Bridges in Medicine Healthcare

"Dr. Krakow has done it yet again with his new book, *Life Saving Sleep*. By revealing the flaws of commitments to mind-body dualism among professionals and in healthcare systems along with one-size-fits-all conventional practice of sleep medicine, Dr. Krakow exposes how bad sleep and canned managed care medical approaches are harmful to your whole being. Among other things, sleep disorders are inflammatory and linked to many metabolic disorders, especially in the brain. *Life Saving Sleep* is a hands-on work setting a new gold standard that systematically and comprehensively helps you spot the harmful myths about and the helpful science of whole health sleep medicine. If you or people you know and care about have sleep breathing disorders, insomnia, nightmares, restless legs and more, then *Life Saving Sleep* is **the** path to begin a journey to sleep health healing. Here is to rest and recovery!"

  Michael Hollifield, M.D.

  Director of Novel Therapies Unit, Long Beach VA Healthcare System

  President and CEO, War Survivors Institute,

  https://warsurvivors.org/

"As a psychologist who manages a practice with six clinicians and often works with sleep disorders, I found myself at one of Dr. Barry Krakow's training events. This was a pivotal moment for me as I was enlightened to the intricacies of sleep and a multimodal approach to treating sleep disorders. I felt a rush of promise as I knew he had information that would aid a number of my clients, but also help me personally. I, much like my clients, had been suffering from a sleep disorder for years prior to this event. I have now been a patient of Dr. Krakow's for several years. Although I had seen numerous sleep specialists before, he was the only one who was able to help my upper airway resistance syndrome (UARS). That chance encounter has forever changed my life's course as well as those that I treat in therapy. He approaches his clients with compassion, awareness, and knowledge unmatched by his peers. If you are looking for someone to listen to your sleep difficulties, look no further. He is on the frontier of changing the way people understand and treat sleep problems. It is time to listen, learn, and be changed."

  Brooke Roberts, PsyD

  Licensed Psychologist, Owner of Santa Fe Psychology

"Dr. Krakow has taken his many years of clinical and research experience in sleep medicine and has written a clear and understandable analysis of the causes and treatments for all sleep disorders that is perfect for anyone troubled with sleep problems. Most of us who practice comprehensive sleep medicine know it is the "poor stepchild" of medicine, poorly understood and treated by the vast majority of care givers whether medical providers or therapists, even though there is excellent treatment for virtually all sleep disorders. Dr. Krakow's book gives patients suffering from these conditions the knowledge necessary to ask the right questions and go beyond this ignorance in order to get appropriate and effective care."

Aaron B. Morse, MD, FCCP, DAASM

Medical Director, Sleep Health MD, www.sleephealthmd.com

To My Beloved, Jessica Lorraine, the editor-in-chief, whose inspiration and love as well as her wisdom, understanding, and knowledge made this book a reality.

ALSO BY BARRY KRAKOW, MD

Conquering Bad Dreams & Nightmares
(coauthor Joseph Neidhardt, MD) 1992

Insomnia Cures 2002

Turning Nightmares into Dreams
(designed and edited by Jessica Krakow) 2002

In the Swing (coauthor Jack Hardwick, PGA) 2006

Sound Sleep, Sound Mind 2007

Figures on Chapters 5, 6 & Appendix A by Illustrator and Graphic Designer Maverick McCarthy
Design and Composition: Edge of Water Designs, edgeofwater.com
Copy editor: Paul Tabili
Cover Design: Angela Panas

The information contained in this book is not intended to serve as a replacement for professional medical treatments or psychological therapies. Any use of the information in this book is at the reader's discretion. The author and publisher disclaim any and all liability arising directly or indirectly from the use or application of any information contained in this book. A healthcare professional should be consulted regarding your specific situation.

Devices, drugs and supplements disclaimer. Information contained in this book on devices, prescription drugs, OTC medications, and supplements is not intended as formal prescriptions. You must discuss using or discontinuing such agents with your healthcare professionals. The author and publisher disclaim any and all liability arising from the use of listed devices, prescription drugs, OTC medications, and supplements. Because of ever-changing updates on drugs and supplements in general and specifically for agents noted in this work, it is imperative to fully evaluate potential side effects and benefits with the direct and ongoing assistance of your healthcare professionals.

For information about other products and services, please see www.BarryKrakowMD.com and www.LifeSavingSleep.com

Library of Congress Control Number: 2022906259
Krakow, Barry.
    Life Saving Sleep: New Horizons in Mental Health Treatment/Barry Krakow
    Includes index.
    ISBN 978-0-9715869-2-5
    1.Insomnia.2.sleep.3.sleep breathing.4.sleep apnea.5.CPAP.6.depression.7.PTSD. 8.nightmares. 9.anxiety.

Life Saving Sleep

New Horizons in Mental Health Treatment

Barry Krakow, MD

TABLE OF CONTENTS

List of Figures   xvi

Abbreviations & Acronyms   xvii

Navigating the Book   xix

Preface   xxiii

Introduction   Bad and Broken Sleep Attacks Your Mind   1

Chapter 1   Know Your Nemesis by the Proper Name: Sleep Disorders   9

Chapter 2   The Invisible Sleep Breathing Disorder   16

Chapter 3   The Breathtaking Complexity of Sleep-Disordered Breathing   24

Chapter 4   You Can Pass this Diagnostic Test with Your Eyes Shut   32

Chapter 5   Using Science, Not Insurance, to Gauge SDB Severity   44

Chapter 6   An Extremely Potent Medical Treatment Is Just a Breath Away   65

Chapter 7   How to Deal with a Medical System Designed to Frustrate   80

Chapter 8   Alternatives to PAP Therapy   96

Chapter 9   The Kicking and Screaming Sleep Movement Disorders   123

Chapter 10   Erasing Racing Thoughts the Natural Way   148

Chapter 11   Imagining Insomnia Out of the Picture   156

Chapter 12   Sleep-Related Emotion-Focused Therapy:
                 Getting Your Feet Wet   168

Chapter 13   Sleep-Related Emotion-Focused Therapy:
                 Beyond the Shallow End   182

Chapter 14   Sleep-Related Emotion-Focused Therapy:
                 Diving In!   192

Chapter 15   Advanced Cognitive-Behavioral Therapy
                 for Insomnia   224

Chapter 16   Nightmares: A Very Treatable Condition   242

Chapter 17   A Fresh Look at Psychotropic Drugs,
                 Hypersomnias & Napping   261

Chapter 18   At the End of the Day, What Attitudes
                 Are Lifesavers?   281

Epilogue   Dreaming of Super Sleep   301

Appendix A   Troubleshooting Guide: Advanced PAP Pearls   307

Appendix B   Quick Start: Sleep Dynamic Therapy Pearls   352

Appendix C   List of References   366

Index   383

Acknowledgments   396
About the Author   398

LIST OF FIGURES

Figure 5.1	Awake and delta sleep.	45
Figure 5.2	Stage 1 NREM, stage 2 NREM, and awake.	46
Figure 5.3	REM sleep and eye movements.	47
Figure 5.4	Normal sleep breathing and three types of breathing events.	48, 323
Figure 5.5	Hypopnea with awakening.	51
Figure 5.6	Flow limitation with arousal.	53
Figure 5.7	Flow limitation with micro-arousals.	54
Figure 5.8	Delta sleep revisited: how deep is deep?	58
Figure 5.9	Consolidated vs. fragmented sleep.	64
Figure 6.1	Degrees of airway collapsibility.	67, 324
Figure 6.2	PAP-induced expiratory pressure intolerance (EPI).	72, 326

ABBREVIATIONS & ACRONYMS

AASM	American Academy of Sleep Medicine
ABPAP	auto-bilevel positive airway pressure
AHI	apnea-hypopnea index
ANP	atrial natriuretic peptide
APAP	auto-CPAP
AR	allergic rhinitis
ASV-PAP	adaptive servo-ventilation positive airway pressure
BMI	body mass index
BP	blood pressure
CBT	cognitive-behavioral therapy
CBT-I	cognitive-behavioral therapy for insomnia
CPAP	continuous positive airway pressure
CSA	central sleep apnea
EASE	endoscopic-assisted surgical expansion
EEG	electro-encephalography
EFT	emotion-focused therapy
EPI	expiratory pressure intolerance
EPR	expiratory pressure relief
FLE	flow limitation event
GERD	gastroesophageal reflux disease
HGNS	hypoglossal nerve stimulator
IHS	idiopathic hypersomnia
IRT	imagery rehearsal therapy
JHU	Johns Hopkins University
LSOLS	losing sleep over losing sleep
MAD	mandibular advancement device
MDO	mandibular distraction osteogenesis
MMA	maxillomandibular advancement
NAR	nonallergic rhinitis
NBE	national brand equivalent
NCPT	nasal cannula pressure transducer

NDS	nasal dilator strips
NES	night eating syndrome
NREM	non–rapid eye movement sleep
OA	overeaters anonymous
OAT	oral appliance therapy
OSA	obstructive sleep apnea
OSCAR	open source CPAP analysis reporter
OTC	over-the-counter
PAP	positive airway pressure
PAP-NAP	focused sleep study for PAP troubleshooting
PLMD	periodic limb movement disorder
PSG	polysomnography
PTSD	posttraumatic stress disorder
RBD	REM behavior disorder
RDI	respiratory disturbance index
REM	rapid eye movement sleep
REPAP	repeat, rescue, retitration PAP studies
RERA	respiratory effort-related arousals
RLS	restless legs syndrome
SDB	sleep-disordered breathing
SOLO	stop, observe mind, let, observe body
SRED	sleep-related eating disorder
SR-EFT	sleep-related emotion-focused therapy
SRT	sleep restriction therapy
TASD	trauma-associated sleep disorder (also TSD)
TBI	traumatic brain injury
TFI	thoughts, feelings, images
TMB	time monitoring behavior
TMJ	temporo-mandibular joint
TRD	tongue-retaining device
UARS	upper airway resistance syndrome
UV	uvulectomy
UPPP	uvulopalatopharyngoplasty

NAVIGATING THE BOOK

▶ *Above all else, closely read the Introduction and Chapter 1 on sleep quality and how both mental and physical factors cause sleep disorders.* This theme is the foundation of the book.

▶ Physical sleep disorders: Chapters 2–8 cover sleep-disordered breathing; Chapter 9 covers leg movements and parasomnia disorders; Appendix A presents a special PAP Pearls unit for anyone initiating, actively using or struggling with PAP therapy.

▶ Psychological insomnia disorders and cures: start with Introduction and Chapter 1, then, if you choose, skip to Chapters 10–15.

▶ At any point, jump to Appendix B for Quick Start Pearls to rapidly initiate treatment steps with physiological or psychological therapies or both.

▶ Chapter 16 discusses nightmare treatments, including six different ways to resolve disturbing dreams.

▶ Chapter 17 presents drug and sleep information mental health patients rarely hear from therapists or prescribing doctors.

▶ Chapter 18 turns to older and wiser strategies to cope with sleep disorders, including work, humor, prayer, gratitude, and forgiveness. It focuses on daily aspects of your lifestyle, personality, and spirituality.

▶ *A final note on the crux of this book: Sleep often improves with a better mattress, lower room temperature, a dark bedroom, and commonsense actions. This book reveals why none of these steps heal your sleep disorders, whereas genuine cures are closer at hand than you might think.*

"In the evening one lies down weeping, but with dawn—a cry of joy!"

Psalm 30, King David (1040 BCE–970 BCE)

"... the cause of truth is borne by a minority ..."

Rabbi Samson Raphael Hirsch (1808–1888)

PREFACE

A radical paradigm shift in sleep therapy is desperately needed because so many mental health professionals as well as their patients do not understand, let alone recognize, the damage inflicted by poor sleep. At the heart of the matter and without exaggerating, bad and broken sleep may be killing you!

Beyond a shadow of a doubt, bad and broken sleep destroys lives in ways you might never have imagined possible. Adding to the confusion, most mental health providers and, again, their patients still use vague terms to describe sleep problems, such as "sleep disturbance" or "sleep issues" or "sleep complaints" or "sleep symptoms." These superficial terms always miss the point when sleep turns bad. The name of the game is **sleep disorders**, diagnosable and treatable independent disorders that cause disturbances, issues, complaints, or symptoms. Regardless of any other mental health diagnosis or its treatment, disordered sleep is its own very big deal. For decades and to this day, the vast majority of mental health classifications and professional institutions ignorantly mislabel sleep disorders as secondary symptoms that supposedly resolve after the mental disorder is treated.

This "secondary" theory is vigorously disproven in real-world mental health clinics as well as in real-world mental health research. Time and again, patients consistently complain how their mental health treatments, including medication or psychotherapy, do not or did not restore their sleep to anything close to normal.

The American Psychiatric Association added information about sleep disorders in the most recent *Diagnostic and Statistical Manual of Mental Disorders, Versions IV-TR* and *5*,[1] but this type of knowledge takes years or decades to filter down into the clinical practices of mental health professionals, and still much later to their patients. Even though *DSM-5* clearly indicates the strong need for ***independent clinical attention for many sleep disorders*** that occur simultaneously with mental health disorders (FYI, sleep doctors and researchers contributed to this section of the manual), the overwhelming majority of mental health practitioners, including psychiatrists, psychologists, social workers, various therapists, and other types of counseling professionals, do not address sleep disorders in a deliberate, focused, or effective way.

Further neglect of evidence-based sleep disorders medicine is regularly exposed through the jaded lens of media coverage of suicides among military personnel. Though intensifying coverage of suicide helps broadcast the scope of the problem, many tragic stories are described as an "unexpected" death without recognizing an ominous pattern that promptly catches the eye of a sleep doctor but not the attention of most medical or mental health professionals.

The formula for tragedy too often echoes the following: "the young man could not sleep; when he did sleep he suffered nightmares; he was handed a prescription for sleeping pills as well as antidepressants or antipsychotics to further knock him out at night; the pills did not work well, and insomnia worsened; dosages of the pills were increased, or new more potent drugs were added; the pills still did not work; insomnia and nightmares intensified ... and so on." And then the individual committed suicide, yet these journalists never discuss the extreme frustration, dejection, and demoralization caused by the chronic sleep loss afflicting these souls.

Variations of this story invariably depict a plight of intractable nightmares and insomnia. If you were to examine 10 consecutive reports from media outlets recounting the grim and gruesome details of trauma survivors dying by suicide or otherwise dying in their sleep, no less than seven or eight cases will unfold according to this sleepless narrative.

Shockingly, the deceased never seem to have been evaluated by a sleep medicine physician specialist, tested in a sleep laboratory for sleep disorders, or offered proven (evidence-based) strategies to effectively treat insomnia or nightmares. Indeed, there was no recognition of the very complex sleep disorders from which these patients suffered. Their healthcare professionals, who earnestly tried to help, were still looking at sleep complaints as a symptom and not a disorder; as a consequence, they only knew to prescribe more drugs.

In a word, these very real sleep disorders were *invisible* to their doctors.

Thus, psychiatrists, psychologists, therapists, counselors and primary care providers must break out of this conventional wisdom trance while sleep medicine specialists must actively break into this clinical care circle to help mental health patients, nearly all of whom suffer unsuspected, undiagnosed, untreated, and disabling sleep disorders, largely misunderstood and improperly addressed by these healthcare professionals. This change—long overdue—must proceed now!

This radical paradigm change must occur because individuals who suffer serious mental illness, as well as risks for suicide, frequently experience a profound sleep misery indisputably aggravating or directly causing their mental illness as well as their suicidal behaviors. As a sleep medical professional who has specialized in the treatment of sleep disorders in mental health patients for three decades, I believe there is absolutely no excuse for these individuals to be deprived of the best possible (evidence-based) sleep medicine resources and therapies with the hope and reasonable expectation such treatments might edge these desperate souls back from the brink.

Surely, it is time to bring this knowledge to the forefront of treatment for mental health patients. More than enough research implicates sleep disorders as a critical factor in mental illness and suicide—a factor maddeningly under-recognized and untreated.

This book delivers the necessary and decisive sleep knowledge to patients and their spouses, as well as to physicians and therapists, to propel this radical paradigm shift. Ultimately, the objective is to help those in dire straits to find relief from their unrelenting, unrelieved, and tormenting anguish as they grapple with sleep turned unbearably bad.

We must show them how to recover their sleep to regain the rest of their lives.

Barry Krakow, MD
Savannah, GA 2022

INTRODUCTION

Bad and Broken Sleep Attacks Your Mind

Never Underestimate Bad and Broken Sleep

When you lose sleep or your sleep goes bad and eventually breaks down, very few physicians, psychiatrists, psychologists, or therapists understand how your life unravels. You might think they know, but, sadly, they know little about sleep.

One of the greatest knowledge gaps plaguing most healthcare providers is the undeniable science proving sleep is a physical or physiological process. Instead, these professionals automatically believe sleep issues must be largely psychological.

They don't realize sleep is an innate and powerful biological process. By comparison, imagine for a moment how sick you would become if physical waste products building up inside your body were no longer eliminated. Picture how rapidly your health would decline should your kidneys and liver no longer clear toxins from your bloodstream. Sleep is comparable to these biological processes.

Every day, physiological waste comprising toxic biomolecules builds up in your brain. These neurotoxic proteins are specifically linked to dementia and generally act like a poison for which the only reliable antidote is sleep. Your brain literally washes away this waste matter while you sleep.[2] Just as kidneys and liver filter your blood, healthy sleep detoxifies and eliminates waste matter generated in your nervous system during wakefulness.

Sounds astonishing, but some "brain-washing" is a healthy thing.[3]

This waste matter is neither easily detected nor fully understood, making it difficult to pinpoint the harmful impact on your mind and body. When missing out on sleep or not sleeping well just for one night, you may only notice the aftereffects of feeling tired or sleepy. Moreover, because our modern world belittles people with low energy (Red Bull is popular for a reason), you may not pay attention to how your tiredness and sleepiness are caused by the brain's failure to restore itself through healthy slumber. It's not a coincidence normal sleepers experience high daytime energy. Making things thornier, far too many individuals, including friends, family, and coworkers dismiss the power of sleep, which further dampens your own motivation to diligently explore your personal sleep complaints.

Worst of all, you might mistakenly believe the solution is about getting more sleep.

Hear this, loud and clear: the number of hours you sleep is rarely the main cause of sleep problems compared to how well you sleep during these hours.

Got it?

You must focus on *quality of sleep*. You've heard the expression "Quality over Quantity" many times in your life. Scientific research proves the quality of sleep is the most critical component you must address to solve your sleep problems.

When sleep quality degrades, we call it "bad and broken sleep." Much to the detriment of society and to you individually, most healthcare professionals lack appreciation for how bad and broken sleep physically destroys cells and tissues inside the brain and the rest of your body, and how bad and broken sleep destroys your psychological and physiological health, all leading to mental and physical illness. My clinical and research experience highlights the failure of many medical communities and institutions to grasp how sleep disruption produces these debilitating and deadly results.

Even the most ill-fated mental health patients, who traveled down dark paths leading to disability or death, never realized, never considered, or were never offered the potentially lifesaving insight that bad and broken sleep contributed to their decline.

Physical, Physical, Physical

Things are trickier at the professional level where you engage with many medical and mental health experts who spread outsized misconceptions, declaring sleep issues are strictly psychological problems as in "it's all in your mind." We know this perspective is a complete falsehood because *all* sleep problems contain a physical component. Let me strongly restate: **All sleep disorders *always* have a physical factor—*always*—because sleep itself is a measurable physiological behavior originating in your brain.**

Virtually every time you experience something wrong with your sleep, even if convinced you're not getting enough, your brain waves measured by electroencephalography (EEG) are likely to show abnormal patterns. This abnormal EEG means unequivocally physical factors are injuring your brain, and this injury is the experience of bad and broken sleep at night as well as tiredness or sleepiness the next day.

Unluckily, the most common presenting sleep complaints, particularly insomnia, look, feel, and sound like a mental condition, leading many (possibly yourself) to miss the diagnosis of underlying physical sleep disorder(s). Moreover, new capsules of scientific knowledge prove difficult to swallow for those repeatedly told their problems are psychologically driven and who are only offered more prescription medications with no other options.

Consider this example: when you suffer night after night from bad and broken sleep, you know your mind may unravel, spinning out of control with far too many sinister thoughts, feelings, and ugly images in your mind's eye, leading down dark paths of despair, dejection, and desolation. At some point on this morbid path, you lose heart for the things that keep you going in life, and you lose your natural, healthy perspective to cope constructively with simple or complex challenges. Soon, the only remaining mood is melancholy, depression, or emptiness, any of which provoke helpless or hopeless feelings where you might imagine no other option but to stop living.

Guess what? Beyond this obvious psychological distress, serious and harmful physical changes are going on in your brain every single minute you suffer from bad and broken sleep. These physical sleep abnormalities cause much of this dangerous psychological unraveling, so much so most mental health patients can expect clear-cut improvements in their distress after receiving expert care from sleep medicine specialists.

I assure you with accuracy and conviction: being robbed of your sleep aggravates mental illness and suicidal thinking and feelings. In some vulnerable individuals, the dark pall of mental illness and suicidal tendencies emerges just as soon as bad and broken sleep starts destroying already damaged or fragile coping skills.

Yes, it is true the overtly psychological appearance of sleep complaints comes across as a mental disease. Nonetheless, you are about to learn how bad and broken slumber in nearly all cases results from physical destruction to your sleep, a destruction directly causing physical brain damage. Over time, this damage turns out to be more harmful than any psychological injury you may be aware of due to disrupted sleep. To reiterate, the problem lies *within* your sleep itself, not in the number of hours you sleep, which explains how and why quality trumps quantity.

Healthy Slumber Is a Life-Sustaining, Innate Human Resource

When your mind functions "normally" (something not easily defined), you do not respond to life's challenges by imagining an ultimate escape from reality as your best solution. Nevertheless, for individuals susceptible to mental illness and suicidal tendencies, the destruction and eventual loss of quality sleep leads to demoralizing thoughts, desperate feelings, and disturbing pictures in the mind's eye, all spiraling out of control.

How and why sleep could prove so critically important to your mental health is the subject of this book. And if you read the next paragraph in bold letters, it may help you, your loved ones, or your patients to guard against underestimating this natural and potent human resource. Critically, I want you to discern something so innate, so obvious, and so precious about your sleep you will soon realize only ignorance or negligence could explain how so many healthcare professionals do not grasp the potency of sleep disorders.

Never forget: Sleep is a self-preservation function built into every human being. High quality sleep is designed to protect, restore, and make resilient the workings of the mind and body; thus, high quality slumber has a very strong potential to treat mental illness and suicidal thinking

or behaviors, because **sleep powerfully delivers a virtually indescribable form of psychotherapy night after night without being awake or aware of this process.**[4]

As you will learn, the attack on your sleep quality prevents you from gaining consolidated periods of deep sleep. This depth of slumber is most commonly defined by two specific sleep stages, called REM and delta. Technically REM is *rapid eye movement* sleep, and delta is the deepest form of non-REM (NREM) sleep (schematic pictures of sleep stages are provided in Chapter 5). Without lengthy, consolidated periods of REM and delta sleep, your mind and body deteriorate in the short and long term, and this deterioration takes a horrible toll on your mental health. Indeed, research now shows that disruption of delta sleep prevents the brain-washing system from working at its best.[5;6]

So, whatever is destroying your sleep is destroying your capacity for sleep to heal you!

Consequently, what you learn and apply to make sleep whole provides the potential for deeper sleep, often referred to as *sound sleep*, to improve your mental health and, most importantly for some, bring you back from the edge.

Why Sound Sleep Holds So Much Promise

Think of sleep as one of the most natural and potent antidepressant or antianxiety drugs provided by our Creator. Sleep literally alleviates and heals, if not cures, the ills and evils every one of us must face day in day out when we awaken and pursue our lives. Remarkably, once you recover the capacity to normalize and optimize sleep, you can attain a quality and consolidation of slumber so profound it will negate many of the bad actors roaming around in your head and simultaneously renew your spirit.

Forgive me for reminding you, but you must learn and embrace the idea that sleep is not about counting hours each night, although fewer hours of sleep may gauge someone's risk for mental illness or suicide. **The ultimate key is the quality of a person's sleep because sleep quality consistently**

determines how deeply and how long you will sleep. Most importantly, it is high quality sleep that accesses the normal mental recovery capacity inherently built into the neurophysiology of your slumber when you obtain sufficient REM and delta sleep.

In contrast, the decline in quality is almost always determined by the amount of physiologic disruption to your normal sleep physiology. Despite overwhelming and compelling evidence for this physical destruction of your sleep, your perceptions may still lead you to believe it's "all in your head." Paradoxically, you are half right because this physical damage goes on inside your brain, assaulting your mental state night after night, all night long, by depriving you of appropriate and consolidated amounts of the deeper sleep stages. Half right because the assault targets your body as well.

As noted in the Preface, the vast majority of media reports about individuals with mental illness who committed suicide describe patients with very severe insomnia or nightmares or both, for which multiple medications were prescribed and attempted; and, yet no medication was able to solve the sleep problems. And though there are individuals without sleep complaints who commit suicide, research demonstrates those with sleep complaints commit suicide in a noticeably shorter time frame.

On the face of things, how is it that no one in the media, let alone in the medical profession, is asking the simple question "Hey, what gives with this sleep stuff?" My sarcastic reply, "You're killin' me! Oh, and by the way, you're killing your patients!"

How Sleeping Pills Mislead

Think closely about similar stories you've heard. Each of the individual tragedies involved a person who was not getting enough sleep due to bad and broken sleep, and nothing resolved their insomnia or their poor sleep quality despite numerous rounds of prescription drug after prescription drug. Which means something was missed.

Something big was missed!

That something big is almost always physical factors destroying the quality of sleep. Because no one attempting to help these individuals understood the critical distinction between *sleep quality* and *sleep quantity*, their healthcare providers kept upping the dosage of medications believing depression or posttraumatic stress disorder, as two common examples, were the only explanation for severe insomnia. Regrettably, these sincere but ignorant healthcare providers could only perceive the sleep issues as a continuity problem—how to help the patient fall asleep and stay asleep for a specific number of hours.

In many such cases, these healthcare professionals were wrong—dead wrong, sad to say, because considerable research already shows when sleeping pills do not work, another physical factor underlies the deteriorating insomnia.[7-9] Worse still, sleeping pills steer patients and providers 180 degrees away from considering something physical as the culprit, which then worsens obsessions about fixing "sleep duration" or "sleep continuity." All the while, patients are continually injured by the absence of life-enhancing and healing properties from naturally restorative, deeper slumber; this high quality sleep is desperately needed to reverse course and steer you toward recovery and away from mental illness and suicidal thoughts or actions.

Waking Up to the New Sleep Reality

When you suffer the problems of mental illness or suicidal thinking and are not sleeping well, you must assess many new things about your sleep problems, more than you might have imagined. Have you heard the saying, *"you don't know what you don't know?"* Frankly, there are things you don't know that could kill you.

Let's find a place of clarity where you fully understand how to treat your sleep problems. When you access the right treatments, there's an excellent chance you will start feeling better in a matter of days or weeks, and your mental outlook will change for the better as well.

These are not speculations and theories; these are the most advanced and proven ideas on the nature of sleep and mental health. Genuine hope for a new dawn in your sleep world is just over the horizon. First, we'll figure out the problems, and then we'll treat them. Are you ready to move forward to seek your own *Life Saving Sleep*?

CHAPTER 1

Know Your Nemesis by the Proper Name:
Sleep Disorders

Which terms best define your sleep complaints, sleep conditions,
sleep problems, sleep issues, sleep symptoms, or sleep disturbances?

Sleep Disorders, Not Sleep Disturbances

We have a lot of ground to cover and not a lot of time if you are feeling actively suicidal or otherwise in need of urgent help for mental illness. Obviously, you must avail yourself of the assets at your disposal, including family and friends, therapists and physicians, and community, religious, or social resources. I am not recommending in any way to defer other treatments or focus exclusively on your sleep because at this point it is impossible for either of us to know how important sleep treatments will prove for you.

Unfortunately, we cannot gauge, let alone predict, the value of sleep therapy until after you experience some degree of successful treatment of your sleep disorders. Fortunately, the probability of improvement is very high.

We want you sleeping better—*now!* To achieve this goal, you must learn how to understand your *sleep disorders* to gain a quick burst of confidence. This assurance will encourage you to believe sleep disorders are solvable, which will ramp up your motivation; and with clear instructions you will focus on precise targets.

This knowledge will help you leap over the second largest barrier (the first, described in the Introduction, is accepting how *quality* trumps *quantity*), which is the distinction between "sleep disturbances"—the term used by psychiatrists, psychologists, therapists, and other medical and mental health professionals to describe your sleep problems—and the term "sleep disorders," used by sleep medicine physicians and behavioral sleep medicine specialists to precisely define and treat specific sleep conditions.

"Sleep disturbances" only prove useful when a psychiatric disorder is unquestionably the exclusive cause of an individual's sleep complaints (almost never!) or when the term is used to imply something is "disturbing" the *quality* of your sleep, as in someone with chronic pain. That said, both a psychiatric patient and a pain patient are also suffering *physical* EEG changes that aggravate their sleep problems.

These changes invariably damage your REM or delta sleep or both, which occurs through a process specifically defined as "sleep fragmentation" or "sleep frag" for short.[10-12] More to come on this pervasive disruption of your natural sleep quality.

Returning to the contrast between disturbances versus disorders, let's look at two of the most common examples: depression or PTSD patients who report sleep complaints that lead many professionals and patients to imagine depression or PTSD caused the sleep symptoms. These doctors and patients latch onto and hold tightly to the term "sleep disturbances." This approach glosses over the more challenging and relevant nuances and complexities of sleep disorders.

I am strongly persuaded this "sleep disturbance" term is stubbornly overemphasized to the detriment of millions of mental health patients with sleep disorders. Problematically, the term "sleep disturbance" moves us toward concepts about sleep deprivation and sleep duration and away from the core concept of sleep quality. In sum, sleep disturbance is vague, whereas "sleep disorders" indicates to virtually everyone with skin in the game that a precise, definable condition affects your sleep, causing great distress and harm, including the worsening of suicidal tendencies.

In no short order, we want you to abandon all terms like disturbances, issues, complaints, problems, or symptoms. Instead, focus on the sleep disorders gang wreaking havoc and chaos night after night.

The Gang of Four

For more than two decades, we have been spelling out in the scientific literature as well as in one of my books the strong probability that four primary sleep disorders cause the most damage to the sleep of mental health patients in general and PTSD and other trauma survivors in particular.[13-15] It is my strong impression based on research and clinical experience these four disorders are directly or indirectly harming your REM and delta sleep, likely through the mechanisms of sleep fragmentation mentioned above, at minimum. Each of these sleep disrupters attacks your mind and body night after night, likely for years. Your brain, your mind, your heart, your airway, and your sense of well-being are literally under assault. These assaults are very real, very pronounced, and clearly traumatizing. They occur as frequently as every 30 to 60 seconds in your sleep, and you might never know exactly how attacks begin and carry on through the night. Make no mistake, sleep disorders carry a very big and potent stick that is relentlessly pounding on your brain and body every time you sleep or try to sleep.

Two disorders are very obvious: insomnia and nightmares. Indeed, if you suffer posttraumatic stress, the presence of insomnia or nightmares or both provides critical information toward formally diagnosing posttraumatic stress disorder (PTSD).

You might imagine these two sleep disorders are easily and accurately diagnosed. Regrettably, the words "insomnia" or "nightmares" are usually not interpreted as disorders in their own right by mental health professionals or by other doctors who prescribe medications for psychiatric conditions. These doctors or therapists do not see insomnia or nightmares as specific, targetable disorders requiring specific, proven (evidence-based medicine) treatments. Instead, the disorders are viewed with a "one-size-fits-all" mentality for which the current formal dress code comprises medication and still more medication, often proving ill-fitting in far too many cases.

Drugs may help some patients a great deal and should not be discounted, but this book is not about "help"—it's about "potential cure" or at least "near-cure" of sleep disorders. Do prescription drugs resolve the insomnia or nightmare problems? If so, we would predict you are sleeping much better—and feeling much better during the daytime when using these medications regularly. Few people consistently gain such large or long-lasting sleep benefits from drugs.

If you are not sleeping better at night or feeling better during the day, then it is highly debatable or questionable whether pills are generating value. More commonly, individuals notice pills do not yield optimal results, yet when receiving no other treatment choices, they assume the improvement achieved must be as good as it gets.

It is undoubtedly not as good as it gets!

Our research teams and clinical centers have developed advanced techniques for both insomnia and nightmares, reported by the *New York Times*,[16;17] *New Yorker* magazine,[18] and *Time* magazine[19] and published in leading medical and psychological journals, such as *JAMA*,[20] *American Journal of Psychiatry*,[21;22] *Journal of Clinical Psychiatry*,[23] *Journal of Traumatic Stress*,[24] and the *Journal of Nervous and Mental Disease*,[25] as well as sleep and respiratory journals *Chest*,[26] *Journal of Clinical Sleep Medicine*,[23] *SLEEP*,[27-29] and *Sleep and Breathing*.[30;31] Television programs, ABC's *20/20* and *Primetime*, CNN, *CBS This Morning*, and Charles Kuralt's *Sunday Morning*, covered the remarkable benefits from these specific, well-described, and proven treatments for nightmares and insomnia that cure without medications. My prior works describe in depth these new approaches to nightmares and insomnia (*Sound Sleep, Sound Mind*, 2007; *Turning Nightmares into Dreams*, 2002; *Insomnia Cures*, 2002*)*, and now we offer 15 more years of research and clinical experience in *Life Saving Sleep*. Many other colleagues in the field have likewise researched and written about the same or similar treatment approaches.[32-35]

With this backdrop, it will probably surprise you to learn direct treatment of nightmares or insomnia, the most obvious sleep disorders reported by mental health and suicidal patients, are not the two disorders we are most concerned about in this early stage of diagnosis and treatment.

Even though insomnia or nightmares are linked to anxiety, depression and suicidal thinking and actions, both sleep disorders often camouflage deeper and more complex sleep disorders. By analogy, nightmares and insomnia are at the tip of an iceberg, beneath which lies a much more dangerous problem afflicting your sleep. When you bump into an iceberg, you harbor no confusion about the bigger problems you face. Regrettably, with insomnia and nightmares, you could spend months, years, even decades trying to treat these nettlesome psychophysiological sleep disorders and never once suspect something more dangerous lurks beneath the surface.

Recognizing that people like choices, if you prefer to start right away on insomnia or nightmare treatment, please skip to Chapter 10 for the former and Chapter 16 for the latter. However, I strongly encourage you to read through the remainder of this chapter and the next before jumping ahead.

Looking Beyond the Obvious

Take a moment to think about the exact reason insomnia and nightmares are so bothersome. The answer is both conditions disrupt your sleep in the middle of the night, and both distort your mental attitude so severely you may develop problems falling asleep at bedtime. In other words, at the most basic level, nightmares and insomnia thwart or fracture your sleep and cause some of the sleep frag mentioned previously.

Here, then, is a clue to begin your detective work on solving so many riddles about your fractured sleep. Why can't you sleep continuously through the night? What if insomnia and nightmares only appear to break up your sleep? What if, in fact, these two disorders are not the primary culprits? What if something else is breaking up your sleep, and the nightmares and insomnia simply surface around the same time?

Sound strange?

Imagine if something else physical were shredding your sleep into little fragments, but you do not possess the sensing capacity to identify this great destroyer because it only operates as you sleep.[29] When you awaken abruptly, the first thing you remember could be a nightmare, or you awaken and recall nothing more. Now, here's the big key: notice what's missing from the explanation; you are missing the invaluable information from the seconds before you awakened—the data that fully explain why or how you awakened. And it's missing because it is beyond your grasp. You were asleep at the time, so how could you know? You might naturally believe the nightmare woke you, but the nightmare turns out not to provide the fullest explanation.

How do we solve this mystery?

What you hear next might save your life, so please pay close attention. **The truth about nightmares and insomnia is they often run with a larger pack of wolves, and the other two beasts are more vicious and bloodthirsty when they savagely attack your mind and body.**

In more than 30 years of research and clinical experience, physical sleep disorders often fuel nightmares or insomnia. If you do not cut off this fuel supply, things burn out of control despite all the best intentions to help someone address his or her sleep disorders. As you are about to learn, the true and most pressing problems you must overcome—sooner, not later—often remain hidden from view. When so much of your energy is invested in the psychological side of the sleep equation, this physiological side goes undetected. Making matters worse, the physiological side is, in two words—nearly invisible.

Just how invisible?

Sleep Research Pearl #1

In the early 1990s, a 42-year-old, male Vietnam veteran with severe PTSD and horribly violent nightmares walked into a Philadelphia Sleep Center, and a few months later nearly all his symptoms had diminished or disappeared. The flashbacks and exaggerated startle response were nearly eliminated. The gruesome, nightly nightmares about all his friends being killed decreased markedly; bad dreams surfaced only monthly, with far less disturbing content; and, to his surprise, pleasant dreaming emerged. For the first time in years, he could smell diesel fuel, his previously worst trigger that catalyzed severe posttraumatic stress symptoms. Finally, after years of insomnia, he slept all through the night.

Adding to this background, the patient abused amphetamines during Vietnam and was a heavy user of alcohol after the war. In the previous decade, he was hospitalized for PTSD on four different occasions and at various intervals a frequent user of sleeping pills and psychotropic medications. When asked at his four-month follow-up sleep center appointment about the dramatic improvement in symptoms, he attributed the change to "a full night's sleep."

This unusual case history was published in the scientific journal *Psychosomatics* in 1998.[36] Very few people heard about it, fewer still read about it, and almost no one believed it or believed it made sense. Sounding like a cross between a placebo response and a magical cure, it was quietly filed away as an odd anecdote to be ignored, if not forgotten.

Those of us in the know were delighted to see the very first publication on what would eventually prove to be some heavy-duty, all-purpose sleep magic, and I trust you'd like to know exactly how this spell was cast.

CHAPTER 2

THE INVISIBLE SLEEP BREATHING DISORDER

Which sleep disorders do your doctors and therapists overlook,
and what causes these blind spots?

Breathing: The Most Powerful Influence on Your Sleep

What you are about to read boggles the mind. Nonetheless, please consider the following data points. My research teams have conducted more studies on this topic than any other research group. Our efforts produced more than 30 peer-reviewed papers,[7-9;13;14;26;29-31;37-59] including our recent landmark study in *The Lancet*[60] (see Appendix C) as well as more than 50 peer-reviewed abstracts, available through the journal *SLEEP* and presented at the annual scientific meetings of the Associated Professional Sleep Societies (renamed the SLEEP ANNUAL MEETING). These papers and abstracts cover all we're about to discuss. And, recently, several independent research groups have arrived at similar conclusions.[61-66]

In nearly all patients examined in our research, the vast majority were complaining about insomnia or nightmares with a background of diagnosed PTSD or depression, or a history of trauma. Astonishingly, all studies showed the same connections between physical sleep disorders and their sleep complaints, even though these complaints sounded exactly like mental health symptoms.

The pivotal connection was the actual or presumptive diagnosis of a sleep breathing disorder in 80% to 95% of the cases.[7-9;29;42;45;55]

Sleep-disordered breathing is the granddaddy of all sleep disorders. A surprisingly large number of patients with insomnia or nightmares suffer from sleep breathing problems; in fact, growing evidence confirms nightmares and insomnia are caused or worsened by blockages in your breathing at night. Obstructed breathing causes severe sleep fragmentation that destroys sleep quality, and it causes pervasive fluctuations in your oxygen levels. Both factors aggravate or cause insomnia and nightmares.

Think for a moment how important these facts might be for your own sleep problems. If you believe firmly your sleep complaints are best defined by the disorders of insomnia or nightmares—two conditions that strongly persuade doctors, therapists, and yourself to think about the mental origins of sleep issues—you are unlikely to ever consider physical factors such as a sleep breathing problem.

When you travel down this psychological pathway, however, will you find a healthcare professional who understands your REM and delta sleep are under attack? Who will help you realize these physical attacks on your sleep are directly damaging your memory, your mood, and the cognitive skills you need to make sound decisions? Who will explain to you how the destruction of your sleep quality is likewise destroying your capacity to work through emotional distress, preventing you from coping in the healthiest of ways?

What's needed here is a broader perspective to analyze whether something physiological is the true culprit and therefore the missing link that better explains why you cannot sleep or why you feel so lousy when you wake up in the morning. In contrast, the failure to recognize an underlying physical sleep disorder as a major cause of your sleep problems will set back your recovery for months or years, if not decades. Making your efforts still more burdensome, few health care professionals in medical, psychiatric, or other mental health fields know much about what we are about to discuss.

Emphatically, this new perspective needs your urgent attention because what you learn may change, if not save, your life.

Now Take another Deeper Breath

Sleep-disordered breathing comes in three flavors. The first two, obstructive sleep apnea (OSA) or its variant known as upper airway resistance syndrome (UARS), both involve collapsibility of the airway. The third condition, known as central sleep apnea (CSA), means your airway is open but your brain chooses not to breathe. More on CSA later.

OSA and UARS operate through both subtle and gross obstructions of your airway. Ahead in Chapter 5 you can view schematic graphs of this collapsibility.

Whether it's a large collapse of the airway (no breathing, 100% collapse = obstructive apnea), a mid-size collapse (50% collapse = obstructive hypopnea), or a more subtle collapse (~10% to 30% drop in breathing = obstructive UARS-type), your body responds by waking up to breathe normally again. These actions repeated hundreds of times per night shatter sleep and lead to numerous mental and physical symptoms that demoralize and debilitate the unsuspecting individual, who often labors for years without a proper diagnosis.

Disordered sleep breathing sabotages your mind and body through its many disguises. First and foremost, it attacks your brain's normal functioning, inhibiting your healthy "brain-washing" capacity by preventing a continuous state of sleep[67;68] (see the Introduction for info on "brain-washing"). Worse, in some it will block your descent into the deepest and most important stages of sleep (REM and delta),[5;69;70] which are not only necessary to restore your mind and body each night but also are specifically linked to recovering emotionally from the previous day's stressors.[71] Emerging research pinpoints the damage inflicted on individuals who lack sufficient REM or delta sleep or whose REM and delta never consolidate for long stretches in the night.[11]

Take a deep breath—this next point may truly be a lifesaver. OSA or UARS literally destroy your sleep without you ever knowing it!

The Unrelenting Attack on Your Sleep

When you consider all the fatigue or sleepiness or energy deficits, not to mention the pessimism, despondency, and lack of motivation associated with patients with depression and PTSD, it is no surprise such individuals might develop suicidal thinking or even attempt suicide.

What if some portion of this debilitated state is due to the ravages of

OSA/UARS degrading your brain waves? For every night you suffer from OSA or UARS, the very next day you neither think as clearly as you would normally, nor can you cope as effectively with troubling emotions. Now multiply this sequence by 100 nights, or 1000 nights, or 10,000 nights in a row. Anyone would become a zombie with such a massive assault on his or her sleep.

At the simplest level, OSA or UARS patients may perceive themselves as sleeping through the night, believing they grab six to eight hours of slumber by the clock when the more accurate quantity might be two to four hours of sleep. Why is the real number so much smaller? Because the degree of sleep fragmentation produced by these sleep breathing disorders is so pronounced—even though you are "sleeping" right through it—your actual sleep time is drastically decreased, and the quality is severely compromised—a veritable double whammy. Even when you suffer severe insomnia and think you're down to 2 to 4 hours per night, the same issues arise, leading to even fewer hours.

We'll delve into sleep fragmentation later. For now, imagine you just slept 60 minutes, measured by a timer, but your slumber was interrupted every 30 seconds by breathing events. Each breathing event could kick you out of sleep for 10 to 30 seconds or longer without you knowing. Once you subtract this "not asleep" time, you end up with considerably less actual sleep than the 60 minutes you counted by the clock.

We have not even begun to discuss the impact of drops in your oxygen levels set off by these insidious sleep breathing disorders. Every time your sleep breathing falters, usually during a 10-to 60-second interval, there is a change in oxygenation, which we call *desaturation* (when it drops below the norm of 90%) or *fluctuation* (when it drops anywhere from 1% to 4% yet remains above 90%).

Damage develops from either desaturations or fluctuations because this rapid cycling of oxygen levels—up and down—causes cascading changes in biomolecules in your bloodstream.[72] Over time, these changes lead to damage along the inner lining of your blood vessels,[73;74] where blood, nutrients, and oxygen are delivered, and waste products are removed. When these vessels are damaged or compromised, the heart and brain as well as nearly all other organ systems in the body are damaged or compromised as well.

From this basic information, is it now clear a sleep breathing disorder destroys your actual sleep cycle? Can you envision how the rapid and abrupt changes in oxygen levels also cause brain damage and eventually heart damage as well? Unfortunately, ignorance might have led you or your healthcare providers to keep mislabeling these serious problems as insomnia or nightmares without ever considering the greater threat from the real enemy.

For these reasons, a sleep breathing disorder is a dangerous and unrelenting condition for anyone at risk for suicidal tendencies.[75] If you are diagnosed with OSA or UARS, you have it every night, and every single night you are in a veritable fight for your life. Throw in at bedtime the use of alcohol or opiates or even specific psychotropic medications, like benzodiazepines, and now your airway collapses even more, worsening the breathing events and worsening the damage to your brain.

Every night your sleeping brain waves suffer disruption leading to insufficient REM or delta or both. Every night oxygen deficits damage your brain and your heart. Is it any wonder a person could start to lose coping skills in the face of this damage? Is it any wonder critical skills of judgment and decision making, as well as the essential virtues of patience and temperance, could easily slip through one's fingers, leading to disorganized thinking, impulsive feelings, and harmful behaviors?

It cannot be reiterated strongly enough: as nightmares and insomnia emerge so visibly on your mental landscape, few if any professionals encourage you to consider the lurking monster hidden, as it were, in your bed, all the while destroying your sleep night after night.

Detecting a Sleep Breathing Disorder

There's an old adage in medicine: "what you don't look for, you don't see." No truer words could be spoken about sleep-disordered breathing, or SDB for short. These breathing disorders are not difficult to spot when you know what to look for; however, critical and sometimes complex measurements are needed to confirm the diagnosis. These measurements are only available when you are tested in a sleep lab or in some cases with a home sleep monitor. In Chapter 5 you will learn about the necessary technology. For now, let's focus on your own capacity to determine the likelihood of a sleep breathing disorder.

Beginning with the obvious, we'll move on to surprising symptoms you would never suspect as being caused by SDB. If you know you snore loudly, suffer from high blood pressure, or feel unrested or unrefreshed when you awaken in the morning, chances are extraordinarily high you will be diagnosed with OSA or UARS. If you suffer from all three, chances for the diagnosis are right at 99.99%. Suffering just one of these factors, your chances remain at the 80% to 90% range. If you notice any other breathing signs or symptoms, such as someone seeing you cease breathing at night, or you awaken choking or gasping for breath, again your chances shoot upward toward 100% probability.

More important than breathing changes, which are difficult to detect if you sleep alone, certain daytime symptoms strongly suggest disordered breathing is attacking and disrupting your sleep at night.

Common sense predicts you would feel tired, sleepy, or drowsy during the day when your sleep is destroyed at night; one clue would be excess caffeine use to ward off a desire to nap. You might also not be surprised to know your ability to pay attention, concentrate, or access your memory are compromised, especially in the afternoon where again you might reach for a caffeinated beverage to sharpen your wits. All these symptoms so many people complain about (or simply insist must be normal) are exceedingly prevalent in people with SDB.

As this book focuses on mental health symptoms such as anxiety, depression, and PTSD, we must consider their overlap with or impact on sleepiness and tiredness. Is it the psychiatric disorder or SDB or both causing daytime symptoms? Complicating matters, if you suffer from anxiety symptoms, the anxiety itself may corrupt your daytime sleepiness or tiredness and challenge your ability to tease apart what you are actually feeling. The most subtle example of this predicament is found in the person who ordinarily would feel sleepy during the day due to bad and broken sleep at night, yet his or her anxiety, hypervigilance, or other jumpy feelings override the sleepiness, causing the person to report fatigue or tiredness (instead of sleepiness) or report nothing but anxiety.

This cardinal example explains why so many psychiatric patients with suicidal thoughts never receive an evaluation for SDB. In their workup with a psychiatrist, therapist, or other healthcare professional, nearly all of whom have been erroneously trained to believe sleepiness is the only reliable daytime symptom of SDB, a discussion involving a physical sleep disorder (if there is any discussion at all) is swiftly discarded once the symptom of "sleepiness" is denied and the terms "tired" and "fatigue" emerge. As so many depressed patients report tiredness and fatigue, mental health providers in particular lean toward the psychiatric explanation to "confirm" the patient's problems must be psychological[76] and then are more prone to drop the ball on the need for a more in-depth evaluation of sleep disorders.

Unexpectedly Reliable Markers of SDB

We are not even close to done yet. The above items easily predict a sleep breathing disorder. The next few—some common and others less so—merit your attention because their relationships to SDB reveal proven pathophysiological theories or evidence (that is, proof), or as we say, connecting the zzzots. Once you learn these additional risk factors or predictors, you stand an excellent chance of persuading, pushing, inveigling, coaxing, or demanding that your providers order a sleep test for you. Since these striking symptoms are so reliable, let's give them a chapter of their own.

Sleep Research Pearl #2

In the first Sleep Research Pearl, the magical spell was cast with a CPAP machine.[36] Two years later in 2000, we published similar findings in the *Journal of Psychosomatic Research* on 15 PTSD patients with OSA or UARS, treated at the University of New Mexico Hospital Sleep Disorders Center.[37] These middle-aged adults with moderate to severe obesity reported snoring and daytime sleepiness or fatigue, the classic symptoms of a sleep breathing disorder. Although not seeking treatment for PTSD, on a hunch we contacted all 15 individuals a year and half later and discovered nine were using treatment (8 CPAP plus one bariatric surgery patient who lost 110 pounds) and six were not, yielding two different groups to compare. Among the treated, seven of nine patients told us PTSD was better. In the six untreated patients, only one reported PTSD improvement; four described worsened PTSD. Also, nightmares decreased in eight of nine treatment patients compared to only one in the untreated group.

These groundbreaking works prompted us to study the rate of OSA or UARS in PTSD patients. We recruited 44 individuals from a group of crime victims suffering PTSD, nightmares, and insomnia to undergo sleep testing in our sleep lab. *Biological Psychiatry* published this work in 2001, revealing an astonishing rate of 90% positive diagnoses for a sleep breathing disorder.[42] This study was the first use of a special respiratory sensor to more accurately measure sleep breathing, thereby improving the precision in detecting the more subtle breathing events of UARS.

Remarkably, the study included 37 women who were not overweight, which was an oddity at the time because the presence of nonobese females challenged the conventional wisdom OSA primarily afflicted obese men. Nearly half the women did not experience snoring or daytime sleepiness. Nonetheless, moderate to severe OSA/UARS was diagnosed, and a key sleep finding demonstrated a 50% reduction in the normal amounts of REM and delta sleep.

From these works, we coined the term "complex insomnia,"[42] as nearly all the individuals believed their insomnia was strictly psychological and were greatly surprised by the diagnosis of a physical sleep disorder.

CHAPTER 3

THE BREATHTAKING COMPLEXITY OF
SLEEP-DISORDERED BREATHING

*If you display no breathing symptoms, could you still suffer from OSA
or UARS, and what clues would point toward the diagnosis?*

Stumbling to the Bathroom at Night

Why do people wake up at night and use the bathroom to urinate? *Nocturia* is the medical term for nighttime trips to empty the bladder. If you know why so many suffer from nocturia, then you know more than 99% of all physicians in the world, which is an amazing and scary statistic. Even a large percentage of urologists and gynecologists do not know the real reason so many people use the bathroom at night even though it is their business to know and treat the problem.

Get ready for some complex pathophysiology. I will make it as simple as possible, but if you have trouble following, please watch my five-minute video at www.nocturiacures.com.

It is a matter of fact, proven and published more than 30 years ago in the scientific literature,[77] OSA causes you to pee at night; sleep-disordered breathing causes your kidneys to work overtime when you sleep, so you end up with more water to pass. UARS also causes nocturia.[78]

How? Please follow closely as we go through several steps. First, as you try to breathe when your airway is obstructed, it is obvious your chest is working like crazy to get more air inside your lungs. If you imagine for just a moment the awful feeling of choking, you can imagine the incredible tension building in your chest wall, sometimes your belly as well. This tension is the pressure building inside the chest cavity (inside your ribs) as you struggle to suck in air.

Therefore, whenever you suffer from breathing events while asleep—which occurs hundreds of times per night in OSA/UARS patients—chest pressure builds during breathing stoppage or choking or gasping for air. Even a subtle breathing event like UARS increases this pressure inside the chest cavity.

The increased pressure transmits a force against the outer walls of blood vessels inside the chest. Veins are most affected, and the blood is pushed faster through the venous system back into the heart. Imagine a never-ending tube of toothpaste and all along the tube something constantly squeezing it. Note squeezing, not clamping it shut. With each squeeze, toothpaste would be flushed faster and farther along the tube. This SDB process causes more blood flow into the right atrium chamber of the heart, filling up the space with an abnormal blood volume.

As the excess blood supply is continually delivered through the night, right atrium muscles stretch to hold the fluid. This stretching acts as a sensor, signaling a dangerous fluid overload state inside the heart. The right atrium now must react to reverse the overload.

The response is the automatic secretion of a biomolecule known as *atrial natriuretic peptide* (ANP)—the body's own natural diuretic. In other words, the right atrial muscles stretch then release ANP, which makes its way through the circulatory system to the kidneys and delivers a simple message: there's too much fluid in the system, so filter out more water and send it to the bladder!

This natural diuresis means your bladder fills faster than normal while you are sleeping. The next thing you know, you are up to the bathroom once or twice per night, or more frequently.

Few physicians know this pathophysiological connection, so they and their patients presume an enlarged prostate, an overactive bladder, or drinking too much water too close to bedtime are the logical explanations for nocturia.

I drink as much as 32 ounces of water within one hour of bedtime; sometimes I drink 24 ounces of water right at bedtime, and I do not visit the bathroom. What's my secret? Do I have a catheter in place? Do I take some medication that solves the problem? Do I wear a diaper, so I don't need to get up? What gives?

None of the above. I use a device to treat sleep apnea every night, and as you might guess, this device typically known as CPAP (or PAP) reverses the whole cycle. No obstructed breathing in the airway, no excess pressure in the chest cavity, therefore no excess pressure pushing on the venous system, no excess blood flow streaming into the right atrium, no distension of the right atrial muscles, and therefore no release of ANP diuretic into the bloodstream. Finally, there is no additional filtering of water by the kidneys and no excess urine delivered to the bladder. No more nightly bathroom trips because there is no extra urine to excrete.

Notably, during the first night you use a PAP machine in a sleep lab, you often reverse this sequence and do not get up to urinate. Think about how potent PAP must be if on the very first night it erases nocturia.

Although many urologists and even primary care physicians will likely howl at what I am about to state, sleep apnea could prove to be the leading cause of nocturia, with the possible exception of patients who must use medications that also affect the kidneys, for example, diuretics for blood pressure or heart problems, lithium for bipolar illness, or certain diabetic meds. Notwithstanding these medication effects, sleep apnea is probably a greater cause of nocturia than prostate or bladder problems, even greater than drinking too much water close to bedtime. All these things aggravate nocturia and in some cases cause it, but overall, I believe we will one day discover OSA/UARS is the leading cause.

Regrettably, these claims have not been well studied in either the field of sleep medicine or urology, but there's a small clue in the scientific literature offering evidence to show nocturia is more likely due to sleep apnea than other causes. The clue is found in the quantitative connection between sleep apnea and nocturia, which is so precise it leads to precise treatment results. Indeed, published evidence in scientific journals by sleep researchers[79] reveals nearly every sleep apnea patient experiences decreased nocturia episodes and some report eliminating the problem. We have seen such results among patients with coexisting prostate or bladder problems.

In contrast, the fields of urology and gynecology view nocturia as multi-factorial, listing a great many possible causes or contributing factors without much attention given to sleep-disordered breathing.[80] While their emphasis is on behavioral changes, prescribed medications or surgical procedures, they appear to be unaware of the potential for a nocturia cure with PAP therapy.

The sleep medicine perspective on nocturia may seem grandiose, but thousands of sleep doctors routinely observe nocturia cures in their patients following treatment of sleep apnea; and *cure* means zero trips to the bathroom at night, something we see more so with the advanced PAP devices to be discussed in subsequent chapters. You will not find this perspective addressed the same way in the urology or gynecology journals.

Nocturia is extremely common in sleep-disordered breathing patients, whether they suffer from OSA or UARS. In one study we conducted, 80% of our sleep apnea patients reported snoring and 81% reported nocturia.[81] No doubt, other causes for trips to the bathroom exist. But when we are evaluating sleep patients who regularly visit the bathroom at least once per night, these trips correlate very highly with the eventual diagnosis of sleep apnea.

Given the difficulties in convincing physicians to order a sleep test for a patient concerned about a possible sleep breathing disorder, bear in mind nocturia is an extremely relevant symptom that will motivate you and your doctors to dig deeper into your sleep problems.

Morning Headaches: Another Blood Flow Problem

Another complexity is the unusual symptom of morning headaches in sleep apnea patients, which also relates to changes in blood flow, this time in the brain. As you know, you breathe in oxygen and breathe out carbon dioxide, but during sleep breathing events you may not bring in enough oxygen and you may not release as much carbon dioxide. As excess carbon dioxide builds up in the brain, blood vessels inside your head reflexively open wider (vasodilation), which causes increased blood flow. This reflex pushes out more carbon dioxide, but as the flow increases so does pressure inside your head, generating the feeling of a headache[82] or as some describe it, "a band sensation" around the top of the head.

A simpler theory is the struggle to breathe during sleep raises pressure inside the head. Another plausible theory for headaches is the excessive movements and repositioning of the head and neck as the sleep apnea patient attempts to open the airway more to breathe better. These neck movements increase tension in neck muscles, a common cause of headaches.

Remarkably, many OSA or UARS patients with morning headaches find total relief with PAP devices, and usually within the first few days or weeks of successful use. Although less common but still worth mentioning, individuals with other types of daytime headaches like migraines or clusters may improve on PAP. Although a headache problem is less common than nocturia in SDB, there's sufficient research on morning headaches (or the band around the head sensation) to help recognize you could be suffering from OSA or UARS; and it may provide a practical pathway to convince your primary physician to schedule a sleep test.

Digging Still Deeper

We just scratched the surface in revealing the broad impact of OSA or UARS on the mind and body. These sleep breathing conditions unequivocally function as a multisystem disease process, affecting so many different organ systems of the body it is a wonder medical science has taken so long to uncover this monster that attacks our sleep night after night. And to remind you, the outright loss or fragmentation of REM and delta sleep causes or aggravates several other mental and physical symptoms or disorders.

Do not be surprised when most or all of your healthcare providers—practicing medical doctors or mental health professionals—have no knowledge of these crucial connections. Nonetheless, use this list to raise or confirm your own suspicions about the potential for a sleep breathing problem:

- Recent worsening or long-standing poor control of high[83] or low[84] blood pressure
- Cardiovascular comorbidities, including arrhythmias, heart failure and more[85]
- Deteriorating diabetes control[86] or chronic kidney disease[87]

- Fibromyalgia symptoms of muscle aches and pains[88]
- A history of motor vehicle accidents or drowsy driving[89]
- Depression not responding to antidepressants[90]
- Anxiety not responding to antianxiety drugs[90]
- Insomnia not responding to sedatives, whether prescription or over-the-counter[9]
- Chronic nightmares,[45] including but not limited to breathing themes
- Waking at night or in the morning with a dry mouth from reflex mouth breathing[91]
- Acid reflux[92]
- Decreased libido[93] and erectile dysfunction[94]
- Unexplained fatigue[95]
- Simple cognitive changes, like misplacing things or forgetting things, that routinely get tagged as an aging phenomenon[96]
- Obvious cognitive impairment in memory, concentration, and paying attention[97]
- Subtle losses in reflexes, like not catching a glass that's tipping over, or your keys slipping out of your hand[98]
- And never forget that any sense of nonrestorative sleep (poor sleep quality)[99] may be the only thing that points toward a sleep breathing disorder

As a corollary to poor sleep quality, my favorite way to engage insomnia patients on the topic of sleep breathing is to inquire how they feel right after an awakening at night. They usually respond, "You know, it's odd, but I often feel wide awake as if I've finished sleeping even though it's 2 a.m." I then explain normal sleepers don't have such experiences. They wake up, roll over, and return to sleep. But sleep apnea patients literally suffer a rush of adrenalin pouring through their system because of the threat from compromised breathing just before the awakenings; think of it as a fright, flight, or fight response. Many people who hear this explanation are immediately sold on the idea of a sleep breathing disorder because there is no other compelling explanation for why they would awaken at night and feel so alert.[29]

For these reasons, let's restate two key points: (a) it is abnormal to suffer any sort of problem with the quality of your sleep; and (b) it is abnormal to wake up in the middle of the night and feel alert and ready to get going.

For any or all of these challenging connections (challenging because you may or may not be working with physicians or therapists who have digested this sleep knowledge), it would be well worth your time to undergo sleep testing and a trial of PAP therapy (you'll learn in Chapter 6 why the C was dropped from PAP). Despite any preconceived notions or misgivings about PAP, determining how much this therapy improves your health could rapidly enhance your motivation to treat SDB.

From a sleep medicine specialist perspective, we often say, "When in doubt, blow the snout!"

Sleep Research Pearl #3

Why is sleep-disordered breathing missed in so many mental health patients? This glaring omission among healthcare professionals was screaming for attention in the 1990s, so we conducted two separate studies looking for answers. The first, published in 2002 in the *Journal of Nervous and Mental Disease*, reviewed charts on 187 female sexual assault survivors seeking to enter a research protocol on the treatment for chronic nightmares.[55] Using risk criteria from the American Academy of Sleep Medicine (AASM), 168 were strongly suspected of an SDB diagnosis. Their most common symptoms, reported by 75% of the group, were unrefreshing sleep, daytime sleepiness, and recurrent awakenings. Less than one-third, however, reported sleep breathing symptoms like snoring. To confirm our assessment was accurate, we sleep tested 21 of the women, and all were positive for OSA or UARS. Statistically speaking, these 21 were no different than the remaining 147 suspected cases who were not tested.

So, how many of these 187 women prior to seeking treatment from us had been referred to sleep centers for evaluation of a sleep breathing disorder?

Very few were referred, despite 69% having been treated by multiple therapists, 40% receiving prescription medications for insomnia, and 71% receiving prescription psychiatric drugs. In all their professional visits collectively numbering in the thousands over the past decade, fewer than a dozen individuals were referred for an evaluation with a sleep medicine specialist.

Did these professionals miss the diagnosis due to the scarcity of sleep breathing symptoms? Did they miss it because these women's average BMI was only 10 pounds overweight? Or was the diagnosis of sleep apnea simply not on their radar?

In 2006, we published a second work in the same journal comparing a group of "typical sleep center patients" to a group of "trauma survivors."[54] Each group comprised 89 adults, and all 178 cases were diagnosed with SDB in a sleep lab or on a home sleep monitor. Each group comprised 78 women and 11 men, and both groups averaged 40 years of age. Our focus examined the types of complaints these individuals reported leading up to their SDB sleep test.

The presenting complaints (a medical term for what patients complain about at a new doctor visit) were poles apart. Sixty percent to 70% of the sleep center patients reported snoring or someone watching them stop breathing in their sleep. In comparison, the trauma patients reported less than 25% of these breathing symptoms. Likewise, 60%-70% of the trauma group reported insomnia and nightmares compared to less than 20% of the sleep center patients.

Bottom line indicated most mental health patients with OSA or UARS do not notice or suffer sleep breathing symptoms and instead complain about sleep in ways easily slotted into a psychological category. Coupled with mental health professionals' lack of awareness of sleep breathing disorders, a picture emerges for how these patients might not get referred to sleep centers.

CHAPTER 4

You Can Pass this Diagnostic Test with Your Eyes Shut

Can I work with any sleep doctor, sleep lab, or sleep center?

Making the Right Diagnosis the Right Way

Health insurance companies and government agencies use any excuse to save money while attempting to avoid hurting the patient—notice the absence of the term "quality of care." Unfortunately, some institutions and businesses do not support the highest quality of care in many areas of medicine, as is the case in sleep medicine. Generally, new medical discoveries lead to innovative tests, procedures, devices, and medications to greatly improve healthcare, but new stuff is more expensive.

While cost is a huge factor in medical businesses, the economic concept known as "creative destruction" is often a larger component of how change unfolds. For example, new and improved things replace an old thing, like computers replacing typewriters, fax machines replacing postal services, or e-mails replacing faxes. In medical economics, one great example is how outpatient day surgery has streamlined care.

Sleep medicine is currently in the throes of creative destruction, leading to an upsurge in inventors and institutions vigorously exploring how to make sleep testing less expensive, less dependent on the sleep laboratory, and less complicated so more people gain access to diagnostic testing and treatment for sleep apnea. Newer inventions and procedures are emerging regularly in the medical marketplace to treat sleep breathing disorders in various ways.

These changes will lead to positive developments for patients and doctors. However, progress may be slow because sleep medicine is an orphan in the family of all medical specialties. Regrettably, sleep medicine is cast aside by those in power due to the tiresome conviction sleep itself could not possibly be as important as, say, the functioning of your heart or your brain. As you will learn in your own personal sleep quest, the field of sleep medicine is under attack by powerful institutions that do not take sleep seriously. When something comes along to save money, it's a no-brainer to select cheap options without regard to the quality of sleep care.

This little rant was offered because you are likely to be forced into receiving a home or portable sleep test, known in the field as HST, which sounds appealing at first glance. You get tested in your own bed, don't leave home, and presumably sleep more like you usually sleep. One day, all these statements will prove true; hopefully that day will arrive sooner than later.

Right now, for mental health patients, home sleep tests might prove worthless, wasteful, and, worst of all, frequently steer the patient in the wrong direction by providing incomplete and inaccurate information. The exception where HST works well is for those who suffer from obvious or severe OSA, what's known as "classic sleep apnea" involving straightforward complaints of disruptive snoring or related breathing symptoms combined with daytime sleepiness but without other symptoms such as insomnia, depression, anxiety, or PTSD.

HST is not useful when sleep breathing problems are complex. Bluntly, nearly all HSTs are not designed to accurately diagnose UARS, which means as many as one-third of all patients may be told they do not suffer a sleep breathing disorder when in fact they do. Such individuals could be diagnosed with UARS on a regular in-lab sleep test.

What's the difference between home and in-lab sleep testing?

Specifically, a home sleep test does *not* measure sleep.

Wait, what?

That's right; no sleep parameters are measured on nearly all home tests.[100]

To detect UARS, a special breathing sensor known as the nasal cannula pressure transducer (NCPT) is applied in the sleep lab,[101] and the findings must be scrutinized with great precision to detect UARS. Despite the use of these same transducers in many HST devices, UARS output is typically ignored. Making matters more confusing, UARS typically requires sleep data to confirm the breathing event, which is then labeled a "respiratory effort-related arousal" (RERA). And, still more confusing, if there is no sleep data, the breathing disruption is often labeled "flow limitation event" (FLE)

Just to be clear, UARS is the global term for the sleep breathing disorder; whereas a specific UARS breathing event is called either a RERA or an FLE. I apologize for all the abbreviations and acronyms that crop up; I hope you become fast friends with the list in the front of the book on page xvii. Perhaps a bookmark will ease your access.

Notwithstanding this jumble of terminology, the best diagnostic test currently is the *polysomnogram* (PSG) during which you sleep in a sleep laboratory hooked up to 16 to 20 sensors to measure breathing, heart rate, brain waves, and more. Even if you only slept two hours in a sleep lab, it could still yield more complete and accurate information about your sleep than sleeping eight hours with an HST. The superiority of the PSG is obvious because it collects more data, specifically your brain waves, which is why the PSG is the only legitimate sleep test for the majority of mental health patients compared to the portable monitor, which is more accurately defined as a breathing test that often yields inaccurate readings in someone suffering insomnia throughout the night. Many professionals view HST as a screening tool, not a diagnostic test.

In Chapter 9, you will learn how leg movement disorders must also be evaluated by PSG as there are no HST sensors to check these movements.

SDB Severity Is a Misleading Term

To repeat, a portable test does *not* measure your sleep, so it is not a sleep test; it typically only measures more severe breathing events—apneas and hypopneas. These two sleep breathing events are counted and divided by the number of hours slept on a test to produce the standard apnea-hypopnea index or AHI, which is used by all sleep centers and insurers in the diagnosis of the disorder. As you will learn, however, AHI has proven unreliable in many ways, all of which will be discussed in the following pages.

Technically, SDB severity refers to the number and type of breathing events and changes in oxygen levels, but lots of scientific evidence shows these data points are limited and cannot accurately gauge the impact on your mental health.[102] This point is critical because your sleep-disordered breathing may not appear severe based on the criteria (AHI) in the field of sleep medicine. Likewise, the vast majority of mental health patients will discover their OSA occurs in combination with some degree of UARS, which again may be ignored or underestimated by sleep doctors. As a quick reminder, the AHI does not even include the UARS breathing events.

So, what if SDB is a hypothetical missing link adversely impacting your mental health issues or suicidal thinking? The last thing you want from a sleep test is to be confused by the "official" severity level. Quite frequently, standard terms like mild, moderate, or severe OSA used in sleep medicine are overtly misleading and routinely lead astray many sleep disorder patients and their doctors.

Hear this loud and clear: you can almost never know the true severity of your sleep breathing condition until after you treat it! Therefore, the most relevant measures regarding impact are how these breathing events disrupt your sleep and the subsequent influences on your mental and physical health. By treating this sleep disruption, you will personally gauge how much things change, hopefully and usually for the better.

What You Need to Know About Delta and REM Sleep

REM and delta sleep have been brought up for discussion several times, and now we must spell out the nature of these sleep stages. Here, we'll describe the big picture for these deeper sleep stages that reflect higher quality slumber. In the next chapter, we'll review schematic drawings for these sleep stages as well as for sleep breathing events and sleep fragmentation episodes.

Delta sleep is the deepest stage of non-REM (NREM) sleep, and its brain tracing yields a pattern of very slow, relaxed, and smooth activity. By analogy, delta sleep looks comparable to how Brahms's "Lullaby" sounds. These brain waves function as the single most restorative sleep you generate. They are so powerful in keeping you asleep, fewer or less intense breathing events occur in this stage. In delta, it's common to see snoring in SDB patients, then upon moving out of delta and into any other stage of sleep, including REM, snoring worsens and eventually transforms into flow limitations, hypopneas, or apneas.

Delta sleep normally disappears as early as halfway through the night; thus OSA worsens in severity during the second half of your sleep, leading to more sleep disruption and thus awakenings, which is why most with chronic insomnia suffer more awakenings after delta has receded. As we age, SDB often worsens, and delta sleep may prove more difficult to generate. In our clinical experience, unless the breathing disorder is definitively treated with advanced PAP devices (more in Chapters 6–7 and Appendix A), delta sleep may not return among older patients.

These points are somewhat speculative; nevertheless, monitoring changes in delta sleep may prove crucial in determining whether someone is attaining an optimal response to PAP therapy. The absence of delta sleep in a CPAP user signals a likely missed opportunity for greater improvement. When you undergo a second sleep study using a PAP machine, as described in the next chapter, you need to ask your sleep doctor about this exact data point (strong delta, sparse delta, no delta?). Scant delta means you might need an advanced PAP machine as described in Chapters 6 and 7 and Appendix A.

Among those regaining delta, it is a near certainty you would feel more restored and refreshed in the morning and achieve greater periods of sustained energy levels during wakefulness. Other attributes of renewed delta include enhanced memory, mood, and learning capacity, so you can imagine its importance in your sleep recovery.

REM sleep is a different kind of deep sleep, very different from delta. Its rapid eye movements may in fact produce a kind of focus in the mind from which the individual does not easily awaken, which in turn may explain how some people report feeling deeply refreshed upon awakening just *after* a REM period.

REM affects "consciousness" in unique ways. Even though you are asleep in REM, so much mental *and* physiological activity (increased blood pressure and heart rate, to name just two) occurs during this stage, many experts believe it looks closer to being awake than being asleep. We might speculate this resemblance to wakefulness explains why some dreams feel so real. Another distinction is we dream in all stages of sleep, but our most vivid or memorable dreaming activity takes place in REM.

REM is analogous to riding a rollercoaster through highs and lows with a ton of emotion, all with one key exception. In this ride, you are strapped in and so secure it would be physically impossible to lift even an inch off your seat because in REM sleep most big muscles are paralyzed. Thus, you enjoy this wild ride without any fear of achieving escape velocity.

When we talk about nightmares in Chapter 16, we see where REM yields very powerful emotional states beyond those felt on an amusement park ride. It's more like running for your life through a haunted house that's tilting over the edge of a cliff while the ground below shakes from an earthquake and the air above gusts at hurricane wind speed. Such experiences transform into visions ranging from disturbing to horrific, with lots of painful feelings along the way. And, if you were to lose your natural REM paralysis, things become wilder.

Most REM time—when it is 15 to 45 consecutive minutes of well consolidated sleep without interruptions—generates transformative imagery, including satisfying or interesting dreams, and appears linked to many cognitive-emotional benefits for the human mind. Like delta sleep, memory, mood, and learning capacity are all influenced by REM, which also possesses a special function to promote emotional processing.

This mental functioning has been researched in various ways dating back several decades in the field of dream science. Now sleep science is catching up to what dream researchers theorized long ago, and we expect to find highly precise biological mechanisms to more thoroughly explain why and how REM is so crucial to mental health.[10;69]

From all this discussion on REM and delta, it is imperative for mental health patients with sleep disorders to undergo testing in a sleep lab using polysomnography to ensure accurate measurement of these two crucial sleep stages.

Revisiting SDB Severity

Did I mention portable sleep tests do not measure sleep?

The following section elaborates in detail why the portable test fails to assess the severity of your SDB.

What if you suffer a mild or moderate case of UARS? Suppose instead of suffering sleep breathing events every minute of the hour all night long (60 per hour), as in severe OSA, you only demonstrate one UARS breathing event every four minutes, or about 15 per hour? Would each of these two cases make someone feel differently? The short answer is fewer events might mean fewer symptoms.

Nonetheless, the secret to understanding sleep breathing events is their impact on your brain waves. Some patients with very mild and subtle UARS suffer extremely debilitating sleepiness or fatigue.[78] When UARS is effectively treated, they literally believe a whole new life has been breathed into them. I've seen many of these patients who do not meet requirements established by the insurance company or the standards of a government agency for the diagnosis of a sleep breathing disorder, that is AHI ≥ 5 events/hour, yet the patient responds dramatically to PAP treatment, especially more advanced PAP devices.

The most likely explanation for this paradox is sleep breathing events (regardless of so-called severity) prevents the patient from entering delta and REM sleep. Or, when the patient enters these deeper stages, these subtle breathing events kick the patient out of these essential phases of slumber into more superficial stages of lighter sleep.

Another explanation is any breathing event, no matter how subtle, still arouses or awakens a patient from sleep, and this sleep fragmentation (chopping up sleep into little pieces) proves more devastating to certain mental health patients who demonstrate greater vulnerabilities to poor quality sleep and resultant sleep loss. Last, and not the least of these theories, UARS may interfere with the "brain-washing" function of sleep in ways yet to be discovered.

If your sleep goes unmeasured—the innate problem with portable devices—none of this information is collected, and then you never learn how much your breathing disorder disrupts your brain's efforts to sleep and sleep deeply.

Make no mistake it is your brain we are talking about. Your brain must sleep to restore itself, so the next day your mind (which seeks to reside comfortably in your brain) can function at the highest level of cognition. All these facts indicate better sleep will improve your memory, concentration, and ability to pay attention to promote sound judgment and good decisions. This same mind directs your efforts to work with and through emotional ups and downs across the day, and these emotions are more effectively dealt with after a solid night of healthy slumber. These functions are potentially instrumental in moving an individual away from self-destructive thoughts and behaviors.

All the above reveals the science of sleep is plagued by several measurement mismatches, and this point explains how the use of the portable monitors could lead to worthless, wasteful, and wrong information. One day, portable testing will be fantastic. And we hope that day comes soon. The test in the sleep lab is essential for patients with mental health problems or suicidal ideation because we must determine whether or not the breathing events, from mild and subtle to obvious and severe, are damaging the brain and the mind along with it.

A Night to Remember

The sleep test in the lab is not as big a deal as some complain about. The skill of the sleep technologist working on the night of your study makes all the difference. A more experienced, personable, and savvy tech makes you feel comfortable and attends to your needs. Although it's no slumber party, you will make it through the night and sleep for most of it. It's not comfortable at times, due to wires and sensors attached to your head, torso, and legs, but you will get enough sleep for the sleep doctor to accurately diagnose the problem.

The biggest question posed by mental health patients who undergo sleep tests is whether to use their regular nighttime medications? Or should they change medications leading up to the test? The short answer to the second question is "no." Do not change things, because it makes the most sense to see how you sleep while using these drugs, some of which were specifically prescribed to aid sleep.

A much larger issue warrants maintaining use of the drugs during the sleep test, and by now the explanation should come as no surprise. Psychotropic medications—like antidepressants, antipsychotics, mood stabilizers, anxiolytics (antianxiety pills), or tranquilizers, as well as opiate painkillers, and finally sedatives or hypnotics—are prescribed for anxiety, depression, other mood disorders (for example, bipolar illness) and PTSD or pain; however, it is extremely common for the prescribing physician to inform the patient the drug(s) may also help sleep.

What is extremely uncommon is for a prescribing physician to declare your drugs may alter the objective sleep patterns measured from your brain waves; and few prescribers are aware of how these drugs damage your sleep. The best example of this conundrum involves REM sleep. Common knowledge asserts antidepressants show strong biological effects by suppressing REM sleep. Instead of REM appearing as it normally would in four to six cycles of progressively longer duration throughout the night, these medications delay REM to only appear in the final third of the night, or no REM appears at all.

Is the lack of REM a problem? Yes, it is potentially a huge problem for someone with suicidal ideation because even though the individual's depression might improve through the positive effects of antidepressants, the psychiatric community and the pharmaceutical industry have done a very poor job of analyzing the potential detrimental effects of losing out on REM sleep. A growing body of research about REM sleep, as discussed above, indicates it is related to critical, cognitive-emotional functions such as learning, memory, and mood.

As REM is so important, let me repeat theories dating back decades from the dream research literature that defined dreaming and REM as critical elements in how one learns to successfully process or cope with adverse life experiences.[103] Specifically, *emotional processing* is the term for this coping behavior in which a person works with and through emotions on a daily and nightly basis. Many experts have long identified REM sleep as your personal, in-residence psychotherapist that enables this processing during slumber.

In the sleep lab, we measure whether your medications deprive you of REM sleep, and then an informed decision can determine whether a change of medication is in order. Keep in mind this point represents a cutting-edge area that bridges the fields of sleep medicine and psychiatry. In the big picture, very few mental healthcare providers and only a slightly greater proportion of sleep doctors are looking at the function of REM and how it may promote resiliency in your mental health, which means some physicians view the above information as pure speculation.

I concur many of the attempts to integrate ideas about REM and mental health into a coherent and accurate theory are somewhat speculative. However, clinically, having worked with thousands of mental health patients who regularly take psychotropic medications, I am impressed with a pattern where patients who generate more REM sleep, or what we call more continuous or consolidated periods of REM sleep (meaning non-fragmented REM), describe greater improvement in their daytime symptoms.

Finally, making matters still more complicated is the critical paradox from the fields of psychiatry and neuroscience where it has long been established how antidepressants seem to produce the most beneficial effects by suppressing REM sleep. Thus, we have distinct and competing perspectives about REM, which means you may need to weigh the risks and benefits of changing medications with your prescribing physicians while you go through your sleep treatment program.

The same issue applies for delta sleep because the vast majority of psychotropic medications show variable effects, including bumping some out of deep sleep and into superficial stages. For example, antianxiety drugs are well-known to completely eliminate delta sleep and turn the patient's night into 90% stage 2 NREM sleep, which is roughly double the proportion spent by a normal sleeper in this lighter stage.

As above, both delta and REM can be compromised by medications commonly used by mental health patients, and these sleep stage data need to be collected accurately in the lab to help patients fine-tune the best treatment program.

Sleep Research Pearl #4

In 1993, I was most fortunate and grateful to train at the Stanford Sleep Center with Dr. Christian Guilleminault, the pioneering neurologist, sleep specialist, and researcher extraordinaire, who discovered UARS in children 10 years earlier.[104] His research team was in high gear publishing works on UARS in adults,[105] and so I learned of my own problems with UARS. However, doctors make horrible patients, so my ignorance blossomed with, "oh well, it's not OSA."

Nevertheless, the training was illuminating on several fronts. First, I learned the diagnostic criteria used to assess a sleep breathing disorder were not only too vague but frequently led to under-diagnosis or what's termed "false negatives" in medicine, meaning someone really has the disorder but the test isn't finding it.

This diagnostic problem led to a second, more practical revelation on how to measure sleep breathing. Dr. Guilleminault had championed the use of an exotic device known as *esophageal manometry*, basically a feeding tube you swallow into your stomach to measure changes in chest pressure while you breathe. He used this instrument to discover UARS, and only later was the NCPT device substituted as an excellent surrogate.[101]

From this experience, I realized the largest problem facing sleep medicine was the continued use of the old thermistor device, a sensor only capable of measuring apneas and hypopneas; in other words, it only captured the AHI. The use of the thermistor appeared to be the main reason no one was paying attention to the flow limitation events of UARS—you can't see them with a thermistor; you need the NCPT device.

For the rest of the decade, I worked at the University of New Mexico

Hospital Sleep Disorders Center, where we regularly used the thermistor and saw hundreds of false negative studies (AHI too low for the diagnosis, but in reality many UARS events were present). Sleep medicine docs call this condition "low AHI/high RDI," the latter acronym stands for Respiratory Disturbance Index: the total count of apneas, hypopneas plus the UARS events to yield the most complete measurement.

Only one course of action could remedy this problem: place these patients on CPAP and monitor changes in their sleep in the lab as well as in their daytime symptoms. As you might imagine, two opposing outcomes occurred. We made a lot of patients very happy by correctly diagnosing them, and we made a lot of insurers unhappy and frustrated when we kept appealing their decisions to deny these patients coverage for their CPAP devices. Sadly, this narrative has continued up to the present and the foreseeable future, because UARS continues to be ignored by many sleep centers and insurance companies.

CHAPTER 5

Using Science, Not Insurance, to Gauge SDB Severity

Why is the measurement of sleep breathing events and SDB severity inconsistent, inaccurate, and clinically unusable?

Basic Sleep Graphics

To provide a working and practical knowledge of sleep and sleep breathing events, the following figures are drawn as black and white schematics. Instead of exact replicas of computer screen tracings from a sleep lab, countless interactions with patients taught me to use line drawings to more effectively transmit valuable knowledge. This style is an easier way to learn about each stage of sleep, each type of sleep breathing event, each episode of sleep fragmentation, and how all three components interact.

Take note of these three simple instructions:

1. How tall, how fast, and how dense are the lines? (EEG brain waves)
2. How rounded are the lines? (sleep breathing tracings)
3. How much space lies between lines? (EEG sleep fragmentation)

The deepest NREM stage of sleep perfectly matches what you would expect for something so restful and restorative—tall lines and lots of space between the lines. These delta waves exhibit a slow frequency, which means more space between the waves. In contrast to the deepest sleep, being awake yields shorter and faster brain waves.

Figure 5.1 Awake and Delta Sleep

Awake

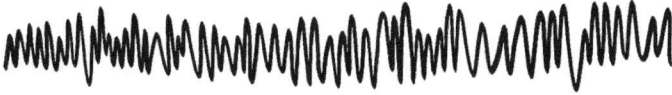

Delta Sleep

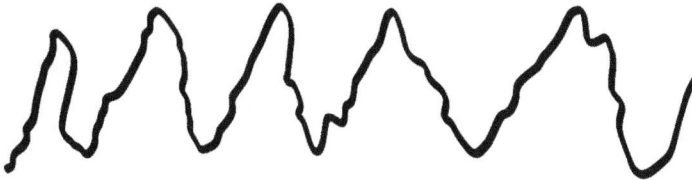

Figure 5.1 The vast difference in brain wave density, highlighted by crowded lines pushed close together while awake, compared to abundant clear space when deep asleep.

The two patterns are easily distinguishable. The shorter, faster frequency waves mirror what's going on at this moment in your brain as you read these words, whereas the taller and slower frequency waves manifest in your brain in your deepest sleep.

In Figure 5.2, two other stages, stage 1 NREM and stage 2 NREM are deemed more superficial sleep. Their lines look a lot like awake, signaling these sleep stages must be lighter. When lines look faster, shorter, and denser you are in some ways closer to being awake than being in deep sleep.

Notice how the top two lines, stage 1 and stage 2, are not as dense as the bottom line (awake). More white space appears between each brain wave in the two stages of sleep. In contrast, the greater density in wakefulness on the bottom graphic make all sleep stages look less dense (again more white space), but white space varies for each specific stage.

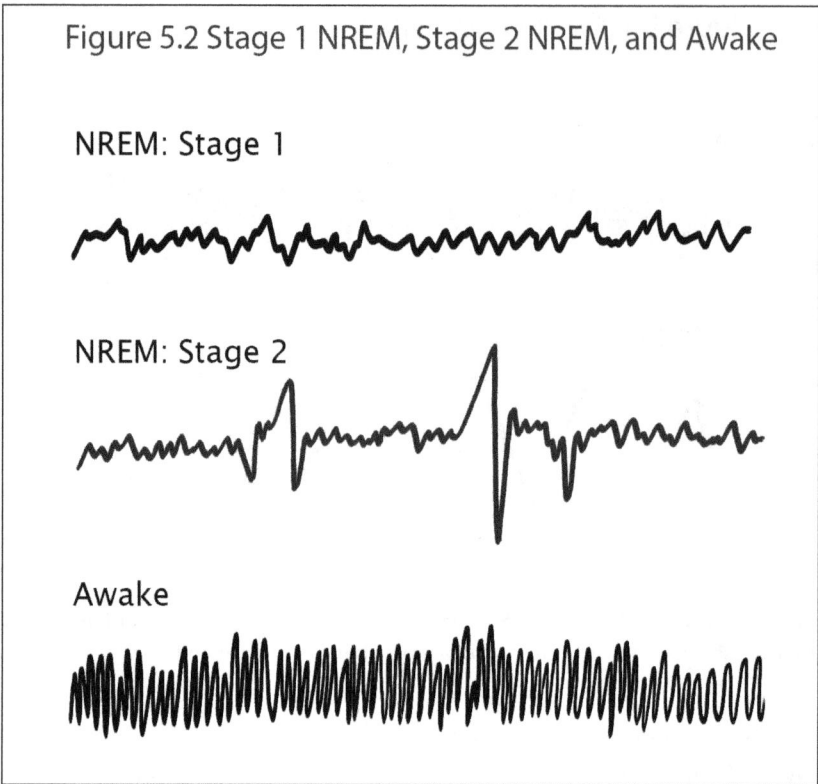

Figure 5.2 Stage 1 NREM, Stage 2 NREM, and Awake

NREM: Stage 1

NREM: Stage 2

Awake

Figure 5.2 In the sleep lab, sleep professionals often require a "fine-tooth comb" to distinguish between awake and stage 1 and sometimes between stage 1 and stage 2, while these schematics show more apparent differences.

REM, also considered deeper sleep by most in sleep medicine, is tricky as REM brain waves only show subtle differences compared to superficial stages. The key to REM sleep is its name, "rapid eye movement."

Notice how the top line of Figure 5.3 might be confused with stage 1 or stage 2 of NREM sleep in Figure 5.2. This confusion is resolved in Figure 5.3 with the middle lines acquired from two sensors attached next to the outer portions of your eyelids. These sharp up-and-down deflections mean your eyes are moving rapidly. Once you spot this activity, REM is identified.

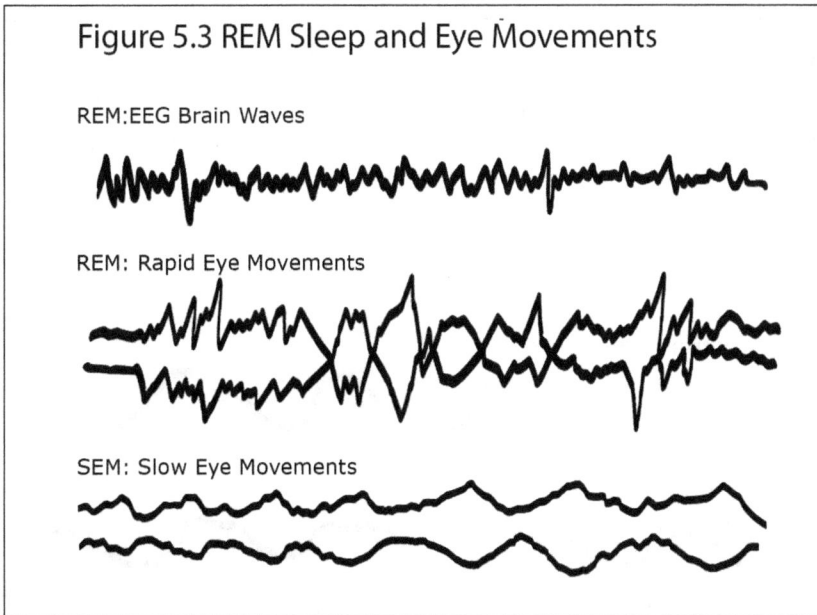

Figure 5.3 REM Sleep and Eye Movements

REM:EEG Brain Waves

REM: Rapid Eye Movements

SEM: Slow Eye Movements

Figure 5.3 Note the rapid deflection of REMs compared to slower eye movements (SEMs). SEM is not REM, but many mental health patients on antidepressants show excessive SEMs of unknown relevance.

Sleep Breathing Graphics

The figures you've been viewing represent normal brain wave patterns found in normal sleep. With sleep breathing waveforms, the shape is the key to spotting normal versus abnormal breathing.

Start with the top line of Figure 5.4, perfectly normal sleep breathing. The top part of its curve rounds during normal inhalation (breathing in). The bottom curve rounds with normal exhalation (breathing out). Look closely at what occurs after you finish breathing out; now there's a relatively straight line, slightly angled upward, leading to the next breath in (rounded curve on top).

This short line warrants its own paragraph, because it has great impact on how SDB develops and how you respond to treatment. This very short line reflects a brief period when nothing is happening. You finished breathing out, but you haven't started breathing in. It is known as the end-expiratory pause. Sit quietly to listen to yourself breathe . . . you'll feel this pause just after you finish exhaling. No air is moving, and then you inhale again.

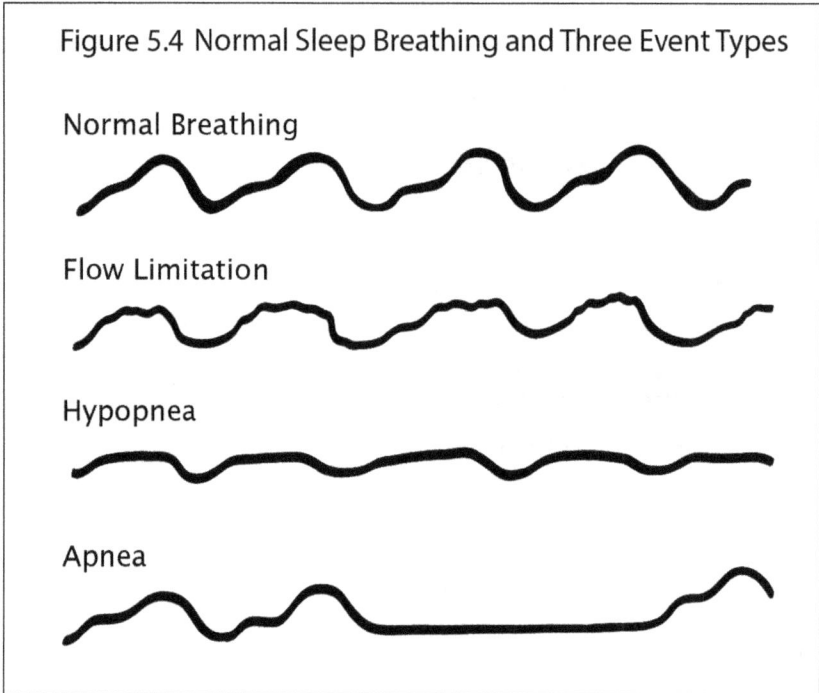

Figure 5.4 Normal Sleep Breathing and Three Event Types

Normal Breathing

Flow Limitation

Hypopnea

Apnea

Figure 5.4 The four shapes range from well-rounded (normal breathing) to extremely flattened. Three sleep breathing events show increasingly severe flattening, indicating increasingly smaller air volume.

Got it? Good, because much more about this little pause will be discussed here and later.

When treating OSA or UARS, the objective is to normalize the airflow signal, which means breathing patterns like the rounded waveforms at the top of Figure 5.4. Anything not rounded is less than optimal treatment (except the brief, flat pause line). Depending on the sleep center you visit, some sleep technologists are not trained or encouraged to round both inspiration and expiration. Logically, eliminating all breathing events during the sleep study should produce rounding, that is, bring the AHI down to zero as well as eliminate all UARS events. Inexplicably, many sleep techs are taught to shy away from aggressively treating the flow limitations, the breathing waveform just below normal breathing. These smaller but not inconsequential events prove challenging to resolve unless using an advanced PAP mode.

Flow limitation, or as named by sleep professionals, *respiratory effort-related arousals* (RERAs) only chop off about 10%-30% of your inspiratory airflow curve.

Notice how most of the curve looks fine; just the very top is cut off. We call this "flattening" because the previously rounded curve flattens from obstruction (collapsing) of your airway. (Hey, now there's a third way to describe UARS events, but thankfully not another abbreviation.) Even though flow limitation was discovered by Dr. Christian Guilleminault 40 years ago, a majority of sleep professionals simply do not pay attention to this component of sleep-disordered breathing.

In clinical practice, this gross disregard of flow limitation events was confirmed on a weekly basis at our sleep center, because we were treating thousands of patients seeking second opinions for CPAP failure. When these individuals tested in our lab, the night started on their current CPAP settings. In virtually every case, flow limitation was easily noticed during CPAP use, which meant pressures were too low. These patients arrived from more than 100 different sleep centers in New Mexico and numerous states in the United States, as well as from Mexico, Canada, and Europe, and none of their CPAP settings were effectively treating the flow limitation.

More telling, they visited us because they identified their own poor responses to CPAP and voiced these concerns to their sleep doctors, which should have provided a clue something was awry in their treatment. We'll return to the problem of unresolved flow limitation in the upcoming chapters, as well as in Appendix A.

The next most severe breathing event, the hypopnea, loses approximately 50% of air volume.

In this picture (Fig 5.4), the hypopnea event has clearly lost a lot of the airflow (almost no rounding). It doesn't look anything like normal rounding on top or bottom, and it's also more degraded than the flattening of flow limitation. Most sleep centers aggressively attempt to resolve hypopneas, but they also must contend with arbitrary rules or policies established by insurers or government agencies in how to define these breathing events.

If it sounds strange to you that nonscientists, policymakers, or business executives are permitted to define a disease, then you would be correct—it's not only strange, but also inexcusable as healthcare policy is now in the hands of people with minimal scientific expertise or clinical interest. Moreover, this policy making directly impacts you and your sleep because these insurance or government "standards" unequivocally lead to substandard care. As we continue, you will see why these policies are not patient friendly.

The most severe of all breathing events are two types of apneas, classified as *obstructive*, when your throat is collapsing, or *central*, for central nervous system, when the brain does not send the proper signal to breathe.

No surprise here. The round shape is entirely gone, a sign of no airflow (Fig 5.4). You might call this a flat line, as when your heart stops beating, but the great news is you will start breathing again on your own after one of these episodes, whether obstructive or central.

Breathing mechanisms are so primal you start breathing again in a matter of seconds. However, the number of seconds may astonish you. Many times, it's "only" 10 or 20 seconds, but in severe cases, a person stops breathing for 30 to 60 seconds or longer. This stoppage is a dramatic shock to someone else sleeping in your bed. In fact, once a wife or husband or anyone else sleeping with you observes just one of these apneic episodes, you better believe the troubled sleeper is promptly if not emphatically told to see a doctor right away.

Regarding obstructive versus central, keep in mind the distinction is detected by the sleep technologist during the study. During an obstructive event, the tech monitors sensors on your chest or abdomen signaling effort or straining as you struggle to draw in air, whereas in central apneas or central hypopneas, these same chest and abdomen sensors go quiet because the brain temporarily turns off your breathing drive. In central events, your airway is wide open; there is no struggle to breathe in because there is no effort to breathe. It's as simple as the brain turning off a breathing switch, again for 10 to 30 seconds, and then turning it back on. If the central apneas last longer, it is usually a more serious condition; however, it is not unusual for most OSA patients to experience a few central events.

Sleep Fragmentation Graphics: The Key to Poor Sleep Quality

We've examined normal sleep stages, normal rounding of sleep breaths, and now abnormal sleep breathing events. The intersection for all these components is EEG sleep fragmentation, the signature component of poor sleep quality. Why is sleep frag so pervasive in SDB? With nearly every type of abnormal breathing event, the brain appears to wake up for a few seconds or longer to return your breathing to normal.

This awakening comes in three measurable forms, and all lead individually or collectively to the destruction of your sleep quality. As a result, 90% or more of the symptoms you develop from OSA/UARS arise from the specifically defined sleep fragmentation episodes shown in the next three figures (Figures 5.5–5.7).

The most obvious would be an awakening (Figure 5.5). You were fast asleep, suffered a breathing event of any sort (apnea, hypopnea, flow limitation), and your brain does not like the experience and wakes you up.

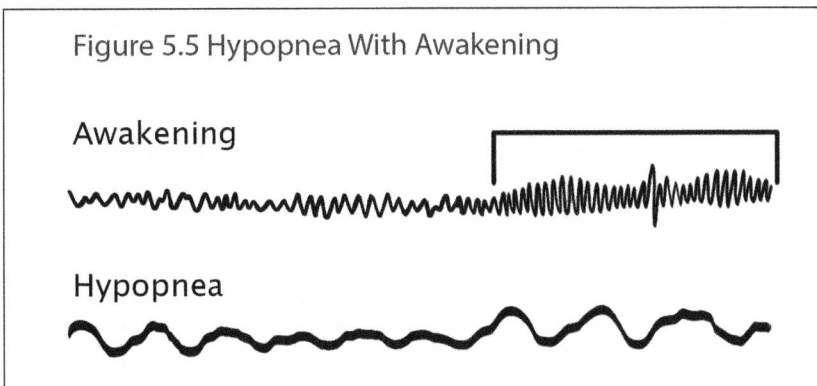

Figure 5.5 Hypopnea With Awakening

Awakening

Hypopnea

Figure 5.5. The bracketed awakening, by the technical definition of sleep scoring, must be at least 16 seconds. Many awakenings last longer, into the two- to three-minute range before you return to sleep.

The top line is the sleep portion and the line below is breathing. Notice how the hypopnea section aligns with the sleeping portion of the brain waves. Then, in the final third of the figure, the brain waves speed up, a sign of awakening. Below this area, you see the hypopnea has been replaced by rounded normal breathing curves. It is not unusual to see these closely aligned patterns where the normal breathing reappears, resuming simultaneously or a moment after the awakening commences.

The full time period of any awakening is crucial to your understanding of the mechanisms of sleep and wakefulness, as well as sleep fragmentation, because most individuals need to be awake at least three minutes before they can remember being awake. This time calibration explains why so many people are confounded by the experience of suffering from a sleep breathing disorder: they simply are not aware of this fragmentation.

The sleep doctor or technologist informs the patient of awakening hundreds of times in a night in the lab while the individual remembers maybe 10 such episodes. In our training in sleep medicine in the 1990s, we would ask the patient the number of awakenings he or she recalled for most nights at home. When the patient said, "two," Dr. Wolfgang Schmidt-Nowara told us to add two zeros to get closer to the correct number, that is, 200 awakenings. Patients were astonished, but the educated guesstimate was useful and accurate enough. I've met many an OSA patient who responded "five" who were in fact experiencing 500 sleep fragmentation episodes during the night, which meant these individuals were arousing or awakening as often as every 30 seconds.

To reiterate, the hallmark of disrupted sleep is your brain waves speeding up, moving you out of sleep and into wakefulness, which can occur in any stage of sleep. And, while some awakenings last perhaps 15 to 20 seconds, any type of breathing event could trigger an awakening lasting several minutes, which becomes one of those dastardly awakenings in the middle of the night from which you find it impossible to return to sleep.

This episode epitomizes how and why you feel so awake and alert upon awakening as discussed earlier; the increase in brain wave activity is also accompanied by increased heart rate and blood pressure. With all this brain and heart activity, you literally feel wide awake, yet typically have no awareness of what woke you up—until now!

To make absolutely sure you appreciate sleep frag, look back at the tall and slow delta waves that look so widely spaced apart compared to being awake where space between brain waves appears miniscule (Fig 5.1). This distinction is a crucial point of context because no matter whether your episodes are caused by sleep breathing or leg movement events, this greater density of the EEG is the clearest evidence you are no longer asleep.

Adding up all these sleep fragmentation episodes means you are subtracting real sleep from whatever hours you believe you are receiving. Moreover, the disruption of sleep means you are going to cycle back and forth between superficial stages (stage 1, stage 2) and being awake instead of creating the opportunity to descend into the deeper stages of delta and REM.

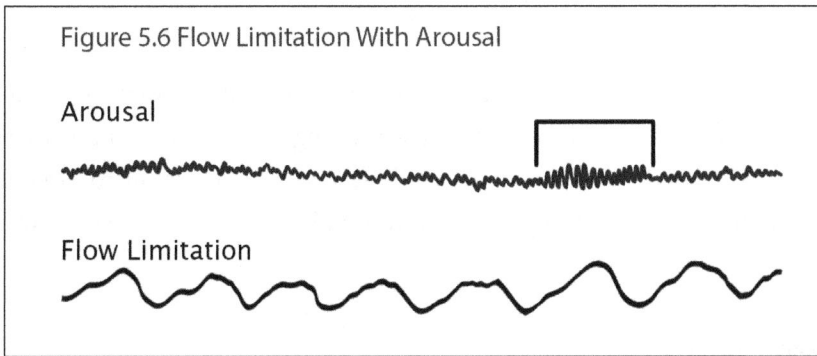

Figure 5.6 Flow Limitation With Arousal

Arousal

Flow Limitation

Figure 5.6 Arousals last from three to 15 seconds, but notice arousals still show the same increase in density of the EEG waves consistent with a waking brain.

Next up are the arousals. Notice how the breathing event shape fits the pattern of flow limitation, and the arousal (under the bracket) is less than 15 seconds—shorter than an awakening. Nevertheless, the length of sleep fragmentation episodes does not always predict the severity of damage because the larger problem is the qualitative disruption to your sleep. That is, you still end up cycling back and forth between light sleep and being awake instead of generating delta or REM. Even the smallest arousal produces damaging effects simply by preventing you from reaching these deepest stages of sleep.

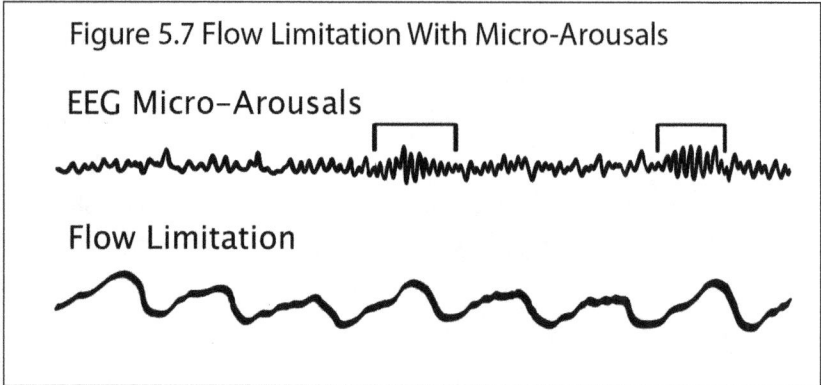

Figure 5.7 Flow Limitation With Micro-Arousals

EEG Micro-Arousals

Flow Limitation

Figure 5.7 The smallest arousal is a *micro-arousal* and usually lasts for 1.5 to < 3 seconds.

In this final sleep frag episode, a flow limitation breathing event is occurring with the classic flattening shape. Twice during these abnormal breathing patterns, the EEG darkens for a couple seconds, and these micro-arousals (under the brackets) while of very short duration still disrupt sleep quality.

Special Categories of Awakenings

Technically, in sleep laboratory medicine, an awakening is arousal activity that lasts 16 seconds or longer. I use the term *technically*, because if you were only aroused 16 seconds, chances are extremely low you would remember these "awakenings." You could be aroused on the EEG tracing anywhere from one to three consecutive minutes and still not realize you were awake. Said another way, you might have brief awareness of being awake, but once you fell back asleep, there's a very good chance you would not remember this brief awakening period.

In other words, you could be waking up all night long in the sleep lab due to awakenings, which due to their length are fracturing your sleep even more than the briefer arousals described above (< 15 seconds). Knowing this information is very useful for establishing your goals in treating sleep-disordered breathing because you would like to eliminate as many awakenings and arousals and micro-arousals as possible during the night.

When we move from physiological sleep disorders to psychological disorders, most commonly insomnia, we'll pick up on the awakenings issue again. With insomnia, the awakenings clearly last longer and are clearly memorable and vexing to the individual. For most insomniacs, it proves enlightening to learn about both shorter and longer forms of awakening, because knowledge about your specific brain activity during sleep leads to a more precise treatment strategy to eliminate these periods of wakefulness.

Finally, when you consider this concept of sleep fragmentation, keep in mind its stark contrast with sleeping and breathing normally, where no disruption should be occurring. Nonetheless, at some sleep centers you may be told you suffer "spontaneous" arousals or disruptions, meaning there is sleep fragmentation without apparent cause. With greater scrutiny, these so-called spontaneous events turn out to be UARS events, that is, the flow limitations or RERAs. As noted above, this problem of untreated flow limitations was widespread in our second opinion cases, so it's likely to be relevant to your care if you are struggling with PAP therapy.

Regardless, once a person is treated for OSA/UARS, the number of sleep fragmentation episodes should drop dramatically because the airflow has been normalized, which means sleep disruption decreases dramatically. All these improvements eliminate the need for the body to react to bring your breathing back to normal because your breathing already returned to normal by using PAP.

Current Problems with Sleep Quality Measurements

By presenting these figures all together, you have been educated on the basics of sleep stages, distinguishing light from deep sleep, the main abnormalities of sleep breathing events, and the way in which your brain waves are disrupted by this abnormal breathing. In current clinical practices, this knowledge constitutes the most widely used information for measuring sleep fragmentation and thereby helping a patient to understand how sleep quality has been compromised.

One final point is needed regarding these depictions. Unfortunately, to reiterate, the sleep medicine measurements in use are at best arbitrary and at worst border on misleading. When something is measured, you would like a measuring stick with lots of precision. You want to include as much data as possible about what you are measuring when you make your final calculations, and ultimately, your treatment decisions.

Believe it or not, none of these steps are actually taken in the standard practices used in the field of sleep medicine. In statistics, the problem boils down to mistakenly transforming continuous variables into categorical events. Here's a gross example using the concept of height. How would you measure someone's height if the tape only included markings for feet but not inches? Over time, the measure would be as follows: "a little over five feet, a little under six feet, nearly five and half feet," and so on. You get the picture—it's not very precise. Now place this same measuring device into the hands of a tailor or seamstress who is making you a new suit or a new dress. While the professional would probably learn to eyeball things very well over time, how would things work out in the hands of an apprentice just learning how to measure with this incomplete system? A sad sack of clothes?!

For a lot of reasons, the field of sleep has accepted very broad, forced, and decidedly unscientific definitions of sleep patterns in measuring sleep fragmentation episodes, sleep breathing events, and even several aspects of sleep itself. These messy measurement systems lead to considerable clinical confusion in attempting to evaluate and treat sleep patients.

AHI Tunnel Vision

The two best examples are how to score a sleep breathing event (for example, hypopnea or flow limitation?) and how to grade the level of sleep quality (do sleep stages accurately describe depth of sleep?).

First, the hypopnea versus flow limitation distinctions are a very big deal due to the arbitrary ways in which insurance companies choose to cover the costs of PAP machines for patients with OSA/UARS. If you suffer from UARS exclusively, several insurers and, notably, Medicare refuse to acknowledge the condition actually exists. Despite all scientific evidence, Medicare ignores flow limitation events. The problem has deteriorated so much, the American Academy of Sleep Medicine has attempted on multiple occasions to rewrite its definitions for hypopneas, hoping to make the term so broad it would encompass at least some of the flow limitation events. Thus, using these methods, they attempted to make it easier to score a larger AHI.[106] However, this approach, while potentially successful in the short term, led to more confusion as sleep professionals eventually and ill-advisedly learned to overlook the entire concept of flow limitation. Over time, "tunnel vision" has developed in the field of sleep medicine such that AHI is the only visible measuring stick despite its severely flawed components. Sadly, RDI is rarely applied.

This illogical and forced gap in knowledge proves disastrous when taking into account how sleep professionals prescribe PAP therapy to treat OSA/UARS, which will be discussed in the very next chapter and in Appendix A. We will also describe how a huge number of individuals never effectively resolve insomnia issues when their sleep breathing disorder is only partially treated due to these misguided perspectives on flow limitations.

Sleep Depth Conundrum

In the second example, sleep quality metrics are much more difficult to resolve because an enormous amount of data are either missing from the observations or, simply, the data have been condensed into imprecise if not vague categories that we currently label as sleep stages. Yet, one would imagine clinically meaningful gradations between sleep stages must exist, but not only are these subtle markers ignored by most sleep doctors, but also sleep researchers rarely investigate this measuring issue.

In the following example involving three sleep patterns, you'll see how one cutting edge researcher is trying to solve this problem.

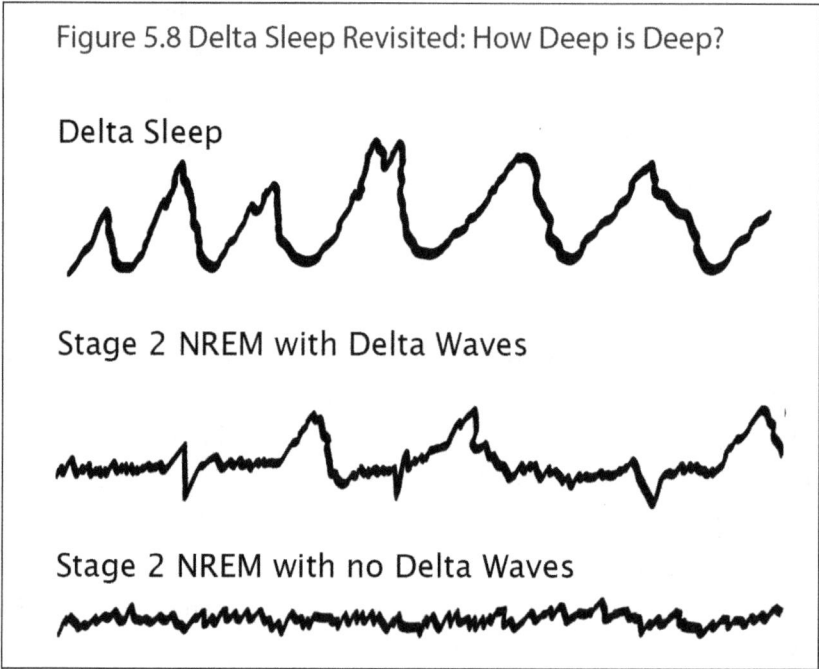

Figure 5.8 Delta Sleep Revisited: How Deep is Deep?

Delta Sleep

Stage 2 NREM with Delta Waves

Stage 2 NREM with no Delta Waves

Figure 5.8 Sleep is deeper if delta waves manifest in another stage of sleep like stage 2 NREM even though current standards do not express the greater depth.

First, consider a delta sleep period with tons of big, wide waves (the deepest sleep). Second, consider a stage 2 NREM period with occasional delta waves but not enough to be called delta sleep—a somewhat deep stage but not as deep as delta. Third, consider a sleep period of stage 2 NREM sleep with no delta waves, a stage not as deep as delta and also not as deep as the stage 2 with some delta.

What's the problem? The delta period with lots of delta is scored delta. Stage 2 NREM with no delta is scored stage 2 NREM. So far, so good. But what do you call the stage 2 NREM that also shows delta waves? It's clearly in between the first two stages, and scientific evidence clearly shows it's a deeper period of sleep. Yet, in the field of sleep medicine there is no clinical term for this stage of sleep, which means we are losing the measurement of how deep this person is sleeping.

A research colleague in Canada, Dr. Magdy Younes, is working to solve this problem by creating a new staging system.[107;108] He's already had success demonstrating actual depth of sleep can be divided into nine distinct categories that are measurable and correlate highly with an individual's objective and subjective experiences. In this example, the stage 2 with delta waves is clearly defined as a deeper stage of sleep. Hopefully, this type of research disseminates into the clinical world so patients receive more accurate and complete information about the quality of their sleep. Check out Dr. Younes' company, *Cerebra*, for more information.

Show & Tell

Do you see how these schematics make the points about normal sleep versus sleep fragmentation as well as normal breathing versus breathing events? In many ways, you now know as much as a sleep doctor or sleep tech in terms of the general nature of these data points. Moreover, you must appreciate the subjective nature of these scoring and measuring techniques, which foretells how all data points are susceptible to wide and varying degrees of interpretation.

In our lab, we showed our patients their computer graphics the morning after testing so they could see what their breathing events looked like and how sleep was disrupted. We point out the different apneas, hypopneas, and flow limitations, and show how this latter event is often the most common finding in mental health or suicidal patients who present with complaints about their sleep.

It is highly motivating for individuals to actually see their breathing disruptions and sleep fragmentation, after which many are eager to get back in the lab to try positive airway pressure (PAP) therapy. One of the biggest motivators is their immediate acceptance that treating sleep breathing will radically decrease, if not eliminate, waking up in the middle of the night.

This looks like a real and immediate cure for this form of insomnia, so most are willing to jump at the chance.

Oxygen

Oxygen is relevant to any discussion about breathing and sleep breathing. Large oxygen drops mostly occur with severe sleep breathing disorders. These drops are harmful and dangerous, which is one reason they receive more urgent attention from the sleep doctor. In particular, these drops more severely damage brain and heart tissues, which can lead to declining cognitive function that looks like dementia, or the triggering of cardiac arrhythmias such as atrial fibrillation, or the worsening of heart failure and coronary artery disease.

Normal oxygenation rests above 90% depending on your elevation. At 5000 feet, a normal level for one person asleep might be 90% all night with occasional drops to 88% or 89%, whereas at sea level, we expect to see values in the 93% to 97% range during sleep.

In severe OSA, some patients' oxygen levels drop not only into the 80% or 70% range, but in REM sleep they may drop into the 60% range or lower. Technically, these drops are life-threatening, but I say *technically* because we see people in the sleep lab with severe oxygen desaturations, yet based on their history they have been sleeping this way for a decade.

The term *life-threatening*, more often than not, means long-term impact. Short-term impact, though, is crucial among cardiac cases in particular as the greater the oxygen drops, the greater the risk for heart rhythm malfunctions (arrhythmias). Then again, we see patients who suffer known cardiac conditions for decades, so they may have been sleeping this way for the same period. Nonetheless, in these cardiac patients we recommend treatment interventions as soon as possible. In rare cases in the sleep lab, we contact emergency services for a patient suffering serious cardiac events.

Unfortunately, some doctors outside the field of sleep medicine imagine these patients just need oxygen therapy, but oxygen can only raise oxygen levels, while doing next to nothing for the sleep fragmentation caused by the sleep-disrupting breathing events.[109] Thus, brain damage may continue from the sleep frag even though oxygen levels may be raised with supplemental oxygen.

Which brings up a very interesting research finding on the nature of oxygen drops. Is it worse to suffer low oxygen levels continuously or worse to experience oxygen repeatedly going down and then back up? A stable low oxygen level, say at 82%, is called *hypoxia*, whereas desaturations refer to the up and down swings over the course of 30 seconds, dropping oxygen from 92% to 88% and then back up to 92%. Dr. David Gozal researched these two scenarios in rats and found more brain damage from the up and down oxygen desaturations compared to a very stable but low hypoxia state.[110]

I like calling these oxygen desaturations another version of fragmentation, that is, oxygen fragmentation, as it often runs in tandem with the brain activity we call sleep fragmentation. Bottom line, both sorts of fragmentation are bad for health, heart, and brain (and rats!) Both are just as likely to impact mood, memory, and emotional regulation and processing. When OSA/UARS is treated, you will reverse both the oxygen and sleep fragmentation; and, the greater the consolidation of both oxygen and sleep patterns, the greater the improvement in symptoms. The degree to which you reverse REM and delta fragmentation (turning them into REM and delta consolidation) will prove paramount in knowing how effectively you are responding to PAP therapy.

As we move on to the treatment of OSA/UARS with PAP, you will learn how this technological invention is a proven game changer with the potential to dramatically uplift, if not save, your life, especially when you experience firsthand how PAP provides an additional boost by decreasing both insomnia and nightmares. Don't worry if you've already tried and quit PAP, we'll discuss plenty of alternatives in Chapter 8.

Sleep Research Pearl #5

In 2003, we opened our own community-based sleep center in Albuquerque,

Maimonides Sleep Arts & Sciences, and immediately renewed our battles with insurance companies. Insurers provide valuable services, but they also employ convoluted reasoning to decide what qualifies for a sleep breathing disorder diagnosis, leading me to spend two decades in numerous dialogues, including phone calls, letters, and e-mails to medical directors, which led at various times to acceptance of the UARS diagnosis, confusion about the diagnosis, or rejection with no appeals allowable. In a nutshell, these institutions paid exclusive attention to the AHI and had great difficulty considering the third sleep breathing event—flow limitation of UARS, let alone RDI.

Within months of opening, we met Claire, a 43-year-old single mother desperately seeking help for debilitating fatigue and sleepiness seriously compromising the quality of her life and her kids. She suffered intermittent suicidal thoughts when coping skills deteriorated. Remarkably, she held a job as an admin assistant at a local hospital but took more sick days than the average employee and was placed on probation three times in the previous eight years for poor work performance. Two sleep studies at two different sleep centers in town alleged no diagnostic findings. One sleep doctor suggested sedating medication for depression; the other doctor recommended Ritalin for an energy boost. She tried sleeping pills and antidepressants but feared stimulants; nothing improved her symptoms.

Claire's case turned into our Patient Zero in providing the fullest explanation for the deficiencies in sleep lab testing. In the years ahead, we helped several hundred patients who had not been diagnosed or not been treated due to by-the-book sleep testing. Claire's case was exceptional as she showed the ultimate "not even close to standard" conventions for a diagnosis of a sleep breathing disorder, not even UARS. There was plenty of sleep fragmentation on the study we conducted, but the breathing irregularities nearly required a magnifying glass to detect. To be absolutely clear, her AHI was *Zero!* In discussing and showing her the results, we explained no insurance guidelines anywhere would label her condition a sleep breathing disorder.

Despite subtle breathing findings, I still wondered about a CPAP trial given all my recent experience at the University along with my prior conversations with Dr. Guilleminault. We spelled out to her how the test results did not meet any criteria for UARS even though the airflow signal did not look normal to my trained eye and that of my top-notch sleep technologist, Dominic Melendrez, who ably assisted us in opening the new center. I informed Claire we could potentially write a letter to an insurer to get coverage for CPAP, but only after it proved to work in decreasing her symptoms.

She was motivated to try one of our loaner CPAP devices, as back then and to this day many people try CPAP, give up, and donate their devices so they don't go to waste. My optimism was muted in this case because I had never before seen an airflow signal so close to normal, but yet not precisely normal, in a patient with such obvious sleep fragmentation. I was perplexed and felt compelled to suggest her case might turn out to be one of these enigmatic hypersomnia disorders where stimulants are in fact a good treatment. Nonetheless, in light of Claire's 20-year struggle with no other medical or psychiatric conditions conclusively established, she and I both wanted her to give CPAP a go.

Stunned is the word of gross understatement describing my reaction when Claire returned a few weeks later and said, "You have saved my life." Tears welled up in me. You wouldn't believe the difference in how she looked, how she talked, and how she felt from just a month earlier. It was not the first and surely not the last time when I pointed to the device and acknowledged, "CPAP saved your life!"

Relative to Claire's story, first check out the bottom of Figure 5.9 that schematically depicts her EEG at diagnosis, then scan the top portion showing the relief she gained by using CPAP.

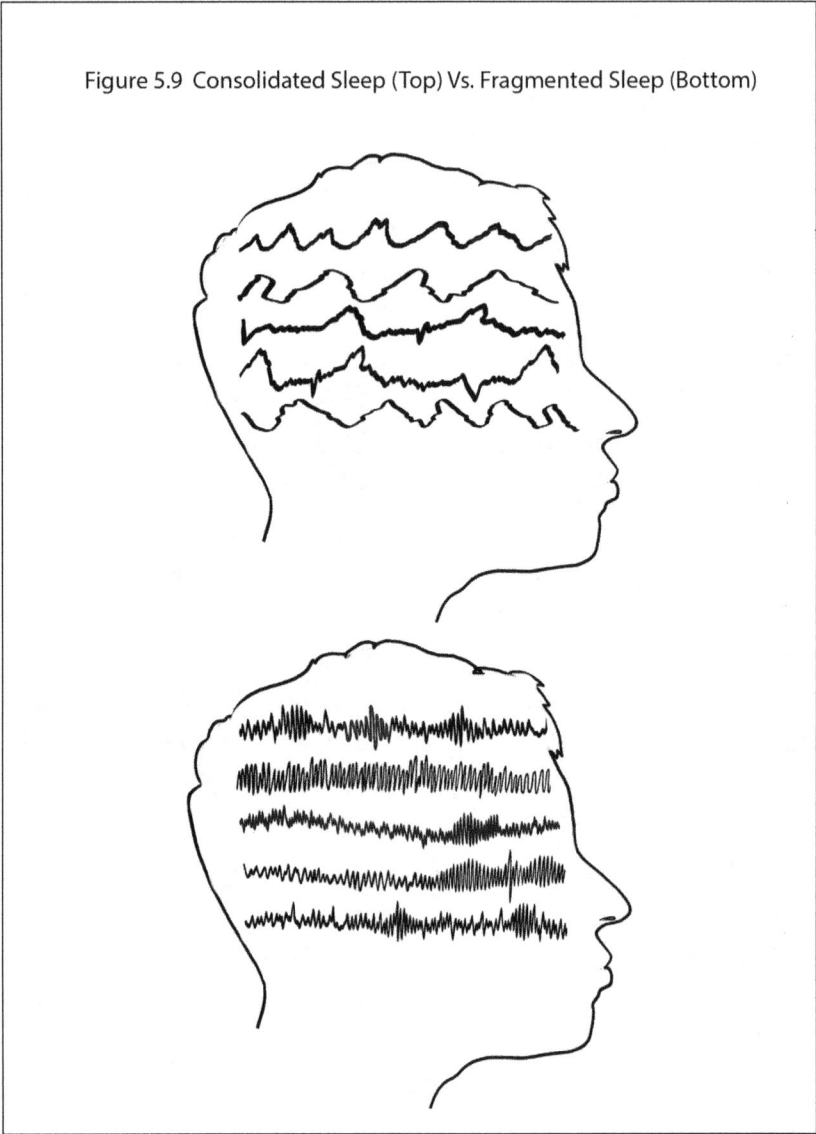

Figure 5.9 Consolidated Sleep (Top) Vs. Fragmented Sleep (Bottom)

Figure 5.9 Two drawings of brain waves demonstrate the sharp contrast between well consolidated sleep (top) and the intense sleep fragmentation of bad and broken sleep (bottom).

CHAPTER 6

An Extremely Potent Medical Treatment Is Just a Breath Away

Why are advanced PAP technologies so much better than CPAP and so much more relevant to mental health patients with OSA, UARS, or CSA?

To PAP or Not to PAP

PAP therapy for SDB comprises three parts: small air compressor device at the bedside; tube running out of the device delivering pressurized air; and, the mask worn on your face receiving pressurized air to keep the airway wide open. "Wide open" is key because many sleep labs do not raise pressures enough to effectively yield a fully patent airway. Instead, they only eliminate apneas and hypopneas but not the flow limitation events of UARS that still cut off up to 10% to 30% of air volume. Sometimes, flow limitation might only be a 10% drop-off, but only by treating UARS can the airway be optimally opened.

Pressurized airflow sensations and mask comfort are invariably the major factors affecting successful use of PAP. Nowadays, mask issues are easier to resolve because the marketplace and related technology have generated a large array of designs to address the considerable variation in nasal and facial shapes, as well as bony contours that require more specific fitting. (See Chapter 7 and Appendix A for tips on mask fitting.) Though mask issues turn out to be a deal breaker for some, the largest nonstarter revolves around pressurized airflow sensations, which could prove easy to resolve if your sleep center is willing to test and prescribe an advanced PAP technology machine.

Many sleep centers only prescribe CPAP, where "C" stands for continuous—one pressure setting used all night long whether breathing in or out and regardless of sleep stage (lighter versus deeper) or sleeping position (side, back, prone). The robotic reliance on CPAP is highlighted by scientific studies conducted more than 30 years ago showing airflow is naturally normalized with dual pressure—greater pressure breathing in and lesser pressure breathing out.[111]

Let's repeat this information in a different way as it is crucial to your progress. Your airway can collapse when you are breathing in or breathing out. For these reasons, you must have positive airway pressure opening up your airway every second you are asleep.

Now let's look at one more schematic, on the next page, to give you a broad view of what this collapsibility looks like. Dominic Melendrez first drew these pictures for our patients 20 years ago.

Notice the bottom row: normal rounded breathing is what the sleep tech would see on your sleep study when PAP therapy has perfectly normalized airflow. Now look to the right of the normal airflow curve to view the schematic of your airway in cross-section. Do you see all the white space? This space reflects zero collapsibility; the airway is fully open, and a normal amount of air passes through into the lungs.

As you move up the figure, each successive breathing event collapses the airway with increasing severity. Flow limitation shows less airspace (first signs of collapse) than normal but more white space than a hypopnea. A hypopnea shows less airspace (greater collapse) than flow limitation but more white space than an apnea. Of course, an apnea shows virtually no space (almost full collapse).

To clairfy your PAP goals, you would like to persuade your sleep professionals to treat not just your AHI, but your RDI as well. Ideally, using the RDI term conveys your desire to treat all 3 breathing events.

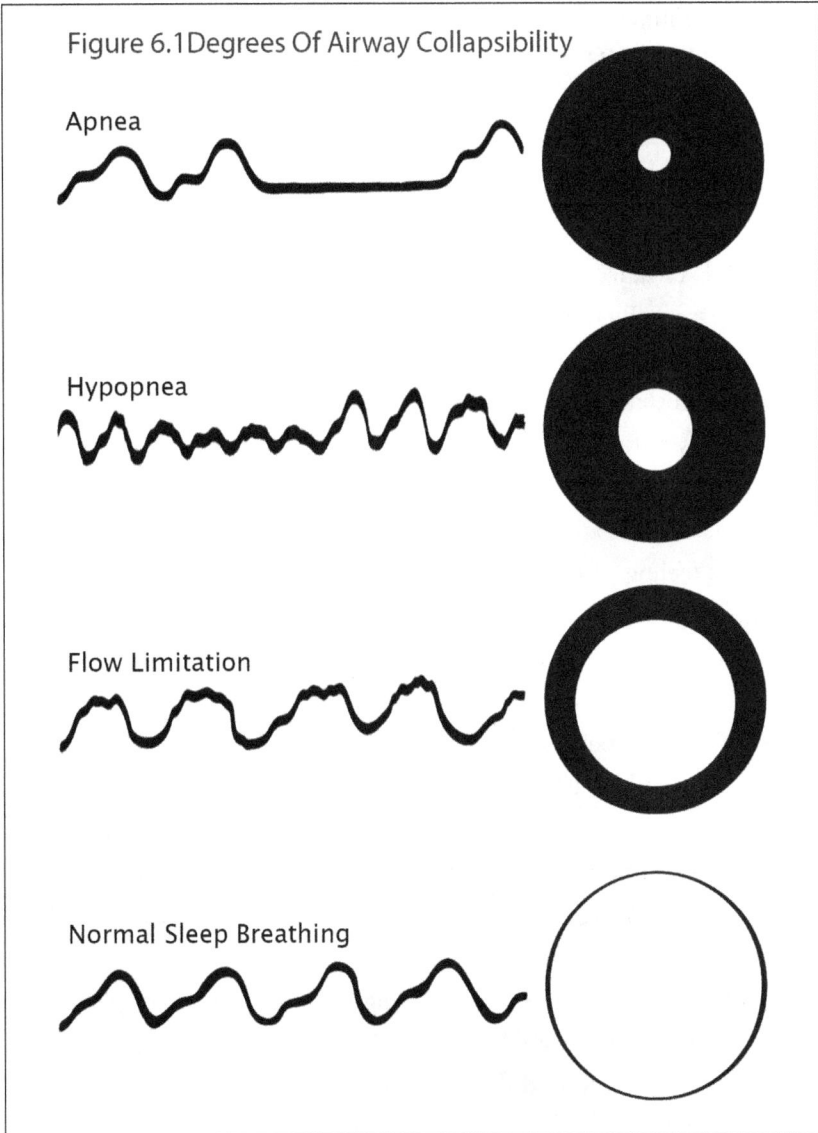

Figure 6.1 The lines on the left side depict tracings of three types of sleep breathing events along with normal airflow last. On the right side, this normal breathing shows a wide open space just as if you were looking down into the bottom of the throat. Moving up the chart, each breathing event shows greater narrowing of the airway space. The apnea shows the greatest collapsibility.

As we continue the discussion, keep these four pictures in mind to better understand how CPAP succeeds or fails in treating OSA/UARS.

How CPAP Fails

The CPAP fallacy derives from the conventional wisdom fixed pressure should work equally well on inhalation and exhalation, contrary to evidence-based medicine. Instead, dual pressure systems known as bilevel are more natural, comfortable, and effective therapy.

Bilevel is critical for mental health patients because their underlying tendency toward anxiety adds to or triggers palpable discomfort on fixed CPAP. Discomfort and distress arise when trying to breathe *out* against an obvious feeling of too much air coming *in*, whereas a two-level system (bilevel) drops the pressure as you breathe out, and the discomfort and associated distress often disappear.

More later on resolving this discomfort (including a special figure). For now, please remember the above point as it is nothing short of a lifesaver given how mental health patients routinely fail CPAP devices. In fact, the failure rate was so high at our sleep center, which specialized in the care of mental health patients, we virtually ceased prescribing CPAP in 2005, more than 17 years ago. Instead, we prescribed only bilevel devices. Quite relevant to your efforts, we noticed bilevel was not only more comfortable, but also the dual pressures yielded a higher quality of sleep, particularly, greater consolidation of REM. Most relevant to insomniacs, bilevel more consistently eradicated middle-of-the-night awakenings.

Since 2009, we used only advanced bilevel devices possessing built-in auto-adjusting algorithms to detect changes in your breathing and adjust accordingly. These machines do not need to know whether you are sleeping lighter or deeper or on your back or side. They simply detect a need for higher pressures by the way you breathe at any given moment. On your back or in lighter sleep your airway is more collapsible; the device senses this vulnerability and increases pressure, just as in delta sleep or a side position it will lower pressure due to greater airway stability.

As the prime example, essentially all patients need higher pressures in REM sleep. The auto-adjusting devices do not detect the presence of REM; rather, the algorithm simply detects your airway experiencing greater collapsibility. Once detected, the pressures automatically increase. Please refer to Figure 6.1 again: when a normal airflow curve deteriorates to flow limitation or hypopneas due to entry into REM sleep, the auto-adjusting algorithm is designed to detect whatever degree of collapsibility must be corrected.

Keep in mind, these devices use their own built-in pressure transducers (like the ones described earlier on the diagnostic study) to determine whether or not your airway is wide open. When not fully opened, the auto-adjusting algorithm detects flow limitation events of UARS and modifies the pressure settings.

While some sleep centers prescribe auto-adjusting devices, in our opinion they may translate the word "auto" too literally, believing the computer program is like an autopilot. It is not a perfected autopilot, and therefore you may not obtain great results just by starting to use one. The auto mode serves as a crucial framework within which you still may require testing with the auto device in a sleep lab, during which an experienced sleep technologist manually overrides the auto function to fine-tune the pressurized air settings. This kind of testing, known as *lab titration*, provides a more nuanced starting point for the patient, which then increases potential for more substantive improvements in airflow and quality of sleep.

For these reasons, testing and in early phases of treatment retesting in the sleep lab (known as re-titration or REPAP)[53] is the most expedient means to promote comfort and faster adaptation to the device. This repeat testing achieves greater clarity in gauging long-term therapeutic settings to produce the highest quality of slumber, the likes of which you might never imagine possible until you experience an advanced PAP device.

If there were a theoretical way to experience the benefits of an auto-adjusting, dual pressure PAP therapy device *before* you ever tried using it (say, a magic wand), then greater than 99% of all sleep apnea patients would insist on using this mode of treatment.

PAP therapy is truly a modern miracle of medical science. I use an auto-adjusting, dual pressure PAP device every night, and it has completely altered my life for the better for many years, even more so than my initial use of standard CPAP and auto-CPAP devices 20 years ago. If by way of this magic wand you could sense the experience of what advanced PAP does to your sleep, your mind, your energy level, and your mood, you would be clamoring for this device faster than you could catch 40 winks.

A relatively small caveat is all PAP devices are not necessarily easy to use at the outset. It is not impossible to use or technically difficult, but because it is foreign, cumbersome, and has a high hassle factor in the early going, you must commit to an earnest effort for several weeks, sometimes several months, and occasionally more than a year to smooth out your relationship with the device. In the first few days or weeks, the relationship often manifests as a love-hate thing for a sizeable number of sleep apnea patients, who struggle to adjust to the process.

"Finesse you must" is a great motto for learning to use PAP because if you are not attentive, precise, and diligent in the first few weeks, it may never blossom into the beautiful and rewarding relationship it offers to regular users.

That said, your very first night in the sleep lab could produce the boost you need to take this *sleap* of faith, because there's a good chance you will "taste" a difference in your sleep quality. In some cases, it might be the surprise of your life if you were to sleep all through the night, or not wake up to use the bathroom, or you were to dream more than usual, or awakened in the morning feeling more refreshed or energized than you felt in a long time. Any of these experiences may and often do occur; at our sleep lab patients received benefits in 80% to 90% of first-time usage in large part because of the use of advanced, dual pressure, auto-adjusting PAP devices.

Nonetheless, to reiterate, if your sensitivity to all the equipment, the pressure, mask, headgear, tubes and so on overwhelms or distracts you, please temper your expectations until you gain more comfort in using the device. Patience is the operative word for sleep apnea patients. There is, however, a way to speed up the process, as you'll read about in the introduction to Chapter 7, coming up soon.

A Running Start

Unlike most other sleep centers in the United States and around the world, we prescribe maybe one or two CPAP machines—per year—and almost always because the patient wants a less expensive device or an insurer forces the issue. Among thousands of patients we treat, most receive newer advanced technology devices, operating as "smart" machines as described above to auto-detect changes in your breathing and respond accordingly.

For now, it is important to learn a more technical explanation for making the switch from CPAP to other devices because it may provide a running start on your treatment by avoiding CPAP altogether in the sleep lab or at home.

To refresh your memory from one minute ago, the problem with CPAP is the single-level air pressure remains constant all through the night, thus providing this same pressure regardless of breathing in or out. If your CPAP is too high, then the pressure sensation is decidedly uncomfortable when you breathe out. In very sensitive individuals, low CPAP pressure still provokes feelings of discomfort or distress during expiration. Touching on a fine point, auto-CPAP is no better. It changes your pressures along a range from low to high, but it never lowers your pressure when breathing out (although some newer auto-CPAPs provide very minor and usually inconsequential relief on expiration).

This problem on exhalation is usually termed *expiratory pressure intolerance*, or EPI, or just *pressure intolerance*. As patients rarely report pressure intolerance while breathing in, we prefer "EPI" to clarify the problem occurs when breathing out.

In Figure 6.2, look very closely at the two curves. On top, everything is normal, rounded curves breathing in and out, and there is the short, relatively "flat" pause line between the end of expiration and the beginning of inhalation.

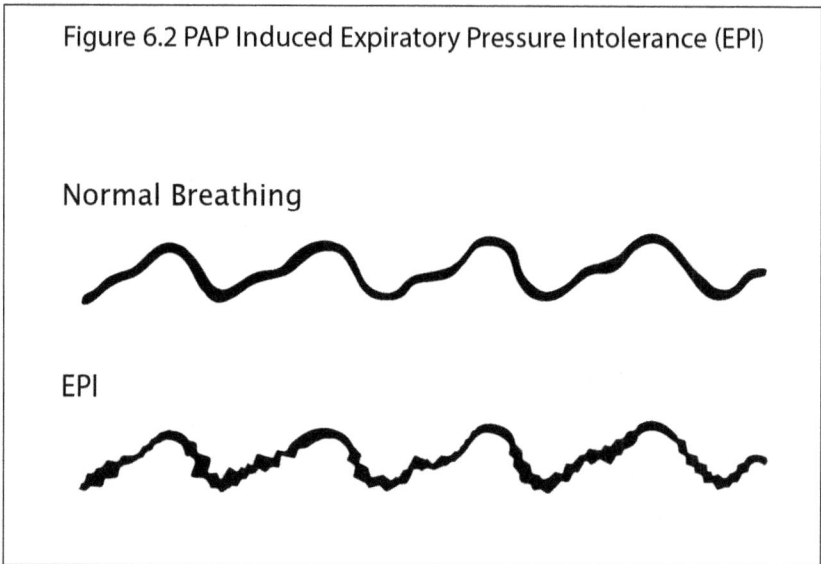

Figure 6.2 PAP Induced Expiratory Pressure Intolerance (EPI)

Normal Breathing

EPI

Figure 6.2 Expiratory pressure intolerance (EPI) is a subtle change on the airflow tracing, and the sleep technologist must be trained to accurately identify EPI and to adjust pressurized air accordingly.

On the bottom tracing, notice two changes. First, the pause line is basically gone, and second, the expiratory limb looks ragged. Inhaling still looks rounded on top, but breathing out shows these two changes, actually abnormalities. From the knowledge gained in working with thousands of CPAP failure cases, these lines appear to be the objective corroboration of EPI. We've published on this finding and included graphics demonstrating the pattern.[39] Most importantly to your efforts, when patients switch to bilevel modes, these expiratory irregularities usually disappear as exhalation returns to normal.

Bilevel is more comfortable for most sleep apnea patients because the feeling of lower pressure while breathing out aligns closer with your natural breathing experience. When bilevel is coupled with "smart" technology— auto-adjusting pressure algorithms—that's auto-bilevel or ABPAP, one of the most advanced devices on the market. Another auto-bilevel type device is called adaptive servo-ventilation or ASV. Not only will ASV auto-adjust and provide two pressure levels, it also applies a "backup rate" to engage the sleep apnea patient to breathe at a more regular rate, which for a surprisingly large proportion of mental health patients turns out to be necessary and highly beneficial to their sleep. ASV is the very best option if you suffer from CSA, the central apnea problem mentioned earlier.

To be absolutely clear, ABPAP and ASV devices are easily capable of bringing your AHI all the way down to zero as well as dramatically reducing your flow limitation events (RDI<5).

ASV is an exceptionally important advance in technology for PTSD and other anxiety patients who may never adapt to CPAP, BPAP, or even ABPAP devices. By comparison, ASV possesses a noticeably distinctive capacity to treat the most subtle breathing events, the flow limitations of UARS, while simultaneously preventing discomfort when pressures might have otherwise felt too high on exhalation. In other words, we see the best results resolving EPI on ASV.

In many OSA/UARS cases, an anxious response to PAP arises during sleep itself; the individual's brain rebels and briefly ceases respiration despite a completely open airway. These stoppages are the clear sign of the central apnea disorder, with "central" referring to central nervous system, that is, the brain signaling not to breathe. Many of our PTSD and other anxiety patients could only use ASV because they developed extreme discomfort or central apneas or both while using any other form of PAP. Unfortunately, most insurances create large hurdles to obtain ASV by declaring only the presence of central apneas warrants their use. However, in our clinical experience, we are confident persistent or pervasive EPI should qualify as another criterion to merit use of ASV.

Making the Most of Your Night in the Sleep Lab

In the sleep lab, gaining a good night of restorative slumber on your first PAP attempt is often a matter of technology, technologist, and time. *Technology* means you will be provided opportunities to test out newer devices, which may be challenging because many sleep labs never use them. *Technologists* are the sleep techs who connect all the sensors on the night of the study and monitor you and all these sensors for the duration. More importantly, the sleep tech serves as a coach, guide, and educator rolled into one to help you through the night and gain the best results. Things such as tweaking how the mask fits on your face or helping you work through your frustrations with a good joke at 3 a.m. are priceless, and more so, the sleep tech must recognize whether or not your breathing is normalizing in response to the pressure settings.

Is the airway wide open, and is sleep quality as good as it gets? If not, then you will find yourself in a situation comparable to being given only one pain pill for your backache when two pills are required. In sum, if the tech doesn't come close to normalizing your airflow signal, you may not wake up feeling much better.

To restate, the greatest lapse in the field of sleep medicine is the neglect of the UARS breathing events (flow limitations), which often require advanced technological solutions, especially ABPAP or ASV. Specifically, refer to Figures 5.4 and 6.1 and notice how the airflow curve must be rounded to achieve normal sleep breathing, that is, no collapsibility. Moreover, when this airflow curve rounds for sustained periods of the night, REM and delta sleep are likely to emerge for lengthier uninterrupted periods even though this sleep test could be your first exposure to PAP.

Think of it: on your very first therapy night, you have a great chance to generate the powerful stages of sleep (REM and delta) that will not only improve sleep quality and decrease middle-of-the-night awakenings, but also yield the incredibly satisfying sensation of refreshing sleep upon awakening in the morning. Many people wake up from PAP for the first time and declare they have experienced their best sleep in 10, 20, or 30 years.

Technologically, again please appreciate all PAP modes are equipped with pressure transducers, so it is relatively straightforward to monitor and treat flow limitation breathing events all night. Regrettably, many sleep labs do not make this connection because of their relative lack of interest in UARS, or they follow the scientifically invalidated conventional wisdom that dictates

CPAP should be adequate for virtually every patient. For all these reasons, the more you know about advanced PAP machines as described further in Appendix A, the better prepared you will be to discuss these options with your sleep professionals.

Time is of the essence during a sleep test as only so much can be experimented with on the very first night of PAP use. With a great sleep tech, you could find:

- The best fitting mask that feels comfortable without leaking
- The best PAP pressure delivery mode that suits your breathing patterns
- A close approximation of the best starting pressure settings to normalize your airflow signal as much of the night as possible
- The identification and treatment of EPI should it interfere with your PAP response

All these factors create considerable potential to generate clear-cut intervals of consolidated sleep on the very first night of treatment.

Applying the Right Kind of Pressure

While the most important pressures you need from a PAP device are settings that normalize your airflow curve when you breathe in and out, long before you arrive at the lab you might apply pressure of your own to achieve superior results on your maiden voyage. Literally, investigating sleep labs prior to seeking care is a smart strategy. Calling on the phone or completing a website contact form, you simply ask whether a center diagnoses or treats UARS and whether advanced technology is used in the lab (for example, BPAP, ABPAP, ASV). If they cannot answer these questions directly, then they are most likely inexperienced in these methods. Try the next one on your list. If your list is limited, then be sure to schedule an appointment with a sleep doctor or other provider at the center to discuss any of these points before testing.

Often, things boil down to finding the best sleep tech at the facility. The best sleep tech might be the only person who works effectively in addressing

UARS and knows how to apply advanced technology to resolve stubborn UARS events by carefully monitoring the airflow curve generated from the pressure transducer. Even if a sleep lab has an average track record, just this one sleep tech might be able to provide the services you need because he or she appreciates the necessity of "rounding" the airflow curve as pictured in Figures 5.4 and 6.1.

This perspective is crucial to your well-being as individuals with mental health problems in general and PTSD or anxiety problems in particular would like and expect to receive care in ways distinct from how classic sleep apnea patients are treated. The probability is so high you will exhibit UARS components to your breathing disorder, you will need the right technology, the right technologist, and the right amount of time to discover the best PAP device, and you may need to persuade the staff caring for you to go the extra mile.

This outlook will make waves, but waves flow out and then they flow back in, meaning sleep center staff should already know or be willing to gain familiarity with the difficulties you may experience trying to use PAP and should have plans in place to help patients troubleshoot.

Consider the alternative: if you start with low-grade technology like CPAP, work with an average sleep tech who does not know about UARS, and you are not given the proper time to work through any obstacles on the first night of PAP testing, then the frustrations you experience will be so great you might give up on PAP therapy and give up on treating the sleep breathing disorder within a month or a week, if not a few days. Such an ending would be tragic as you would have missed out on the strong potential to experience far-reaching improvements in both insomnia and nightmares just by using a PAP device.

Focusing on gaining the best, advanced sleep therapy as soon as possible is an optimal guiding directive because currently there is nothing else in this world that can increase your sleep quality to this degree and this rapidly. There are other options, but most of them are mediocre or simply above average compared to this new, advanced gold standard.

An overarching theme put forward in this book details how sleep and oxygen fragmentation destroy your sleep quality, trigger insomnia, and aggravate nightmares, and thereby corrupt your memory, coping abilities, and mood, all of which may worsen suicidal ideation and behavior.

Somehow, some way, we must find a path to start you on the best type of PAP therapy as soon as possible—your life may depend on it!

Sleep Research Pearl #6

At the opening of our sleep center, we experimented with CPAP, auto-CPAP, C-Flex, and EPR (expiratory pressure relief), the latter three each providing small degrees of auto-adjusting capabilities. Many of our patients received prescriptions for these modes, and I was using auto-CPAP from 2002 to 2005. However, we were very disappointed in the results. The majority of the mental health patients were not adapting well, universally complaining about breathing out against the airflow, and rarely was anyone obtaining fantastic results from any of these modes.

One memorable day in 2005, Dominic and I were scrutinizing sleep study tracings of the airflow signal. The question plaguing us was a simple one: "If patients are complaining about breathing out against pressurized air, then does it show up in some way on the airflow tracing?" Typically, when reviewing their sleep studies, we noticed flow limitation was not resolving consistently with these devices; sleep fragmentation was evident in many forms, notably a lack of consolidated REM; and, overall sleep quality was exhibiting neither normal proportions of sleep stages nor consolidated intervals of sleep time. So, it wasn't a surprise patients were receiving scant benefits.

On this day, we zoomed in on the airflow tracing in a patient using C-Flex, a device that pauses pressurized air on expiration. Though this mode was providing comfort, patients were not benefiting. On the breathing out phase, or what we call the *expiratory limb* of the airflow curve, the signal was not normal, as if the cessation of pressurized air was inducing an expiratory flow limitation.

For whatever reasons, we had not been looking closely at the expiratory limb until we noticed this abnormality on the C-Flex patient. We quickly pulled up a study on a regular CPAP patient and were surprised by an obvious irregularity on the expiratory limb. We asked ourselves whether this "jumbled" or "raggedy" appearance was depicting the patient's discomfort with pressurized air while breathing out. Or, was the patient not just uncomfortable, but "fighting" the air coming in?

See Figure 6.2 to review this depiction.

At the time, we were testing a few patients, including myself on bilevel, so we pulled up one of these studies and were stunned to see what we had been missing all along. The airflow curve was rounded on *both* inspiration and expiration.

The full sequence of events immediately came into view. Patients fighting air pressure on CPAP were regularly demonstrating this abnormal pattern on expiration that matched their physical complaint, commonly described as "it feels like too much air." Fighting with air produced the odd-looking expiratory limb in Figure 6.2. All that was needed was lower air pressure when breathing out, which then normalized the expiratory limb to its rounded shape. Bilevel solved both problems. It resolved discomfort by lowering pressure on breathing out, but not too low, so normal rounding of expiratory airflow is still achieved.

The take-home message was the expiratory limb turned out to be much more important than we imagined, and to this day we are surprised at how long it took us to spot this abnormality, as well as how many sleep professionals still seem to be ignoring it. From that moment in 2005 on, we chanted, "bilevel, bilevel, bilevel." By 2008 we saw how auto-bilevel (ABPAP) actually rounded the expiratory limb better than standard bilevel, and then the mini-miracle occurred in 2010 with ASV when we saw not only greater roundedness on the expiratory curve, but also patients were declaring they had never experienced so much comfort with any prior device. The telling quote from many individuals, including myself, says it all: "Sometimes I can't tell whether there is any air; it just feels like I'm breathing on my own."

———·———

Key Pointers for New, Active or Struggling PAP Users

Once you receive your PAP device, a lamentably convoluted process, I encourage you to repeatedly comb through all the tips and Pearls in Appendix A to aid in your troubleshooting. For now, please go directly to the next chapter and read the first section on the Pearl of all Pearls to rapidly enhance your adaptation experience with PAP.

Also, if struggling with PAP early on, be sure to read Sleep Research Pearl #7, which describes the procedure we invented known as the PAP-NAP, a day- or nighttime experience specifically designed to troubleshoot and resolve numerous PAP obstacles.[112]

CHAPTER 7

How to Deal with a Medical System Designed to Frustrate

Should I use my health insurance to obtain a PAP device, or is it better to avoid insurance and pay out of pocket?

The Pearl of All Pearls in Using PAP

Before we take up the business of PAP, let's discuss imagery distraction, a game changer for as much as 90% of patients attempting to start PAP. This Pearl is a two-for-one deal, and the first part involves your natural inclination to synchronize your breathing with the flow of pressurized air. Don't! It doesn't work.

When you breathe to harmonize or get in rhythm with PAP airflow, you will find it nearly impossible to adapt to the pressure sensation because the machine rebels against your efforts. The auto-adjusting devices like ABPAP and ASV work through their own algorithm to detect how you breathe and then respond accordingly. If you are "over controlling" your breathing, trying to match it with this pressurized air, the machine no longer operates as intended, and the ensuing disharmony feels sufficiently uncomfortable to prevent sleep.

So, how should you breathe when starting PAP? Do everything possible to avoid paying any attention to the device, mask, and, most importantly, the pressure sensations. And the best way to succeed is to picture things in your mind's eye as if daydreaming, or what we call *imagery distraction*. Pick something pleasant and relaxing or even boring, not something unpleasant or stressful. If you know how to daydream, then technically that's all you are doing. Daydreaming about a sunny beach with waves lapping on the shore is all you might need. When you use your mind's eye and engage with the pictures you see, your body and your mind no longer react to the pressure sensations, and the device does its magic.

When we learned the value of this technique, it was a game changer for thousands of patients who were reporting initial difficulties with adaptation to PAP, including those using CPAP or auto-CPAP as well. Personally, it was a game changer for my first PAP efforts 20 years ago. If you need more elaboration on these instructions, Chapter 11 is devoted exclusively to the use of mind's eye imagery, so please review the information there if you struggle with the pressurized air or if you are uncertain how to distract yourself from these sensations.

The Business of PAP Therapy

Life with PAP therapy would be considerably easier if your doctor wrote a prescription for your device and you filled at a drug store. Then, you start treatment at home as if PAP were just a pill you swallowed with a glass of water every night at bedtime. As you might imagine from the degree of complexity and precision described so far, to find the right machine and the best pressures to treat your sleep breathing problems is not a straightforward task. The business side of buying, renting, or leasing the device and all the supplies needed for proper functioning also proves complicated, convoluted, and sometimes unfriendly.

Making the mess more frustrating, most sleep doctors and sleep medical centers are not directly involved in the equipment phase of your experience even though their PAP expertise is greater than anyone else on the planet. Only about one in seven sleep centers sell PAP devices. Instead, you must work with durable medical equipment (DME) or home medical equipment (HME) companies.

What goes on in far too many DME and HME companies is nothing short of scandalous regarding quality of care as measured by success or failure in teaching sleep apnea patients to adapt to and use a PAP machine. These companies are consistently subpar in how they coach sleep apnea patients to achieve regular PAP use. If you are lucky to find a DME or HME directly linked to your sleep center, you gain a greater chance of finding the support and expertise you need to succeed. You often achieve better results if you find a specialized DME/HME working exclusively with sleep equipment.

The majority of sleep centers avoid selling DME because of the potential for a conflict of interest. These alleged conflicts are concerning to sleep professionals and their centers because they fear government regulators will swoop in and cry foul. This specific problem, arbitrarily manufactured years ago by Congressional laws (Stark Law in particular) to prevent doctors from routinely selling PAP equipment, is one of many bureaucratic entanglements that can lead to shoddy customer service as sleep professionals battle with DMEs to manage cases. Conversely, DMEs often battle with sleep centers. Overall, dealing with DMEs has consistently proven to be the weakest link in the sleep medicine industry, the one area of universal complaint from every other player in the game, and the one system for which no one has ever attempted a fix.

Sooner or later, you might have trouble dealing with your DME. At some point, many people with additional resources go elsewhere to find their PAP medical supplies, even forgoing their insurance coverage out of sheer frustration.

Finding a Good Sleep Tech

A good sleep tech knows more and possesses more experience than the smartest respiratory therapist at most of these medical supply companies. (Often, a great sleep tech knows more than the sleep doctor!) While respiratory therapists are very bright people, they almost never acquire the vast in-the-trenches expertise in coaching patients to use the PAP device, yet most DME/HME companies employ (often by legal requirements) respiratory therapists to set up devices for sleep apnea patients.

Let's say a respiratory therapist sets up two or three patients several days in a week. This scenario amounts to five to 15 hours of experience per week, so maybe 250 to 750 hours per year of hands-on exposure. Yet, most sleep techs spend 1500 to 2000 hours per year working only and directly with sleep apnea patients. To boot, most of their experience occurs while the patient is trying to use the PAP device during sleep in the lab. Respiratory therapists typically possess close to zero experience observing the use of PAP therapy in a sleeping patient unless they actually worked as a sleep tech at some point.

Which one would you choose to help you start PAP? Don't bother answering; you have no choice. Insurance companies and DME/HME companies as well as government regulators have created barriers in many regions of the country that make things nearly impossible for sleep techs and sleep doctors to directly work with their sleep apnea patients in the equipment side of treatment.

Notwithstanding the rant, which I hope encourages you to turn a skeptical eye toward these lackluster business entities you must encounter, you still must find a DME/HME to get started and to maintain essential PAP supplies for as long as you use your device, assuming you do not or cannot pay out of pocket.

I want you armed with the right details and the most precision about the equipment so you feel more confident in asserting some degree of control over the transactions with these companies.

Masks: How Businesses Mask the Problem

Beyond the PAP device and pressure settings, a mask is the second most critical element for adapting to PAP. You must realize the market for mask technology is exploding: virtually every patient can find a mask that fits well without leaking or causing discomfort or pain. If you are willing to pay out of pocket, you can purchase custom designed masks from companies now emerging on the sleep medical landscape.

Sounds logical so far, but a struggle immediately arises in mask fitting because insurance carriers are not able to pay for every mask you wish to try out, which means you need to find ways to test-drive masks in your early attempts at using the device. In past years, this step was easier as you could try out a lot of masks in the sleep lab on the first titration test you completed.

But, as the insurance companies and government regulators continue their efforts to gut sleep medical center operations by foisting home sleep testing on more patients, now you may only experience a couple of looks at fewer mask styles, depending on the service provider. Moreover, new pandemic rules also limit the number of masks you try out.

Some home sleep testing is conducted through primary care facilities, where the choice of masks would be further limited. Sleep medical centers also conduct home sleep tests, but depending on the business model, they may still refer you to a DME/HME with the expectation these companies will solve your mask issues. At the DME/HME, the expectation is for you to choose the "right" mask despite never having gained the opportunity to sleep with it, much less lie down in a bed to test the fit and the leak. It is no wonder sleep apnea patients report so much difficulty in adapting to and regularly using PAP.

No doubt, better variations will emerge as more people complain about this limited service model of care, which is both dumb and expensive because it leads to so many people failing PAP therapy. The system is made more problematic by insurance carrier rules offering coverage for a new mask every three to six months. In the big scheme, we appreciate their paying fully or a portion for your masks, but short- and long-term your best bet is to develop a "mask inventory." That is, select a different mask every time you use your insurance coverage; then, over time, you'll have a stock of mask styles you can continue experimenting with until you find one or two that work well for you. Finally, in the current adversarial healthcare climate where the powers that be want to force costs down without regard to maintaining or improving quality of care, you may need to shop around and pay out of pocket for masks over the Internet or through other resources.

Masks and Mask Liners: One Size Does Not Fit All

Some time ago (less than a decade), the belief was most people would do best with the "perfect" mask. Now so many masks are near perfect, you are better off learning to sleep reasonably well with several different styles of masks and maybe sleep perfectly with one particular brand or style. Then, as things change, you might discover the "newest" mask on the market could turn out to be something entirely different and now "perfect" for you.

I started out using nasal pillow masks that fit into the nose, and wore them successfully the first four years of PAP. Then, they caused pain inside my nose, and I switched to the full face mask (FFM) covering nose and mouth. I thought my sleep was great with the nasal pillows, but to my surprise, I discovered sleep was noticeably better with the FFM.

Still, with the full face another wrinkle needed to be ironed out: I could not sleep for more than a week with this bulkier system without it causing bruises, soreness, rashes, and redness on my face, which brings us to the next solution.

There are mask liners and other padding devices that can alter your experiences with certain masks, notably over-the-nose masks and FFMs, so much so a mask you previously could not imagine wearing soon becomes your favorite. These liners are designed with soft cotton-like materials, and nasal pads are made from a rubbery material. Either the liners or pads can be inserted between the mask and your skin to prevent irritation to your face. The RemZzzs mask liners and Pad A Cheek products are two of the best products on the market. Once I started using them, I could wear the FFM for months at a time without any worrisome marks on my face—marks that all but disappeared with my morning shower.

In general, I favor the RemZzzs as the best mask liner available, but they require finesse and precision to get them to work well each night. I am exceedingly fastidious about my sleep (shocker, I know!), so the RemZzzs are perfect for me. Many of our patients prefer RemZzzs as well, but many others need something simpler like Pad A Check because it just snaps onto the mask and, voilà, you're done.

Mask liners and mask leaks are often related. Sometimes, you can use a mask liner to solve a mask leak problem. Again, the RemZzzs may provide superior results. Regardless of which mask liner you use, the key is to ensure greater comfort, eliminate any irritations to the skin, and, as feasible, obtain a secure mask seal to reduce or eradicate any leak. Occasionally, the liner causes leaking when not properly placed or just doesn't seem to fit a particular individual.

These liners and nasal pads are critical to your efforts if you suffer from mask-induced pain. It should be unthinkable to use a mask and suffer pain, leaks, or discomfort. It will take time tweaking things and an observant sense of when to be more finicky in solving equipment issues. In the long run, your efforts will make a huge difference.

An addendum to the above is the recently released memory foam mask from ResMed. It has already proven a game changer in its short time of availability. The cushion is so soft yet sealable, it solves both comfort and leak problems for many individuals, and it appears better than just about any other combination system on the market. The memory foam mask does not work for everyone, but it does work very well for a sizeable number of individuals who could never get both leak and comfort resolved. Its only caveat is that it sometimes aggravates puffiness of the skin under your eyes.

A second addendum involves the emergence of the Bleep Basic and Eclipse DreamPort series that fits directly to the openings of the nose through a connector. Its claim to fame is the connection is so strong, no headgear whatsoever is needed. I've been impressed with the Basic version's male-female plastic connecting system and am eager to see the new Eclipse metal model, set to go to market in 2022, using a magnetic connector that simply attracts both ends to seal the system in place. If they can solve some of their earlier problems with leak and noise, these nasal port systems are likely to be game changers.

Fine-Tuning Your Way to a Great Night of Sleep

You have your equipment (assuming you've gotten this far) and are trying to use the device every night at least a few hours at a time. This phase is most crucial because you are largely on your own compared to all prior steps. You are the one responsible for cleaning the machine, masks, and tubes. You are the one setting up your device each night before bedtime. You must correctly place the mask on your face and keep it on during the night. So much rests on your efforts now, and if something goes wrong, it is all too easy to become frustrated or disgusted with the process.

Two time-tested rules to follow during this early start-up phase will improve your chances for success.

First, if you think there is something wrong—anything at all—and I mean the tiniest little snag with your mask or tubes or pressures, then *it's wrong!* Do not, I repeat, do not imagine you need to adapt to something. While some mask or pressure sensations require adaptation on your part, by ignoring little issues in the early going that do not resolve in short periods of one to three hours or one to three days at most, you are almost invariably dealing with a glitch in the way your system was set up.

It is extremely common for a user to repeatedly misfit or misalign his or her own mask on the face during the first few days or weeks when starting out on a PAP device. Do not be afraid of perfectionism when it comes to making the system comfortable. Pain is a deal breaker, and even discomfort can set you back weeks or months. Being a stickler has its advantages in the early going.

Your Inner Perfectionism Versus Pragmatic Solutions

Thus, the second rule—*perfectionism.* Just consider for a moment you must learn to apply this mask to your face after having slept 20 or 40 or 60 years, your whole life, without ever wearing a mask at bedtime. It is not just that you need to properly position the mask; you need to properly position the mask every single night you use it, not to mention possibly readjusting the mask or the headgear that holds the mask a few times during the night. You actually must pay attention to how the mask material seats over your nose or over your mouth or against your cheeks or forehead and, of course, your skin.

Each night, though, is a new night. Just consider that the hair on your head or face grows every day, which means the headgear that holds the mask may need to be adjusted every few days. Or, what if you use hair rollers at night; will the mask still fit snugly without causing pain or discomfort on your face or the back of your neck or top of your head? And consider oddities such as washing your face squeaky clean before bedtime, which may actually cause the mask to slide off, whereas going to bed with some oil or lotion on your face might promote traction or gripping for the mask to seal better.

Are you ready for all these tweaks?

Being obsessive-compulsive for the first few weeks is the ideal way to approach PAP therapy. The good news is, once you figure out these details, you will solve most of these problems in less than five minutes a day, and soon it will amount to less than one or two minutes before bedtime to make sure the machine and mask are operating in a way that's best for you.

Even the durability of this equipment is suspect. For example, you probably should replace your mask every three months. Some masks are manufactured with disposable cushions and are covered by insurance for monthly replacement. Many patients may not realize or pay attention to this critical detail, or their DME or HME company does not apprise them of this option, which is ironic given these businesses earn more by selling mask cushions.

Nonetheless, changing cushions once per month improves mask comfort and the likelihood of using the mask regularly. And, if you possess fair or sensitive skin or you suffer from diabetes, you may need to start from the outset with RemZzzs or nasal pads to prevent facial skin abrasions or bruises on the bridge of the nose. Even though these items cost a bit more money out of pocket, as insurance carriers do not reimburse them, these add-ons could yield the critical difference between success and failure given the extra comfort offered in the beginning and throughout treatment. Personally, success in regular long-term use of an FFM occurred only after the application of RemZzzs mask liners. My level of comfort these past several years on an FFM using these mask liners is a testament to how this little tool produces a big impact.

More recently, I have gained still more consistency with the ResMed AirFit F20 memory foam mask. I have also tried out Bleep masks, both plastic and magnetic versions and am looking forward to the continued evolution of these products. Indeed, many masks are frequently upgraded or redesigned through new innovations.

Yet another factor is cleanliness, so often taken for granted by patients using PAP. It truly makes a difference to clean your equipment every single morning, hang it up to dry, and then start each night with freshly cleaned gear. Whether you use soap and water or vinegar and water—whatever solution cleans off the grease and grime—it's a small effort with a large reward. The cleanliness factor is also about building a routine and generating positive reinforcement about the experience. Good habits produce good results, and cleaning is essential because the mask and tubes build up grease, grime, and perhaps some bacteria every single night. It makes sense to clean every morning.

Even the headgear holding the mask in place accumulates grease or grime from the back or top of the scalp or hair. This headgear should be cleaned to prevent scalp irritations, including acne. In all these examples, you will see the dirt, the grease, and the grime coming off in the water in which you wash the equipment, and seeing this junk should motivate you to wash it every morning, although headgear may work fine with once per week cleaning.

Note, the new memory foam masks cannot be cleaned with water; instead use a baby wipe without alcohol.

Pressure Perfectionism

The ultimate finicky scenario arises from your PAP pressure settings. Gaining good support from your sleep center and sleep techs is essential to address your pressure needs and sensitivities. With PAP, the pressure settings can be adjusted at precise levels with changes as small as 0.2 units. These measurements are known as *centimeters of water*, but it is easier to just say units of pressure. When you go to the lab, you might be tested at pressures such as 15 over 10 with a bilevel machine, meaning it gives you 15 units of pressure breathing in and 10 units of pressure breathing out. You or the sleep tech or both might believe the titration (adjusting the pressures in the lab at night) went fairly well—maybe better than that. You might feel good the next morning, which would be a great sign for an easier adaptation to the machine as well as gaining benefits sooner than later.

Nevertheless, what if 15/10 (the way to write bilevel pressures) are actually not the optimal settings for you? What if you actually need 15.4/10.6? How are you going to discover the necessity of this little pressure tweak? By analogy, you would like this step to be similar to a psychiatrist fine-tuning the dosage of your medication. Instead, here you may need to return for repeat titrations (REPAPs)[53] in the sleep laboratory to produce the optimal response, because this approach is the only way to most accurately treat the flow limitation events of the upper airway resistance syndrome that are measured on the pressure transducer. To be sure, it is the only known way, outside of trial and error, to round the curve optimally.

What if you are not getting support at the sleep lab or the DME/HME regarding minor pressure tweaks? Then you will need to experiment on your own.

I personally tested this theory a number of times in my own sleep lab and learned without question small changes of 0.2 to 0.4 units of pressure affect the way I feel in the morning and throughout the ensuing day. It is likely these changes will manifest in the first year of use, because it is difficult to find optimal settings when you first apply PAP therapy. Moreover, as time goes on, things change: you age; drink more or less alcohol; suffer other medical or psychiatric conditions; or, have difficulty controlling nasal congestion. Any or all these factors impact your pressure settings. Of course, the biggest one is change in weight.

As a special consideration, be sure to check out the information in Appendix A regarding the use of the OSCAR software, which might prove useful in your efforts to fine-tune small pressure changes on your own.

Overall, you are not obliged to rush back to the sleep lab every single time you experience health changes, although returning to the sleep lab is a very good idea for big changes. The most important point, then, is you need to pay close attention to the issue of pressure settings, whether something needs to be changed on inspiration or something on expiration. If it doesn't feel right, you will need to experiment very gradually through trial and error to determine whether a small change enhances your PAP response.

Obviously, all changes can be accomplished more easily when the sleep medical center or the DME or HME company vigorously support your efforts. Yes, I'm suggesting "the squeaky wheel gets oiled." But I also want you to gain perspective about all these questions and clarifications you may be seeking answers to in the first few weeks or months; this gathering of information will give you tools and skills to resolve 90% of the problems yourself.

You will also develop more clarity about when and from whom you need to ask for help as new problems arise, whether the problem relates to masks, cushions, tubes, testing, pressures, leaks, or data assessment. You will discover and apply so much information, soon enough it will take two to five minutes before bedtime to manage your treatment program to get the best possible results.

Fail-Safe Maneuver

When things are not going well, the most important set of instructions to embrace is the "less is more" approach. There's nothing written in stone that you must use your PAP device every night, all night long as soon as you get your machine. There are a few insurance carriers using rules to threaten patients with a loss of coverage for the device if you do not use it four hours per night for five nights per week, but in general, most of these entities recognize some need a longer time to adapt as well as more coaching along the way.

With this backdrop, *it is okay to start out wearing the device just a couple hours and even skipping some nights.* Obviously, we do not want this approach to be the long-term goal, but a substantial minority of patients needs to go slower for a few weeks or months in trying to build up to every night, all night use of the machine.

It is absolutely fine to take the minimalist approach because there can be no question some people who push along too far and too fast acquire a strong distaste for the PAP device and then give up within a few weeks or a matter of days. Recognizing these pacing options proves invaluable to those who discover the initial struggle is greater than initially imagined. Just like the saying "slow down and take a deep breath" to deal with daily life stressors, so too, in starting PAP, "slow and steady wins the race!"

Temporizing Recommendations

Oh, how I wish you could have already started your PAP! Still, given your need to digest all this material and the countless steps necessary to engage with one of your primary care providers, be it a medical doctor or mental health therapist, after which getting all your tests and finally getting your shiny new device through a DME company, it's not realistic for me to think any but the most brave hearted would have already passed these milestones and started PAP. Instead, we know from current practices in the field of sleep medicine, weeks or months roll by before you finally receive your PAP device, so please take note of two practical instructions in the interim.

First, though it takes time for your PAP to arrive on the scene, waiting around and losing momentum is not a great option. That's why the very next chapter provides additional ways to begin treatment of SDB without PAP, and they often provide meaningful results. In other words, if you embrace this SDB paradigm from everything you've learned, why wait to get better? Don't! Read Chapter 8 and get started treating your SDB tonight. Or, if so motivated, schedule an appointment ASAP with a sleep center or with your primary care physician to refer there.

Second, **when the PAP device is in place, keep in mind there's a large troubleshooting guide at the end of the book in Appendix A** that will coach you on a multitude of steps to overcome every obstacle you can conceive of that might interfere with your efforts. In particular, Appendix A addresses certain fine points about using ABPAP or ASV, which are the devices I encourage virtually all mental health patients to pursue once they've been diagnosed with OSA or UARS. Please, please, please make regular use of this guide as it will teach you a variety of tips, pointers, and steps you will rarely come upon through other resources.

Sleep Research Pearl #7

Before our eyes were opened to the need for advanced PAP to solve the riddle of expiratory pressure intolerance, we worked closely with our Regional Medicare medical director, Dr. Lynne Hickman (1936–2012) to invent a new procedure, the PAP-NAP to address EPI. The idea, born from the frustrations of mental health patients failing PAP so quickly, was to create a new test-drive, daytime napping procedure, where we could apply PAP without all the wires and sensors used in a standard sleep study. The PAP-NAP offered a one-to-one patient–sleep tech encounter for a few hours of troubleshooting. The procedure included coaching and specialized care in helping psychiatric patients adapt to PAP.[112]

The beauty of the PAP-NAP is the gradual style where each aspect receives prolonged attention and desensitization. The individual begins with 30 minutes or longer finding comfortable masks and headgear, then, while sitting bedside, the patient holds the mask (not strapped on) to the face to test pressurized air. Only after comfort is achieved, the headgear is strapped in place. After further time adapting, the patient tries the whole thing lying down, lights still on. You get the picture. Eventually the individual agrees to lights out and spends an hour or two hours lying in the sleep lab bed using the PAP device at low pressure.

Regardless of whether the individual falls asleep, the endpoint is all about helping the patient appreciate his or her successful use of the device without triggering anxiety. Ninety percent of individuals who undergo a PAP-NAP pursue PAP soon after. Not every patient succeeds, but keep in mind the procedure was used initially on individuals who declared they would never use a PAP machine—ever!

Later, we looked for special circumstances in which to apply the PAP-NAP. Louis was in his early sixties when we met him in 2011. Ten years earlier, he failed CPAP at two other facilities, then at our center initiated bilevel and then auto-bilevel with so-so results. Louis was never seen regularly as he spent only a few months each year in New Mexico; he lived and worked in two other states for business and personal reasons. Around 2014 at a lengthy appointment, he was ready to throw in the towel. In addition to lack of benefit, he reported air swallowing from PAP (discussed at length in Appendix A under the term *aerophagia*). He also suffered GERD (gastroesophageal reflux disease), a common trigger for air swallowing, although even when reflux improved he still suffered a bloated stomach from PAP.

Overall, his frustration was enough to quit PAP; however, his greater frustration with horrible daytime impairment due to awful sleep quality at night provided the motivation to try something new. I suggested a PAP-NAP to give ASV a whirl.

That day, upon completing the PAP-NAP, he expressed no enthusiasm for the device, though he described ASV pressures as gentler and noticed less air swallowing. The procedure lasted three hours, of which only 1.5 hours were lying down in bed. Despite the lack of persuasive evidence to move forward, he agreed to try ASV. During this time period, we were seeing more patients purchase ASV out of pocket when they did not qualify by insurance standards. Louis anticipated his insurance hassles would never resolve during his short stay in New Mexico, so he bought a used ASV online.

We did not hear from Louis until 2016. Work kept him out of state for two years. He scheduled a routine follow-up, and I was delighted to see how well rested he looked at the appointment. Turns out he'd been using ASV faithfully the whole time. No further episodes of air swallowing occurred, and he was extremely satisfied with the quality of his sleep and greatly improved daytime sleepiness and fatigue.

The PAP-NAP is an excellent example of how personally tailored medicine (the wave of the future in healthcare) makes a huge difference. My team and I take pride in hearing how hundreds of sleep centers all over the United States and beyond now use the PAP-NAP procedure as needed.

Sometimes, a center using PAP-NAPs indicates more open-minded sleep professionals are involved in the lab operations.

Last, my colleague and senior research collaborator, Victor Ulibarri, the most instrumental sleep technologist in our development of the PAP-NAP, recently published an update in the journal *Sleep and Breathing*.[113] Among patients who underwent the procedure, the most relevant predictors of successful long-term use of PAP therapy were those who demonstrated decreased emotional aversion to the mask and pressurized air and those who increased their motivation to consider a home trial of PAP directly after completing the PAP-NAP. Common sense or a little reflection explains these unsurprising findings. Yet, the PAP-NAP, while ideally suited for mental health patients who might be leery of PAP therapy, has received little support and occasional antagonism from a few elite and academic circles in the professional sleep community, a sad commentary on the state of affairs in the field of sleep medicine.

CHAPTER 8

Alternatives to PAP Therapy

If I cannot adapt to PAP, or if I refuse to try PAP, what are my options?

PAP therapy is one of the greatest inventions of medical science, but some people just cannot or will not use it. Which means other options might provide at least partial treatment of your sleep breathing condition instead of no treatment at all. We will review these possibilities, from the simplistic and inexpensive to more complex and costly. Many options can be used to jump-start your treatment as early as tonight.

That said, nearly all these options suffer from one highly relevant drawback, namely, the failure to fully address flow limitation, the discrete breathing event linked to the UARS variant of OSA. Failing to completely address these more subtle breathing events frequently yields a suboptimal response. While this point impacts each person uniquely, nevertheless, it's worth reiterating partial treatment is preferable to no therapy at all.

Nasal Hygiene

To solve a sleep breathing disorder, your nose must work well; and the better the nose functions, the better the PAP response. If you select an alternate treatment, the nose still must function well. Complicating matters, sleep-disordered breathing itself causes friction in the nasal and oral airway that increases inflammation in the mucosa (the inner skin that lines your nose and the rest of your upper airway). This inflammation provides a fertile ground for allergens and other irritants to trigger *rhinitis*, the condition of obstruction in the nose due to congestion and related symptoms. Both allergic rhinitis and nonallergic rhinitis are common in SDB patients.[114] Upper respiratory tract infections are also more common in OSA/UARS patients.

Due to human tendencies, any type of nasal congestion, stuffiness, or runny nose (whatever the cause) is so common, it often leads to "normalizing one's behavior." Once you suffer from nasal congestion long enough, you believe whatever degree of congestion you suffer from must in fact be normal. You may develop mouth breathing because the congestion is chronic, yet not realize you are mouth breathing.

Does it sound odd that people would not notice partially blocked breathing during waking hours? It is odd, but it's also a human trait for the mind to steer away from such conditions. Instead, we simply adapt to the way we breathe even when we are suffering from a stuffy, runny, or congested nose on a daily basis.

Arguably, breathing—the critical and unrelenting function of the living human organism—defies close self-monitoring unless a true urgency develops, like choking or coughing. Later, when we discuss the emotional side of sleep problems, you will learn about a more detailed reason for the lack of attention to breathing, but here's the short story: many of us do not or will not reflect on our breathing because it scares us.

Notwithstanding, virtually every treatment you apply to improve nasal breathing will instantaneously improve sleep breathing. Some proven treatments actually decrease apneas and hypopneas, while others enhance sleep quality. Just by starting a nasal breathing treatment, you could start sleeping better.

Treating Allergic and Nonallergic Rhinitis

Allergic rhinitis (also known as AR or hay fever) is most widely known due to seasonal nasal blockages. Most with seasonal allergies try out OTC medications or nasal sprays or are prescribed a more potent medication or nasal spray. Nonallergic rhinitis (NAR) is the trickier of the two types of congestion because it is more difficult to diagnose and treat. Learning about AR first makes it easier to understand NAR.

AR treatment is straightforward; you start with simple cleansing like nasal saline rinses or full neti pot washes or other lavage equipment. You might experiment with different products ranging from standard saline and sodium bicarbonate solutions to xylitol rinses. Not only will you gain relief, but also you will learn about what else might be needed and eventually whether NAR is clouding the picture. Here are three treatment keys:

- These simple therapies may cure (truly cure) the entire problem of allergic rhinitis.
- If they improve AR without curing it, then more treatment is necessary.
- If they worsen (that's right, worsen) stuffiness, runny nose, or congestion, then NAR is the larger issue, necessitating a different approach.

You must develop a zero-tolerance policy about nasal breathing problems: everything should be assessed and reassessed when relief has not achieved 100% improvement.

The impact of rinses or washes occurs within one to three weeks tops, and often in one to three days. Conversely, an adverse reaction, like NAR, may occur immediately. Get into the habit of discussing nasal sprays with your primary care physician, or consider an alternative healthcare provider to explore nontraditional options. An allergist may be useful for more persistent AR problems.

OTC pills are useful for many AR sufferers, but the OTC nasal spray Afrin (oxymetazoline) should be avoided as it triggers rebound congestion in the majority of regular users. Your plan may also include prescription pills and nasal steroid sprays. For many years, I found nasal steroid sprays coupled with Nasalcrom (cromolyn sodium) spray to be consistently more effective than any other type of medication on the market, prescription or OTC.

Nasal steroids are plentiful. Most notably, Sensimist is an OTC nasal spray with a new mist-delivery system that appears to send the steroid medicine higher up into the nasal passages and sinus tissues. Among patients switching from other nasal steroids to Sensimist, we hear many reports of greater improvements with this new delivery system. As there are so many nasal steroid sprays, discussing the best ones for you may require a more detailed conversation with your primary care physician or allergist.

For nonallergic rhinitis, recall Thomas Jefferson's quote about government—to paraphrase, "least is best." NAR is a problem of overstimulation. For example, if squirting something as benign as nasal saline into your nose worsens congestion, then the problem is NAR. This sensitivity increases your vulnerability to more nasal obstruction.

NAR is distinctive because it manifests as stuffiness or runny nose or congestion or any combination, yet it almost always does not share the same allergy-like symptoms of itchiness or sneezing, except when you suffer both AR and NAR, a common co-occurrence in those with sleep-disordered breathing. To assess, ask yourself whether congestion, stuffiness, or runny nose occur when exposed to:

- Changes or dramatic swings in weather
- Changes or dramatic swings in temperature
- Wind blowing in the face

With affirmative answers to one or more of these patterns, we presume the presence of an NAR component. Moreover, most NAR sufferers report symptoms year-round, not just seasonally.

Most primary care providers know little about NAR and therefore generally assume AR must be the issue. Numerous allergy meds, including nasal steroid sprays, are then prescribed. Among thousands of patients seen at our sleep center, of which well over half suffered from NAR alone or AR+NAR, it was extremely rare for the NAR component to have been treated, let alone diagnosed in the past by another doctor.

This statement means virtually all cases of NAR were failing other treatments currently in use. These reports of failure tipped us off to the presence of NAR.

Years ago, scant treatment was offered for NAR because no well-described or consistently successful treatments were available; moreover, the condition was frequently dismissed as psychosomatic, that is, caused by anxiety, which is likely to be partially true.

Nonetheless, from the sleep medicine perspective, we realized PAP is "wind blowing in the face," which aggravates NAR. Indeed, some NAR patients should not use PAP at the outset. We learned this lesson the hard way, when two such patients developed raging sinus issues within a week of starting PAP. In other words, NAR needed treatment beforehand so nasal passages would be cleared up first.

The great news is both older and newer treatments for NAR are available, and in the past decade antihistamine nasal sprays have demonstrated great benefit. At least two versions are available now (azelastine, olopatadine) under brand names Astelin, Astepro, or Patanase, and more of these sprays will be forthcoming because they are so potent in the treatment of NAR. I would venture between 70% and 80% of our patients using these sprays are experiencing a complete resolution of NAR symptoms. One of the most common responses we receive from our patients is "No other nasal spray ever produced this level of success."

Again, an important reminder that AR and NAR are very common in SDB, therefore the average patient at our center was using the combination of Sensimist and Astelin, the same combination I've applied for myself the past several years.

Last, the drug ipratropium (brand name Atrovent) is also coming into regular use for NAR. It is an anticholinergic spray, on the market for nearly 50 years, but its use as a nasal spray for NAR is more recent. Typically, when an antihistamine nasal spray does not provide benefit for NAR, the patient switches to Atrovent. With either of these two prescription nasal sprays (azelastine or ipratropium), we see success rates exceeding 80%.

A couple of final tips are worth noting. First, if you suffer from reflux, it increases your chances of suffering from NAR. Moreover, many NAR patients suffer silent reflux,[115] so they don't realize the reflux is happening, yet it's causing NAR instead of the heartburn that would be expected. Such suspicions can only be evaluated by use of a fiber-optic tool to examine the esophagus and upper airway. Gastroenterologists and otolaryngologists perform these procedures.

Second, recent studies on xylitol nasal sprays show an impact on NAR. You've probably heard of xylitol in chewing gum to make it "sugarless" and that it actually helps prevent dental cavities. This same activity likely works on the mucosa lining in your nasal passages. The xylitol nasal spray seems to change the chemistry of the inflamed nasal tissues. This inflammation could have been caused by AR and NAR or OSA and UARS. By changing the chemistry, the tissue reverts to normal and is now capable of using its natural defense systems to fight off bacteria that cause or aggravate the inflammation. Moreover, xylitol itself may make the mucosa less "sticky," yet another way to prevent bacteria from triggering more inflammation. In my limited experience with xylitol, patients with both AR and NAR are describing improvements with these nasal sprays.

To close this discussion on rhinitis, it is imperative to appreciate not only how crucial it is to keep your nose clean and clear while using PAP or any other treatment, but also of near equal importance, you must appreciate your astronomically high risk of suffering from AR or NAR or both, because sleep-disordered breathing patients show much higher rates than patients without these sleep disorders.

Please keep this final point in mind: while there are occasional reports of patients completely eliminating AR and NAR with the use of PAP, a more likely scenario is finding the best independent treatment for AR/NAR so that PAP works better. A large majority of individuals with OSA/UARS will notice clear-cut benefits in their sleep by aggressively and effectively eliminating any and all nasal congestion issues.

Nasal Dilator Devices

Tonight, start using nasal dilator strips (for example, Breathe Right or the national brand equivalent (NBE) often sold at a lower price) and continue every night regardless of your congestion status; your nose often functions better with nasal dilator strip (NDS) therapy. I use an NBE nasal strip every night with my PAP, and if on rare occasions I forget, I feel less refreshed than when I had used one.

These gadgets come in either internal or external forms, the latter most widely known as Breathe Right or the NBE versions often seen on the noses of professional athletes. NDS therapy is both an independent as well as a supplemental treatment. We conducted research on NDS and found it successfully reduced insomnia symptoms in 75% of patients suspected of suffering mild OSA or UARS.[43] Of 40 patients in the NDS treatment group using strips nightly, 30 patients saw meaningful improvements in insomnia severity after one month. In the control group, which only received education and no NDS, there was little to no change in insomnia.

The bottom line is nasal dilator strips seem to treat sleep-disordered breathing in and of themselves, although in most cases we presume a patient would need more than just NDS. NDS therapy also serves as a great starter program because it engages the individual in treating OSA/UARS, after which a more active approach with advanced devices may be chosen. Remarkably, the combination of NDS and PAP produces its own benefits, and many patients will not use PAP without first putting a nasal strip on the nose.

The three main points to remember about NDS include:

- Shortly before using the strip, wash the nose with soap, then rinse and dry.
- Without delay, place the strip *below* the bony bridge of your nose.
- Remove the strip in the morning with soap and water or a steam shower.

With the internal devices, usually called nasal dilators, the goal is to insert the tool into the nose. It remains in place and expands the internal nasal valve area, which thereby decreases nasal resistance and increases air flow. Many gadgets are on the market but are rarely researched, which is not to say you would not find benefit from a device were it to fit well and did not fall out during the night.

AIRMAX is one model that alleges its insertion climbs higher into the nasal cavity and thus provides a larger decrease in resistance and greater improvement in airflow. With all internal dilators, there are questions about potential discomfort as well as reliability of remaining in place. An individual may end up trying different dilators to find the right fit and comfort level. My experience with AIRMAX has proven beneficial for short naps or in combo with PAP.

If you need a starter treatment before committing to PAP, tools like nasal strips or internal nasal dilators are worth the investment to gain some relief from your sleep breathing problem. Once you achieve a bit of success, your motivation increases to consider more sophisticated treatment options.

Oral Dental and Tongue Devices

Some of the most sophisticated devices to treat OSA/UARS include gadgets fitting inside your mouth to either prevent the tongue from falling to the back of your throat or that thrust your lower jaw forward to open up the back of the airway. Some devices do both, and the most researched and widely used devices are known as *oral appliance therapy* (OAT) or *mandibular advancement devices* (MAD). This treatment approach is a veritable godsend for a sizeable proportion of patients who are unable or unwilling to use PAP therapy as their first treatment strategy upon receiving the diagnosis of OSA/UARS.

Numerous oral appliances have entered the marketplace, and all possess similar features in fitting over the teeth, using your dental arches for anchoring. The best devices are custom molded to your teeth and therefore must be designed and manufactured in a dental lab, which leads to costs frequently in excess of a thousand dollars.

Many of the original OAT devices were bulky and created a cramped space for the front half of the tongue. That is, the two pieces fitting over your dental arches provided very little space between the upper and lower parts. More recently, designers are creating more space for the tongue to glide forward through an opening in the front part of the device, closest to the backs of your lips.

On the other hand, most dentists avow the position of the tongue in normal breathing "rests" against the roof of the mouth while you sleep. So, a problem arises when OAT users cannot teach themselves to keep the tongue in this position during sleep. Instead, the tongue may thrust forward in an unconscious attempt to unblock the crowding in the back of the throat. Moreover, depending on a person's sensitivity, a cramped sensation may arise with OAT/MAD due to a feeling of having nowhere to rest the tongue. Claustrophobia may ensue, after which the individual may rip out the device.

As you can imagine, the fitting of OAT requires precision, not only to improve the way it opens the airway to help you sleep, but also, and perhaps more importantly long term, how the device fits to remain in your mouth all night without causing serious side effects. The upshot is you want a dentist who regularly works on fitting OAT devices. In fact, you might ask whether the dentist has fitted 100 patients or more before selecting who performs your fitting. Some dentists may dabble in this area with the utmost sincerity, but there is a lot of finesse required to get it right without causing pain in the teeth, movement of the teeth, problematic changes in the bite, and worst of all, problems in the jaw, notably the temporomandibular joint. A history of TMJ usually precludes OAT.

I used OAT for three very successful years in the late 1990s, and then in the fourth year the results faded, so I switched to PAP. During my OAT use, the main side effect was a change in bite such that my back molars no longer touched. This open bite was noticeably worse in the morning, making it difficult to eat crunchy breakfast like toast or granola. Later in the day the effect diminishes, but when I ceased use of OAT it took six months for the bite to return to normal.

Virtually everyone who uses OAT develops bite problems, but these effects can be lessened by practicing a specific exercise each morning to pull the lower jaw back into place. All you need for this exercise is a thin, short piece of malleable plastic. First, you slide the plastic so its front side (that is, facing forward) fits against the back side of your upper middle front teeth. Then, slide up the lower front teeth to press against the backside of the plastic to hold it in place. You know you are doing it correctly when you feel the pressure of this exercise tugging your lower jaw back toward its original location. If you hold this bite position on the plastic for five to 10 minutes, it noticeably lessens the bite problem. Sitting on the toilet and reading the morning news is a good time to get it done.

To more easily grasp this idea, you could insert your thumb into the positions described above, but long term, the malleable piece of plastic works better, and some dentists will make a similar contraption, like a very small retainer, to resolve this issue for use each morning.

Tongue-retaining devices (TRDs) are making a comeback because it seems so logical to move the tongue forward to open the airway, and newer devices seem to work. As you would guess, the fitting process is a lot more hit or miss compared to OAT because the tongue is not a static or rigid structure like dental arches. Most TRDs work to create a suction cavity so the tongue remains forward; there is still the problem of keeping it in the mouth all night. Most TRDs build a seat for the teeth and lips, which at least in the early part of the night seems comfortable and stable. Whether the person easily keeps the device in place all night is far less likely than a well-fitting OAT device.

TRD is cheaper than a custom-built OAT device, and it might be a worthwhile place to start for some, but it is not likely to serve as a long-term solution. Even OAT may only be useful for a few years because of the side effects to the bite or TMJ joint or, as is often the case, the worsening of the OSA/UARS.

All in all, OAT and TRDs may be worth your effort for long-term use if you do not see yourself exploring PAP. And many individuals using these devices for several years have made tremendous gains in their sleep quality. The American Academy of Dental Sleep Medicine is a resource to help locate experienced sleep dentists (https://www.aadsm.org/).

Nose, Throat, and Sinus Surgery

If you lumped together all the surgeries attempting to treat OSA/UARS, you would be immensely disappointed with their long-term benefits. Said another way, the average surgical patient is typically going to need to try something else, usually PAP, anywhere from six months to six years after undergoing a sleep surgery, although this point is rarely emphasized in the scientific literature.[116]

Some surgeries provide substantial benefits and should be considered by specific patients in personally tailored circumstances. However, a tremendous volume of relatively useless surgery is performed on sleep apnea patients, which results in minimal benefit or, in a large number of cases, tangible harm by worsening sleep apnea or creating new obstacles in those trying to subsequently use a PAP or OAT device.

The record of sleep surgery failures is not widely known in the medical community, because surgical research has often defined success as a 50%

reduction in breathing events. In comparison, a PAP treatment routinely eliminates 90% to 95% of breathing events.

That surgery is not comparable to PAP therapy should raise your level of suspicion when considering these procedures. Moreover, if you chat with a surgeon about potential techniques, do not hesitate to inquire about the number of patients who were cured of sleep apnea and the definition of "cured" in such discussions. Do they take into account the flow limitation type of breathing events?

While beneficial surgeries are available, I am starting this section with considerable caution because it is quite common to encounter vast numbers of second opinion patients who were promised the moon and the stars by surgeons. Instead, they find themselves in a black hole with few benefits and much muddled thinking about the nature of and treatment for sleep-disordered breathing.

That said, four common categories of traditional surgeries can help:
- Nasal surgeries involving the septum, turbinates, or polyps
- Oral airway surgeries involving tonsils and possibly the tongue
- Sinus surgeries
- Jaw surgeries expanding the upper or lower portions or both

These surgeries may show positive outcomes because they resolve specific blockages in the airway, or they contribute to a more aerodynamically healthy system, generating smoother and larger air volume for use of PAP or OAT. Unfortunately, many surgeons conducting procedures on sleep patients may communicate simplistically about how the "airway is likened to a tube: remove the blockages and more air gets through the tube." Schematically, as you saw in Figure 6.1, the airway can be viewed as a tube, but its functioning is far more dynamic and complex than a simple tube.

To clarify, if this tube perspective were accurate, two common procedures that cut out the soft palate tissue and uvula from the back of the throat would have high rates of success. The two procedures, uvulopalatopharyngoplasty (UPPP) and uvulectomy (UV), to an untrained eye yield a postsurgical airway noticeably more spacious. This surgical step seems logical because a crowded airway in the back of the throat is a telltale sign of a patient likely to suffer from sleep apnea. But looks and results are deceiving—both UPPP and UV demonstrate conspicuously low success rates, not to mention making future attempts at PAP more difficult. Thus, decreasing blockage in the airway is only part of the picture.

The real story is the dynamic nature of the upper airway, a system involving the head and neck and more than 20 specific muscles or muscle groups that collectively function in harmony to keep the airway open while lying down and sleeping. This system also includes the impact of the throat, including bone, cartilage, fat, and soft tissues. Many surgeries fail because they do not account for the dysfunction of the airway musculature that persists after the removal of a particular blockage. For this single reason, few surgeries cure sleep apnea; they may prove beneficial, but they are not really attacking the whole problem.

In contrast, consider the impact of a sinus procedure. Nowadays, there are numerous in-office or day surgeries to open up sinus passageways. Or more extensive surgeries may be needed for complex, chronic sinusitis. These surgeries directly target frontal, maxillary, ethmoid, or sphenoid sinuses as needed. Here's the remarkable thing about sinus surgeries: you do not breathe through your sinuses, yet I have encountered patients in which sinus surgery and sinus surgery alone completely eliminated sleep breathing disorders.

How could sinus surgery produce these results? The best answer is the poorly functioning sinus cavities were not effectively draining in normal fashion, which then caused profound and chronic inflammation of the nasal passages. By resolving the sinus problems, a stronger than anticipated improvement in nasal breathing ensues, leading to greater normalization of airflow and potentially a cure of a sleep-disordered breathing condition.

In a related scenario, consider patients who start nasal steroid sprays to treat their sinus conditions and quickly discover how much better they sleep.[117] In each of these cases, the blockage in the sinus cavities was severely impacting the nasal airway. As a result, aggressive treatment of sinusitis led to a dynamic change in the nasal breathing flow.

Similar results may occur with surgeries that straighten the septum in the nose (septoplasty) or shrink the turbinate structures (turbinoplasty), which are the air filtering tissues on the lateral walls of the nasal passages. Over time, turbinates swell in response to many irritants (allergic or otherwise), and shrinking the size of turbinates may smooth out passages to favor what is called the laminar flow of air through the nose. So, yes, removing a blockage is an essential feature of upper airway surgery, but the critical question is whether the improvement in sleep breathing is just a matter of gaining air volume or is also about reducing the turbulence in the airflow caused by the turbinates?

For the same reasons, surgeons cannot predict the degree of benefits from tonsillectomy. Even when someone has horribly enlarged tonsils, no guarantee is offered that removal will dramatically decrease OSA/UARS, although in children large improvements are common.[118] If you looked at the obvious blockage caused by tonsils, you would surely predict marked improvement from removal. Unfortunately, it is not so. Again, more is involved; as one example, the airway musculature may exert a disproportionate impact on airway collapsibility regardless of the size of the tonsils. The whole system of airflow from the nose into the bottom of the throat and finally down into the lungs must be taken into account.

In sum, I have purposely limited my discussion of the traditional or most common surgical interventions because they should not be the primary approach to treating sleep apnea, except when a specific blockage in the nose and perhaps the tonsils seems to hamper an individual's use of PAP. No doubt, some patients insist on surgery first, while others need surgeries as a crucial step to make PAP viable.

Notwithstanding the information discussed above, to be fair let's take the surgeons' viewpoint to appreciate how they are helping sleep apnea patients. They argue surgery reduces breathing events by 50%, therefore every night you suffer 50% fewer breathing events; whereas if PAP reduces 90% of breathing events yet you only apply PAP half the night (and the 2nd half of the night features greater SDB severity), then by arithmetic alone the surgery was a better choice. This argument is entirely valid and worthy of consideration for specific patients.

To reiterate, I am not advising you to veto surgery; I would hope most patients work diligently at PAP therapy from the outset because among those who finally gain optimal results with the device, it is my experience they would never choose a surgical option unless they were guaranteed the same results from the surgery. And I will guarantee there are very few such guarantees! Conversely, as some surgeries make PAP use easier, by all means, these surgeries should be considered in timely fashion.

The failure of surgery to favorably influence the problem of flow limitation is one big reason why these procedures have a ceiling on how much improvement you might gain, but advances in surgery may yet solve these problems.

Last and not least, asking about potential problems regarding a specific surgery you are considering is the most important question to raise with your sleep surgeon. All surgeries have risk of bleeding and infection, but I'm referring to additional complications[119] as well as side effects,[120] all of which you should know about before going under the knife. For example, if a procedure might impact your speech or swallowing, it is imperative to understand more details about such risks beforehand, and these points are relevant to the additional surgeries described next.

Specialized Surgeries of the Jaw and Dental Arches

The most interesting and useful developments in the surgical fields include sophisticated procedures such as maxillomandibular advancement (MMA), endoscopic-assisted surgical expansion (EASE), and mandibular distraction osteogenesis (MDO). MMA has been around for decades because it is used to repair damaged or deformed jaw structures in trauma patients or in children or adolescents with congenital jaw abnormalities. MMA provides miraculous cosmetic improvements, and these changes eventually led to the recognition of how a marked expansion of the airway led to improvements in breathing.

MMA has been the most widely used treatment of last resort in patients who could not tolerate any other options. Some people, mostly young adults, opted for MMA instead of trying out any other therapy as they were hoping for a definitive cure.

The MMA procedure literally means both the upper (maxilla) and lower (mandible) components of the jaw are intentionally fractured so each can be pulled apart as well as pulled forward. These radical changes, as would be expected, markedly increase the volume of air descending into the airway.

The other two procedures, EASE and MDO, are emerging as innovative developments; both are less surgically invasive while attempting to yield improvements similar to MMA.

EASE focuses exclusively on the upper jaw, or maxilla, with the objective to widen the floor of the nasal cavity to permit greater airflow. A metal distractor is implanted into the hard palate, situated horizontally between the two sides of the upper dental arch. After insertion, a screw is manipulated by millimeters over a two-month period, during which the added force of the distractor is causing outward movement in the maxilla, which causes the nasal floor to expand. Once expansion is complete, the distractor is removed.

Although research is sparse, a paper published in 2019 by Dr. Kasey Li, the pioneer of the technique, revealed an average 70% reduction in breathing events and noticeable improvements in daytime sleepiness in nearly 90% of the 33 patients who underwent EASE.[121] Several of these patients still used their PAP machines, and no data were provided regarding changes in flow limitation.

MDO reflects the use of a distractor on the lower jaw or mandible, which by widening should lead to some expansion of the airway in ways similar to a patient undergoing MMA. Again, the use of the distractor is less invasive, and no attention is directed at the upper jaw. MDO research focuses exclusively on children, although I have spoken with dentists who believe the procedure will be used in adults.

To reiterate, many of these patients still require the use of PAP therapy, and the question remains as to the impact on the UARS component of sleep-disordered breathing. Nonetheless, the emergence of distraction osteogenesis, which simply means applying pressure to move bone into new positions, appears an exciting and promising new pathway to treat SDB, and I trust future research will look more closely at the impact on flow limitation.

Weight Loss

Weight loss is a remarkably useful strategy when the goal is to reduce the severity of OSA, but an impractical approach, if the goal were to cure OSA. Besides, obesity under any circumstance is a difficult condition to treat, and the most consistent results are to lose, regain, lose, regain again, and continue on that pathway for years. For weight loss to be a legitimate strategy, two things must be abundantly clear from the outset:

- What is the realistic goal for targeted weight loss in the short term to reduce the severity of sleep breathing events?
- Is the weight loss program either a well-proven system or at least one that merits a trial run due to widespread anecdotal evidence?

Remarkably, if you set a goal for a 10% decrease from current weight (lose 30 pounds if you weigh 300; lose 20 pounds if you weigh 200), there is a huge probability you will reduce the severity of your sleep breathing events, which often proves noticeable to the sleeper. Then again, if you are starting at 350 pounds and lose 35 pounds, the conundrum is you may only drop the number of breathing events into a range from extremely severe to, you guessed it, still extremely severe. In other words, in terms of your overall health, you still need PAP, and you need it right away.

Another question is whether a 10% weight loss will improve oxygen drops caused by breathing events. Weight loss reduces the amount of hypoxia time (constant O_2 level < 90%). For obese OSA/UARS patients, hypoxia is frequently in the 80% range and much lower during REM sleep. Both oxygen desaturations and hypoxia may improve with weight loss and are important metrics to follow closely if weight loss is the only strategy.

While this 10% method is accurate and fairly reliable when you achieve the target, if you are starting out with a severe OSA condition and severe oxygen desaturations, a weight loss strategy is not only unrealistic but also tantamount to medical malpractice should your doctor prescribe this approach over PAP initiation.

A weight loss strategy must realistically account for how bad things are at the outset. Patients with mild to moderate OSA with minimal oxygen desaturations and hypoxia are the best candidates for weight loss, notwithstanding the next critical topic—what's known in science as "the rate-limiting step."

Most weight loss systems are ineffective and unreliable and rarely cure obesity. Numerous reasons account for the difficulty in losing weight, but the largest factor is the failure of medical science and related treatment programs to fully grasp the nature of obesity, including its predisposing factors and, ultimately, its primary causes.

Though it is relatively true anyone could lose weight if they correctly counted calories and ate the correct amount of food to gradually lose fat, the core problem in obesity is its psychological underpinnings. I could write a book about this aspect and hope to one day, but in a nutshell, nearly every obese patient will admit to "emotional eating."[122] Therefore, if you taught someone how to cease this specific behavior, then a very large majority of obesity patients would lose weight and would do so with a relatively clear mission compared to the ups and downs of dieting. They would also find themselves more capable of keeping off the weight as they would have learned how to combat emotional eating.

In suggesting the need for a reliable weight loss system, note that any system theoretically could work as long as it included some counseling or related therapy that specifically addresses the emotional eating component. Hypothetically, Weight Watchers, NutriSystem, Noom, Jenny Craig, and many other dietary approaches, such as keto, paleo, vegan, vegetarian, and Mediterranean, could prove effective by providing a lot of structure as well as recommended changes in eating habits and nutrition, but again most systems fail in the absence of counseling or therapy directed at emotional eating. Even something as drastic and immediately effective as bariatric surgery subsequently fails when the patient neglects to address the cravings triggered by emotional eating impulses.

Practically, one of the best programs out there is free; it's called Overeaters Anonymous (OA), which while not directly offering an emotion-focused therapy system, still includes a 12-step program that typically evokes strong emotional connections to the problems you are dealing with as you attempt to heal yourself. Whether you drink too much, use illicit drugs, are repeatedly engaging in risky and promiscuous sexual encounters, or you are unable to stop eating, a 12-step program is continually asking of you to hold a mirror up and reflect on who you really are, what you really feel, and how these insights about yourself provide new direction in your life.

In the second half of this book, you will learn a great deal about sleep-related *emotion-focused therapy* (EFT) and how this potent tool treats severe, intractable, drug-dependent insomniacs. For now, keep in mind most people with insomnia, or nightmares, or mental health problems, and all the above, suffer regular difficulties in managing their emotions. This deficit in emotional processing skills, otherwise known as *emotional coping capacity*, is extremely common in our society, but in particular, it is all but universal in people who suffer obesity, as evidenced by the nearly universal complaint of emotional eating. Thus, a strong correlation between very poor coping and very unhealthy weight gain is inextricably linked.

If someone entered an EFT program and successfully learned new coping skills, almost automatically this individual would recognize emotional eating situations and therefore would possess a potential to cease or at least curb emotional eating. It is not unheard of for such patients to enter into very advanced forms of psychotherapy and subsequently gain refreshingly new motivation to take better care of mind and body. As a result, these individuals start losing weight for no apparent reason, that is, without some special plan to lose the weight. Instead, their appetite changes because it is no longer triggered to the same degree by emotional eating impulses. The stomach no longer needs to be filled up to the bursting point to resolve the "emptiness" feelings inside the tummy (and elsewhere), and therefore eating becomes a more natural experience, as in eating what you need and not what you want.

Taken together, I rarely recommend anyone use a weight loss strategy as an initial treatment for sleep apnea unless the individual is suffering a mild OSA/UARS problem and has detailed a very exacting regimen to combine weight loss and a gentle exercise program. Even then, I usually beg them to consider an EFT component because I know their likelihood of failure will be much higher without EFT.

Unfortunately, obese patients are most suited for PAP, given the limitations of nearly all their other options, save bariatric surgery. Moreover, PAP has the distinct potential of a rapid response, including feeling noticeably better after just the first night in the sleep lab. As many mental health patients gain weight from psychotropic medications that cause or aggravate obesity, it's a crying shame these patients are reluctant to try PAP, especially as improvements in sleep quality can lead to better emotional coping.

Nevertheless, when PAP is not an option for the obese OSA/UARS patient, metabolic bariatric surgery might be an option to consider,[123] or a more conservative step involves adjustments to one's sleep position.

Positional Therapy

Positional therapy, usually trying to sleep off of your back, is highly overrated and almost never leads to anything close to a cure. However, many patients in select circumstances profit from repositioning themselves during the sleep period, and if such an individual is reluctant or unable to attempt a more expensive therapy like PAP or OAT, learning to reposition is certainly worth a trial and may yield moderate to marked improvements.

The oldest version of a position change system is sewing tennis balls to the backside of a sleep shirt; presumably the discomfort of rolling onto your back will cause you to change to any other position. Unfortunately, the device does not work well.

Now, more technologically savvy devices have been developed in the past few years. Night Balance, manufactured by a leading PAP supplier, Respironics, uses a belt to sense when you are moving to your back, after which a vibration occurs in the belt. Over time, the patient learns to recognize the vibration stimuli and move into a different position. This stimulus-movement response appears to occur on a relatively unconscious level.

Night Balance has been tested in scientifically designed research studies and has yielded improvements including, most importantly, decreased daytime fatigue and sleepiness in the large majority of cases. The only caveat is the research was conducted on a select group of individuals whose OSA was unquestionably worse on their backs, a condition labeled *positional OSA*.

The above point raises the salient issue of how different breathing events manifest in different positions. For example, it's obvious when the problem is your tongue collapsing into the back of your throat, then lying on your back probably aggravates the problem simply by gravity. Therefore, avoiding your back is a good thing. But this view is too simplistic because plenty of patients suffer apneas (complete breathing cessation) lying on their side or stomach. In other words, you can suffer all types of breathing events in all positions.

If you were fortunate to suffer the majority of severe breathing events only on your back, then the position-change device could provide marked improvement, but most do not suffer this black-and-white degree of SDB. Moreover, even when you do show a preponderance of apneas on your back, you could still suffer a great many hypopneas and flow limitations on your side. And, as you hopefully recall from the earlier discussions on sleep quality, each event type does not necessarily predict how poorly you sleep or how badly you feel the next day.

With this backdrop, it is imperative to appreciate when you move off your back, you might see little to no improvement if your flow limitations are still causing severe sleep fragmentation. This singular point explains how positional therapy is sometimes misapplied by suggesting to specific patients they should feel fantastic when they move off their backs. In some cases, the individual might need more intensive repositioning, namely, greater elevation of the head via a wedge or, in extreme cases, a hospital bed or a sleep chair.

There are other devices on the market, and you can research them and try one out. Remember, though, these devices do not cure OSA or UARS, and therefore whatever you gain, do not overestimate its impact on SDB. You will probably need more treatment whenever you are ready to move forward.

Hypoglossal Nerve Stimulator (HGNS)

A nerve stimulator (an electrical wire) involves three components. The controller is implanted under the collarbone, and then two sensors emerge from this device. One sensor travels to the ribs to monitor breathing, while the other sensor travels under the jaw to the hypoglossal nerve that controls tongue function.

With this combination of input and output, the rib sensor detects your inspiratory breathing cycle to time the neurostimulation to the tongue in rhythmical fashion. In the most relevant description of research on the device, known as HGNS, a surgical procedure is required to implant the wires, which then takes a month to heal, after which the device is activated. In a small sample of patients in one study, all of whom suffered moderate to severe OSA, everything improved for the measures of breathing events, oxygen desaturations, arousal index, and objectively measured sleep quality in the form of decreased stage 1 NREM, increased REM sleep, and overall increased sleep efficiency. And daytime sleepiness and functioning also greatly improved.

The main drawback in outcomes was the absence of any cures. When breathing events were cut in half, which is clearly a marked improvement, the patients still suffered from sleep apnea, just of a lesser severity, but sufficient to still warrant restarting use of PAP therapy if they chose to. On the other hand, the patients clearly reported improvements in daytime symptoms, including depression.

Side effects appear to be minor in terms of skin irritation or numbness or tongue abrasions, which occurs due to tongue movements across the teeth. Unfortunately, the device does not seem to work as well in patients with morbid obesity (BMI > 35) or those with excessive crowding in the oral airway, this latter finding related to the greater complexity of the anatomical obstruction in certain patients.

Perhaps the most interesting thing about HGNS is patients activate the device when they go to bed; and in same research study, their patients averaged use for 90% of the night. Therefore, when you compare this high level of use with lower adherence in patients on standard CPAP, HGNS has distinct advantages by gaining a high level of treatment use virtually every night.

It remains concerning the overall improvement may not be much better than a 50% reduction in breathing events, particularly compared to our sleep center's level of success where as much as 90% of patients who filled a prescription for PAP went on to become regular users. With the advanced PAP mentioned earlier, many use these sophisticated pressurized air modes all night long, leading to greater than 90% decreases in AHI/RDI .

Regardless, more recent HGNS data suggest further decreases in the AHI, but the problem with these assessments, as with any postsurgical assessments, is the absence of flow limitation measurements. A decrease in AHI is great, but if flow limitation is not even addressed, as is the case with HGNS and most surgery, then the statements on reduction in breathing events are misleading. I have spoken with representatives of one of the main companies promulgating this procedure and informed them of the necessity to address flow limitation, but we will need to see how they respond to this constructive criticism.

Inevitably, we would anticipate technological advances in this area because one can easily imagine increasing precision over time. In fact, wouldn't it be lovely if such a device proved more effective than PAP? Then, neurostimulation would be at the top of the hierarchy for treating OSA/UARS. Thinking futuristically, it seems likely someone will invent a very small chip embedded in the throat to solve these problems.

In the interim, if an individual could not tolerate other treatments such as PAP or OAT, it is reasonable to argue HGNS is a suitable option and should be considered.[124;125]

Medications

Drugs to treat sleep apnea remain in the experimental stage. According to recent reviews on this topic, nothing comes close to matching the success of a PAP or OAT device or, for that matter, surgery or HGNS. Given the enormous size of the market for sleep apnea treatments, expect large investments from the pharmaceutical industry to find specific receptors in the airway dilator muscles, particularly the tongue, after which medications to treat sleep apnea will likely offer attractive alternatives. Another experimental pathway will look at brain receptors that control breathing. While this research flies under the radar now, in the next 10 years or sooner we should see a rapid increase in research and development.

Until proven drug treatments are available, it could still be useful to consider specific medications in personalized circumstances that may indirectly improve OSA/UARS in a patient unable or unwilling to try PAP or OAT or for whom surgery or HGNS is not an option. We've already discussed drugs working to improve nasal breathing at the top of the chapter, and these should be revisited to address chronic congestion.

As many OSA/UARS patients show their very worst breathing and oxygen drops during REM sleep, there is renewed interest in REM-suppressant medications, notably antidepressants. Three drugs have been researched, Prozac (fluoxetine), Paxil (paroxetine), and Remeron (mirtazapine); the latter was the subject of intense scrutiny after the publication of an initial case series showing marked improvements, but subsequent controlled studies did not prove the drug effective in treating OSA. Still, if a person suffers from a predominantly REM-dependent form of OSA/UARS, an antidepressant pill will conceivably yield some relief. Interestingly, though, these drugs were not necessarily studied for REM suppressant activity; rather, they seemed to target sites in the brain or elsewhere to stimulate breathing. Practically, however, the REM suppression action might have the most potent effect on a specific patient and therefore may be worth a trial.

The caveat, however, must be reiterated that REM sleep is crucial to memory, mood, and emotional processing, so why take a drug that suppresses this highly beneficial stage of sleep? Currently, there are no known answers to this question, though it is worth restating many patients with OSA/UARS do not consolidate their REM sleep very well. In fact, many suffer from severe REM sleep fragmentation due to the breathing events disrupting REM or even preventing entry into REM. Therefore, untreated OSA/UARS patients are unlikely to receive benefit from this fragmented REM or its scarcity. Overall, research is needed to determine whether further suppression of fragmented REM with an antidepressant leads to any sleep gains or daytime symptom improvement.

One angle must be mentioned here; research has confirmed some patients suffer REM-dependent OSA, which means the predominant occurrence of their breathing events is almost exclusively in REM sleep and is linked to daytime symptoms. It could prove worthwhile for these patients, if unable to implement any other strategy, to initiate a trial with their prescribing physician to aim at suppressing REM sleep. As REM-dependent OSA is more common in younger patients, they may be particularly motivated to try a medication instead of PAP.

Stimulants are a different class of drugs used for the problem of daytime sleepiness. Even though we discussed how mental health patients with sleep apnea report fewer problems with sleepiness and more with fatigue, stimulants might work on either symptom. Clearly, a stimulant would not be expected to improve sleep apnea itself, but given the potential impact on sleepiness or fatigue, a fair number of patients would gain improvements in daytime functioning. Indeed, many OSA/UARS patients are already seeking and gaining benefit from caffeine, the world's most commonly used stimulant.

Stimulants are not without side effects, and agitation is one of the more obvious problems due to the drugs speeding up your heart rate or provoking jittery or anxious feelings. Then again, a stimulant may decrease feelings of depression just by increasing your energy level. If a mental health patient were predisposed toward the symptom of depression and less so anxiety, then a stimulant might be a useful option to treat daytime symptoms. In the circumstances of more anxiety and less depression, the stimulant might aggravate anxiety.

A psychiatrist is the preferred physician to prescribe a stimulant because this doctor may be able to gauge better the interplay between the drug and all the symptoms needing to be addressed, but there are sleep doctors who have developed expertise in this area in their own quest to help patients who fail other forms of OSA/UARS treatment.

Among this group of sleep physicians, the general clinical opinion now forming is many patients diagnosed with depression are actually patients with OSA/UARS exclusively or those suffering from both conditions. Either way, the sleep breathing problem has much more influence than previously recognized. Thus, it is possible to see a patient's depression and sleepiness and fatigue all improve while using a stimulant. Although the same results should be achievable with effective sleep breathing treatments, these patients are nevertheless grateful for this unexpected medication treatment option that served them so well.

Another reason stimulants may be useful in the short term is their appetite-suppressant activity. For patients suffering from obesity, a stimulant is not a good long-term solution for weight loss, but in the short term a patient using stimulants for a year or two is afforded more time to figure out a more direct way to treat OSA/UARS while simultaneously losing weight.

Two of the more common benefits of weight loss would be easier or better control of diabetes or hypertension, albeit in some patients blood pressure may rise with stimulants despite the weight loss. If the stimulant improves daytime energy levels, then daytime physical activity and exertion may increase, which may yield further weight loss or, at minimum, facilitate keeping off the pounds recently lost.

Unfortunately, in my opinion, there has been a trend toward more rapid introduction of stimulant medication for patients who are failing CPAP.[126] Unfortunate because these patients would have probably succeeded if exposed to more advanced, dual-pressure, auto-adjusting devices (ASV or ABPAP) as described earlier and expanded on in Appendix A. Still, there can be no question stimulants help some people in the short term when no other treatment is available. A medication such as Ritalin, Adderall, Provigil, Nuvigil, or Strattera, to name a few, just might be the right answer until other therapies can be revised and attempted.

The Horizon

From this point forward, you will be pleased to hear that invention after invention are appearing on the sleep medicine landscape as often as every month. While none might work perfectly just yet, the entrepreneurial spirit is finally invigorating the sleep apnea industry, and assorted options are appearing on the horizon much sooner than previously imagined. In fact, every year going forward I expect yet another moderately effective invention or two to land in the marketplace, and some of these innovations could lead to dramatic changes in the way sleep-disordered breathing is treated.

Here are some innovative products in early stages of development or now on the marketplace. Most have not been extensively evaluated, although scientifically conducted studies have tested some products' efficacy. ExciteOSA by Signifier Medical Technologies retrains the tongue through electrical stimulation to decrease its collapsibility (https://exciteosa.com). The specially designed mouthpiece is worn 20 minutes/day to deliver neuromuscular electrical stimulation. After 6 weeks, it's regularly used twice/week. HVNSleep Pod also uses electrical stimulation (https://www.buyhvnsleep.com), but this device situates under your chin and is designed to detect snoring vibrations. It stimulates throat and tongue muscles to firm up. Micro-CPAP devices are battery operated nose plugs to pull air into your nose, marketed as anti-snoring devices. Several versions are currently available with Airing, a notable leader in development (www.fundairing.com). While some hint at, most do not say it will eliminate the need for CPAP. V-Com, invented by Dr. William Noah at SleepRes (https://sleepres.com) is a tool to insert between mask and tubing to decrease peak inspiratory pressure. The device improves CPAP adaptation and may be removed after a few weeks or months or used long-term.

To be sure, by the time this book is published, I am certain newer procedures or technology will already be available for either clinical trials or in the marketplace.

Sleep Research Pearl #8

These eight chapters pinpointed sleep quality as the single most important component of your sleep. Because you understand sleep quality is a physical thing inside your brain, the sleep breathing disorders fragmenting your sleep (broken brain waves) must be a primary target for treatment. In more than 30 years of clinical practice and research investigations, this paradigm stands out as the missing and decisively pivotal link the mental health community and even portions of the sleep medicine community are failing to embrace when treating mental health patients' sleep disorders.

The largest obstacle to advancing this paradigm is outright ignorance of the high prevalence of SDB in psychiatric patients. Another equally large barrier is the entrenched belief mental health therapies and behavioral sleep therapies geared toward psychological origins must always be the initial treatment pathway.

I did not write this book to declare all must start with physiological assessment and treatment, but I am persuaded a huge proportion of mental health patients, easily more than 50% and possibly as high as 90%, would fare much better by looking at OSA/UARS connections as early as possible in their treatment regimens.

I cannot begin to count the number of demoralized individuals who desperately sought aid at our sleep center as the place of last resort or who enrolled in one of our research protocols after years of failing numerous other therapies. In so many of our research publications, we elaborated on the sad circumstances where individuals went back and forth and around and around with psychiatrists, psychologists, and therapists, as well as conventional sleep docs, all of whom were missing the SDB diagnosis. The time span was often measured not in years but in decades of missed opportunities.

Though it has been a wonderful experience to treat these individuals to improve their sleep and usually their mental health along with it, far too many times, both in the clinic and in our research protocols, we have heard the refrain, "If only someone had given me this information years ago, my life would have been so different."

We'd like your life to be different *now*, and my earnest hope is you can find a shortcut through this tangled web to discern how physiological disorders are fueling your sleep symptoms. Our goal is simple: recover your normal sleep so you can in fact experience *the rest of your life!*

CHAPTER 9

THE KICKING AND SCREAMING SLEEP MOVEMENT DISORDERS

How do I treat restless legs, leg jerks, and parasomnia disorders?

Tossing and Turning

Compared to typical sleep center patients, those with mental health conditions suffer higher rates of movement disorders literally ranging from head to toe. The most common disorders involve movement of the legs, but a close second are parasomnia disorders (arising from your brain); sleepwalking is the most common. Sleepwalking usually is benign, but other parasomnias, while uncommon, prove more concerning, such as sleep terrors (previously called night terrors), REM behavior disorder, nocturnal eating, bruxism (teeth grinding), and the recently described *trauma-associated sleep disorder* (TASD or TSD). Nightmares are the most prevalent parasomnia and are covered separately in Chapter 16.

These physiological conditions are covered here for two reasons. First, as the chapter title suggests, each condition reflects something moving while you sleep. The second and clinically more relevant factor is sleep-disordered breathing is extremely common in all these conditions, and the great news is SDB treatment often partially or completely resolves these disorders. A few exceptions hold, but it is so common to see movement symptoms abate with PAP therapy, it's important to overemphasize this point while you sort out the nature of your tossing and turning or your extra movements during sleep. As before, tossing and turning may signify attempts to reposition your head and neck to open the airway—more evidence suggesting sleep movements are connected to sleep breathing.

We'll start from the bottom and work our way up.

The Basics of Leg Movements

Leg movement disorders are epidemic in mental health patients, and particularly so in those taking psychotropic medications. In my clinical experience, at least 25% to as high as 50% of patients on antidepressant, antianxiety, or sleeping pills, and possibly greater, suffer from these conditions. Yet, their prescribing physicians and psychologists, as well as their therapists, appear oblivious and express scant interest in exploring these symptoms and disorders with their patients.

The ramifications are not as severe as missing the diagnosis of OSA or UARS, but they are problematic nonetheless because *restless legs syndrome* (RLS) and *periodic limb movement disorder* (PLMD) are the second leading physical disrupters to sleep in mental health patients. Their impact is consequential because restless legs and leg jerks may completely sabotage any benefits gained with PAP. Even among patients without sleep breathing disorders, leg movements independently seem to cause or aggravate anxiety, depression, and posttraumatic stress.

Making matters potentially much worse and more serious is the recent speculation linking restless legs syndrome to suicidal ideation. How this connection might arise is unproven so far, but it's worth mentioning for individuals who are at risk or currently suffering from suicidality.

Think of RLS as a frequent irritant in your system, as if a fly were constantly buzzing you despite attempts to swat it away. To take another analogy, suppose you had to scratch an itch all day long as if your skin were always inflamed with poison ivy, but you were unable to recognize the condition "poison ivy"; you just noticed your skin was always itching.

Both scenarios parallel the course of RLS, except these examples reflect external factors, something on your skin needs scratching or swatting away. RLS is more insidious and indirect as the sensations emanate from your own nervous system. The feelings surface in an elusive way, so you may not even recognize you suffer from them. Instead, individuals feel antsy without identifying the antsy-ness coming from their legs. Based on this premise alone, we could expect anyone experiencing RLS to report an increase in anxiety, and anxiety often leads to depression symptoms.

All these descriptions of leg movements strongly suggest a biological process that causes mental illness, and in my opinion, we will one day discover RLS and PLMD are in fact not just physical sleep disrupters but also independent neurologically driven mental disorders. To reiterate, few mental health professionals show any awareness of RLS or PLMD, and patients must wait years or decades until encountering a sleep specialist before proper diagnosis and care are administered.

I wanted to introduce the seriousness of this condition because so much is at stake for so many mental health patients who don't realize they could be suffering RLS and PLMD. Please do not ignore such symptoms, and do be skeptical of any physician unwilling to help you address these disorders.

Now, let's get into the details of these two unusual and overlapping sleep disorders.

Legs and More Legs

Restless legs syndrome comprises the following:
- When lying or sitting, uncomfortable or difficult-to-describe sensations emerge in the back of the calves (or other spots on legs or arms) so unpleasant you must move.
- Movement of the legs, arms, or body eliminates the unpleasant feeling.
- The sensation returns when you stop moving.
- The sensation intensifies during evening or bedtime.
- The feelings prevent sleep at bedtime or trying to return to sleep at night.

RLS is a *waking* condition; it does not occur during sleep, whereas periodic limb movement disorder (PLMD) is a *sleeping* condition with the following aspects:
- Legs jerk or twitch rhythmically (periodically) during the night.
- The leg jerk may be small and barely noticeable, perhaps occurring only in the ankle, or involving dramatic motions in the whole body.

- Each jerk(s) lasts 5-10 seconds or as little as a half second.
- Movements repeat in cycles, say, once every 30 seconds, with cycles ranging from 30 to 90 seconds.
- Movement may or may not provoke an arousal (speeding up the brain waves) discernible in the sleep EEG.
- PLMD's impact on sleep is controversial but often underestimated; it can produce enough disruption in SDB patients to halt PAP use or significantly diminish PAP benefits, or it may produce sleep disruption in patients without SDB.
- If you suffer RLS, you likely suffer PLMD during sleep, whereas those with PLMD suffer a 50% chance of RLS.

RLS can drive a person into a state of mental instability because it is so harrowing to not know what's going on or how to stop it. RLS is easily missed; few physicians are aware of RLS as an independent sleep disorder, and patients recognize RLS as a weird complaint, so they often don't bring it up.

The patient endures the condition for years and compensates in various ways. Many with RLS use drugs particularly alcohol to sleep, which often compounds the problem. Moreover, no small number of patients present to their doctors as potential alcoholics, yet no one brings up RLS/PLMD as a contributing factor until years later.

Many physicians prescribe sedatives, antianxiety pills, or antidepressants for these patients without ever "hearing" about the leg movement part of the sleep complaint.[127] Sedatives are weak treatments for RLS in comparison to well-researched medications. Antidepressants often aggravate RLS or PLMD symptoms. Ironically, both RLS and PLMD cause or worsen anxiety or depression. Both conditions likely cause or aggravate suicidal thinking or actions.[128;129]

Legs and SDB

The greatest controversy about RLS and PLMD is their relationship to

SDB.[130] Many with RLS and PLMD also suffer SDB, especially upper airway resistance, that is the flow limitation events. Many limb movements occur at the end of subtle UARS disruptions.[131] Remarkably, when these patients receive PAP therapy, their leg jerks often decrease when air pressure fully normalizes their breathing. Older research revealed the opposite situation in which a PLMD patient with SDB was treated with a medication to eliminate leg jerks, which then stabilized sleep and virtually eliminated the SDB.

These SDB findings are confusing, so this puzzle requires persistence to find a solution, usually through a sleep center. If we see PLMD in an SDB patient, we are reluctant to treat legs until we've treated breathing. But, if the patient also complains of RLS, then leg jerks are more suspicious. We could start medication before using PAP; then, in the lab we determine whether the drug decreased leg jerks. Or, if the patient reports the drug decreased waking RLS, the sleep test often confirms the sleeping leg jerks decreased, too.

The majority of RLS/PLMD patients are so confused about these movement symptoms they rarely agree to start medication promptly. Patients must return to the sleep lab multiple times before they finally accept the leg movements as an independent disorder needing independent treatment. The most important consideration in SDB cases is whether RLS or PLMD interferes with PAP therapy. In clear-cut cases of restless legs or leg jerks, the proper medication positively transforms their use of PAP therapy simply by preventing the disruption from leg movements that unknowingly was interfering with their use of the breathing mask.

The tragic dilemma in managing RLS/PLMD is mental health patients may already suffer high levels of anxiety, which makes them feel very restless and may lead to tossing and turning at night. In other words, it is a logical analysis to assume anxiety is the problem when in fact many of these people actually suffer from RLS, the real cause of their restlessness, while PLMD is the real cause of the tossing and turning. This conundrum is perplexing and challenging to sort out, even for sleep specialists, let alone mental health providers who are not asking questions about RLS/PLMD. Some patients take months or years to distinguish between anxiety and restless legs.

When Sleeping Pills Are Not Sedatives and the Problem of Augmentation

Fortunately, you only need one drug to treat RLS or PLMD or both. In severe cases, a patient may use two medications or alternate drugs. The list of available drugs is growing with increasing research interest in movement disorders. We'll focus on proven medications.

Dopamine Derivatives. Carbidopa/levodopa, or Sinemet, is the granddaddy medication, having been used to treat RLS or PLMD successfully for decades. It works through dopamine (a neurotransmitter) pathways, and newer derivatives also work on these dopaminergic pathways.

Sinemet or its variations are taken 30 minutes or longer before bedtime, and a repeat dose can be used a few hours later if awakened by leg jerks. A long-acting version may work for some and avert the second dose. The problem with Sinemet is side effects, many of which are minor and often resolve in a week or two. Most notable is nausea or vomiting that may prove insurmountable.

The worst and quite unexpected side effect is the worsening of RLS to earlier in the day. If the drug is not stopped, the restlessness can span 24/7, a distressing experience that directly leads to suicidal ideation or behavior. This side effect, known as *augmentation*, can develop into a psychiatric emergency if the patient becomes mentally unstable with around-the-clock RLS. Typically, the drug should never be used again.

Other side effects include increased risk for depression among individuals with a past or family history of depression. More severe side effects include neurologic symptoms such as further movement disorders like tardive dyskinesia, a condition of involuntary repetitive movements like grimacing or blinking.

Newer dopaminergic agents include pramipexole (Mirapex), ropinirole (Requip), and rotigotine patch (Neupro), which have excellent safety profiles with two important caveats to be described below. You must start with the lowest dosage for about a week and assess impact on RLS, then increase over time. This schedule also reduces side effects. Requip is unique in dosing one to three hours before bedtime. The Neupro patch is placed on your skin once daily at a time convenient to you. One hassle factor with Neupro is the need to change the delivery site on your skin every day for 14 consecutive days. Thus, you can only return to the original site after two weeks, and once again respect the everyday changes on a 14-day cycle.

Although very effective, many patients misperceive the action of these drugs, presuming they are sedatives. By analogy, a better way to understand the actions of these pills is to presume they erase an intense emotion that had been blocking your natural wave of sleepiness. This point will be explained further in the chapters ahead on emotional processing (Chapters 12–14). As a brief example, when someone is anxious, she may not feel sleepy at bedtime. If deep breathing relaxed her and the anxiety abated, we would expect sleepiness to rush in. Patients with RLS likewise suffer blocked feelings of sleepiness due to the restless feelings or sensations popping up at bedtime. Once the drug eliminates RLS, the wave of sleepiness laps upon the shore, and the patient falls asleep. This sequence explains why the medication is taken *before* bedtime, not *at* bedtime.

One huge and growing caveat with dopaminergic agents is the increasing evidence on augmentation (making the RLS worse instead of better) occurring more commonly than previously realized.[132] Some sleep specialists no longer prescribe this family of medications. In fact, this controversy is spreading so widely, some sleep professionals are openly questioning whether use of these drugs constitutes malpractice. To say the least, this is a tough nut to crack because so many people have experienced transformative life experiences by knocking out RLS/PLMD symptoms with dopamine derivatives. While it's true years later they may be forced to switch to other medications, I believe patients should be permitted to make their own choices in healthcare therapies until or unless evidence arises proving these drugs manifest more immediate and serious harmful side effects. Unfortunately, the current climate in healthcare is very cloudy with large storm activity rapidly approaching. The main front moving in is too many mandates and regulations from the top down. Instead, we should be listening to each individual patient to allow for personally tailored medicine, a much more attractive system to weather the looming tempest.

Which bring us to the second caveat. In a smaller number of instances, impulse-control disorder could emerge with the use of dopaminergic drugs, most commonly compulsive gambling, shopping or sexual activity.[133] I have only treated one patient in my career who suffered these compulsive symptoms, and it was undoubtedly a living nightmare for him and his family. Again, though the risk is low, you should know about the potential for such side effects.

Opiates. Another drug category includes oxycodone, the narcotic that raises red flags in many peoples' minds. Please note—treatment of RLS or PLMD almost invariably responds to very low (2.5 mg) to low (5 mg to 10 mg) dosages. These dosages are much lower than used in pain management for a broken bone, where an individual could receive a bottle of sixty 5 mg pills to last one week. For an RLS patient, 60 of these 5 mg pills might last one to four months or longer. A sleep physician would not prescribe more than this low amount except for a rare individual who might require three or four pills (15 mg to 20 mg) per night. In my clinical experience, only three patients ever received a dosing schedule greater than two pills (10 milligrams).

Abuse potential is very low and very rare because the patient typically cannot persuade the sleep physician to prescribe more. Patients can always doctor shop for more pills, but then signs of addiction or dependency show up. As *rare* means it can still happen, patients must be closely monitored by the prescribing physician, and their refills nowadays are tracked by statewide prescription monitoring programs.

Oxycodone is safe, but it produces the troubling side effect of constipation. It also imparts occasional sleepy feelings during the daytime, especially in the first few days or weeks. Nonetheless, oxycodone research has proven the powerful treatment impact on RLS and PLMD. Other narcotics used regularly with leg movement patients include hydrocodone and methadone. Johns Hopkins University (JHU) has extensively researched the use of opiates in RLS/PLMD, and their sleep doctors advocate this therapy as top-line agents. Therefore, to keep current or learn more about opiates, JHU is the place to follow.

One caveat involves the potential for an opiate to depress breathing. In fact opiates can worsen OSA and CSA. Typically, no worries arise if the patient is also using PAP as it protects the airway. Greater caution, therefore, is advised in an RLS/PLMD patient not using a breathing treatment.

GABA Derivatives. The last category, GABA-related drugs, includes Neurontin, Lyrica, and Horizant. In the past decade, we have seen not only an increase in their prescribing but also more evidence revealing greater effectiveness than once thought.

Neurontin is first in line and works well, but a sizeable drawback is the unusual dosing. Each time you take Neurontin, the dosage should never exceed 600 mg, yet some need more than 600 mg for optimal results. In other words, the drug may require other dosing times besides bedtime. When you take 600 mg before bedtime and need more, your doctor raises the total dosage by adding 300 mg or 600 mg, except now you need to take this pill four to six hours earlier in the evening. It might be 600 mg at dinner time and then 600 mg at bedtime. Yet again, if more medication is needed, the next increase of 300 mg to 600 mg could occur near lunchtime.

This timetable is the main barrier, often proving inconvenient, if not unrealistic to maintain. Daytime dosing to treat something occurring at night is easy to forget. You must plan very efficiently, yet if it works well, chances are you will maintain this regimen.

Ultimately, most respond to Neurontin in the 600 mg to 1800 mg range, and this dosage remains on the low to medium side. By comparison, chronic pain patients are dosed much higher at 3600 mg to 4500 mg in a day.

Lyrica, in the same family of drugs, also may work, but frequently causes weight gain, and sometimes rapid weight gain, so most stop using after the first 10- to 30-pound increase.

Horizant is a very efficient drug because it takes advantage of the properties of Neurontin and turns it into a long-acting agent. You take it once around 5 p.m., or earlier or later depending on your bedtime, and it lasts all night. Nearly everyone who uses Horizant reports it works well, but the peculiar thing is follow-up sleep studies do not always show objective improvement in leg jerks. Still, Horizant has proven a useful drug for many patients, albeit its cost prevents widespread use. Horizant also adds the burden of submitting prior authorization to your insurer, which only prevails if you've previously tried and failed two other drugs. Even with coverage, the price still challenges many budgets.

The augmentation effect described above for dopamine-acting drugs also may occur for GABA-acting drugs, though less frequently. Overall, it is important to reiterate, if you start on a medication for RLS/PLMD and things worsen, it is clearly time to consider whether you are suffering from augmentation.

Reminder: augmentation is not always just symptoms worsening but also symptoms moving into an around-the-clock cycle. Most commonly, a person describes RLS in the evening, but with augmentation restlessness now occurs morning, afternoon, and evening. The individual assumes the drug must not be working, starts increasing the dosage, and then daytime symptoms worsen. The around-the-clock scenario is highly distressing as many patients report restlessness so severe they cannot cope and feel as if they are being driven out of their minds. Many suffering severe augmentation could develop suicidal ideation, but unfortunately this problem has not been thoroughly researched.

Like opiates, GABA-acting drugs also cause respiratory depression, therefore the same cautions are advised when using without PAP.

Other medications are prescribed for RLS or PLMD, but those discussed above are well supported by evidence. Sleep specialists keep current on drug research for movement disorders because 10% of their patients suffer from these problems. Unfortunately, many physicians, even some sleep professionals, prescribe benzodiazepines such as Valium or Clonazepam or sedatives such as Ambien, without first using evidence-based drugs. While these third-line agents work very well for select patients, more commonly they yield fair to poor results.

Medication is all you need for an independent movement disorder, that is, no SDB or other sleep disorders are present. With better technology to measure breathing, we see more cases of PLMD interconnected to SDB where sleep breathing requires independent attention. Some patients use PAP therapy *and* drugs to treat both conditions. Therefore, make sure your sleep center uses nasal cannula pressure transducers to detect, score, and diagnose the flow limitation events of UARS. In this way, you will learn whether your leg jerks are independent or related to SDB.

When Leg Jerks Don't Cause Arousals

A frequent controversy in sleep medicine involves the scoring of leg jerks on sleep studies.[134] In the ideal scenario, each leg jerk causes some type of arousal as depicted in the sleep fragmentation diagrams (Figures 5.5–5.7 in Chapter 5). More often than not, many people demonstrate leg jerks without arousals, thus making it difficult to declare the patient is suffering from sleep fragmentation since, well, there is no frag.

Leg jerks without arousals would seem to not need treatment, but therein arises the controversy. What if other forms of arousal occur that cannot be viewed on the sleep study recording? One such arousal was researched by Dr. John Winkelman at Harvard, who has shown a leg jerk will cause a brief spike in blood pressure or increased heart rate even when no obvious cortical (EEG brain waves) arousal occurs.[135] These changes are consistent with an arousal in the autonomic nervous system (the fight or flight control center).

In the lab, the most common circumstances where these issues emerge are with OSA/UARS patients suffering leg jerks. In our experience, we see many flaws in the arousal-based scoring for leg jerks. Instead, we approach these patients strictly on their responses to PAP. If PAP is going well but leg jerks persist, we wait and see. However, if the patient is faring poorly with PAP and still shows leg jerks, we presume these movements are interfering with the SDB treatment.

In this last scenario, more than 80% of the patients who agreed to move forward with leg jerk medications transformed their entire sleep treatment response from something poor or mediocre to something very good to great. We view "invisible" arousals as potentially crucial in patients not faring well. Many were very thankful to be given the option to consider leg jerk medication.

Is There a Natural Way to Treat?

Vitamin and mineral deficiencies have been implicated in RLS and PLMD, but the research is only solid with the element of iron. Low iron storage measured in the lab test known as *serum ferritin* has been closely scrutinized, and individuals with values less than 50 ng/ml often are at risk for RLS or PLMD or both. Recently, this level was raised to 75 ng/ml, although some research suggests even higher levels might be useful.[136]

Remarkably, when ferritin levels drop, it adversely affects the impact of the prescription medications on leg movement conditions. In some, we had to raise ferritin to 50 ng/ml or 75 ng/ml or above before patients noted an optimal response to their prescription drugs. This outcome is especially relevant in helping PAP patients with leg jerks who suffer from air swallowing (aerophagia), a very common side effect caused by untreated leg jerks in OSA/UARS patients. More details on this air swallowing phenomenon are presented in Appendix A, the troubleshooting guide for PAP.

Considering all the discussion about dopamine agents, there appears to be an iron–dopamine connection to RLS. One dramatic report showed RLS emerging in patients with acute blood loss, and the movement symptoms were eliminated following blood transfusions, which must have resupplied the iron levels. In a placebo-controlled study, iron was administered intravenously to patients and resulted in clear improvements in RLS within the first week or two, but over time, the improvements decreased. Of practical interest, you do *not* need to experience anemia to develop a low ferritin level.

More recent research implicates more widespread iron deficiency without anemia. As such, many RLS/PLMD patients undergo evaluations by hematologists to test iron more precisely beyond ferritin levels. Many of these patients benefit from intravenous iron infusions.

Oral iron supplementation is not straightforward. Do not just start iron pills to experiment. First, you absolutely must clarify the serum ferritin level is below 50 ng/ml or 75 ng/ml. Next, if ferritin is low, discuss iron supplements with your primary physician. Most doctors do not know about this connection, so they may be skeptical about recommending iron because testing laboratories frequently declare ferritin of 10 ng/ml as normal.

Nevertheless, doctors are usually familiar with treating anemia patients with iron, and your discussion with your doctor is also important to make sure iron is a safe supplement for you. For example, patients who suffer from thickened blood volumes due to polycythemia, or those with iron storage conditions such as hemochromatosis, can almost never use iron supplements. So, the biggest reason to work with your doctor is to ensure your safety.

Iron supplements cause very distressing side effects like indigestion or constipation or both. Many people stop iron supplements within the first week due to stomach symptoms, so you may need to explore different options. Liquid iron supplements may be gentler on the stomach. You can find liquid iron in drugstores or vitamin stores, but it is usually expensive. Liquid iron is also more dangerous, so you would be advised to not use this form if small children live in your home.

Ingestion of excess iron in a child can be fatal.

For those with difficulty absorbing iron, prescription iron pills are needed. As noted, patients may work with a hematologist to determine why ferritin levels are low or why iron supplements do not increase ferritin levels; and, to reiterate, a hematologist may put you on a program of iron infusions given intravenously, and this therapy proves highly successful, though repeated transfusions are often needed.

Magnesium is the next mineral that shows a bit of evidence for helping leg jerks, based on only one study.[137] Many alternative medicine publications or practitioners proclaim the value of magnesium in solving RLS or PLMD conditions, and yet there is scant support for these claims.[138] In fact, when we have worked with numerous patients making this claim about their magnesium use, virtually all showed leg movements when retested in the sleep lab. This finding does not preclude the possibility that magnesium might work for you, so it is not unreasonable to consider its use, possibly for RLS but probably not PLMD.

Other substances of interest include vitamin D, folate, and vitamin B12. Vitamin D has received the most recent research, and several studies indicate a link between low levels and RLS/PLMD.[139] Checking vitamin D level is advised. Most other vitamins and minerals have not received much attention, so your own attempts would be trial and error at best, although some blood tests may provide guidance.

L-Tyrosine. In the past few years, we have seen surprisingly good results with the amino acid supplement L-tyrosine in about 30 patients (including myself) who were uninterested in taking a prescription medication, had tried and failed to gain benefit from a drug, or had suffered side effects. This amino acid is a precursor to L-DOPA and thus involves the dopamine pathway, suggesting its actions on RLS and PLMD are similar to drugs like Mirapex, Requip, or Neupro.

Dosages typically start at 500 mg, and we have read about and know of patients using levels as high as 2000 mg to 3000 mg at bedtime. Of those who clearly noted benefits, the most common improvements were feeling more refreshed in the morning, decreased daytime sleepiness, and more dreaming during sleep. We have not tested enough patients in the sleep lab to know whether these self-reported benefits of L-tyrosine are objectively corroborated.

One large caveat regarding this supplement is the vast array of alleged benefits it offers. For example, some use it for sleep irrespective of leg movements, whereas others report using it daily as a stimulant to decrease sleepiness and increase concentration. Others report improvements in anxiety and depression, apparently used during the daytime. This unusual list of benefits suggests L-tyrosine is a potent supplement, but without more research we can only mention a few dozen of our patients raved about its value for RLS/PLMD. I am among those who have used the supplement with clear-cut benefit for the past three years with dosages ranging from 500 mg to 3500 mg.

Notwithstanding, L-tyrosine may be problematic for patients on thyroid medications or MAO inhibitor antidepressants, and don't forget, if it is working on a dopamine pathway, perhaps one should be on the lookout for the kinds of side effects seen with Mirapex, Requip, and Neupro, perhaps even the augmentation problem and the impulse-control disorder. Working with a physician who knows your health history is imperative when considering a supplement like L-tyrosine.

Melatonin. Ever since the explosion of OTC melatonin use 20-plus years ago for the treatment of insomnia and circadian rhythm dysfunction, clinicians, researchers and patients have all wondered about its use in RLS and PLMD. Moreover, based on a recent survey, it appears melatonin is one of the most widely used OTC agents for these movement disorders, which is not surprising given the reluctance of so many to add another prescription medication to their already long list of drugs. Yet, according to some, melatonin should not prove effective and may worsen RLS/PLMD, because it inhibits the release of dopamine. Unfortunately, there is not a lot of research one way or another to make a strong recommendation, but it is clear there is a sense of large scale "anecdotal" evidence with so many individuals apparently using this OTC remedy for these specific problems. Hopefully, more research will settle the issue.

In sum, working with a sleep doctor or neurologist who has experience with patients using melatonin, vitamin D, L-tyrosine or any other OTC remedy is your best pathway forward if you want to avoid prescription medications.

How Do Antidepressants Cause or Aggravate RLS or PLMD?

On a sleep test, many patients using antidepressants or other psychotropic meds demonstrate leg jerks (PLMD). This side effect is widely unknown in the mental health community, or if it is known, it is not yet viewed as problematic.

Not all antidepressants cause leg jerks, but many, notably SSRI (selective serotonin reuptake inhibitors) medications, appear to induce leg jerks during sleep.[140] We see a great increase in leg jerk frequency on sleep tests for these patients, yet sometimes without the expected arousals. The conflictual questions arising for poor sleepers are whether they should switch medications to one without this side effect or whether the leg jerks have any impact on sleep? Perhaps the leg jerks were always there, and the antidepressant worsened them.

These issues are not easy to sort through, but mental health patients who use antidepressants must address them in the following contexts:
- Is the antidepressant producing clear-cut improvements in depression?
- Is it worth changing medication to find one yielding more improvement?

137

- Is it feasible to stop a medication to determine the impact on leg jerks?
- Is it feasible to stop a medication and use emotional processing skills (described in Chapters 12–14) as an alternative to antidepressant medication?
- If the medication is working well and should be maintained, would there be a value in adding a new medication to treat the leg jerks?

Many mental health patients and other sleep disorders patients with the combination of SDB and leg movements must sort out whether breathing is the prime culprit. This step may take months.

In one of my first cases with this degree of complexity, two years were needed to help a psychiatric patient taper off three medications while starting her on two new ones and at the same time helping her with PAP therapy struggles. Finally, she selected oral appliance therapy, OAT. The difficulties arose because her medications were helping her depression but also making her sleep much worse with very frequent leg jerks. When her medication was changed, her depression got worse even though her leg jerks and sleep were improving. We saw a large improvement in her sleep consolidation, a decrease in leg jerks, and a decrease in arousals once she was stabilized on a combination of OAT, new medications for psychiatric disorders, and a drug for RLS and PLMD.

For mental health patients, this process takes considerable time and effort, and frequent sleep testing and physician encounters, but the results are well worth it. However, for someone with suicidal ideation or behaviors, this process proves aggravating and demoralizing. For this reason alone, it is critical to attempt to arrange for your sleep physician and prescribing psychiatrist or psychologist to work closely together to speed up the efforts to solve the leg jerk problem without worsening the depression.

Some key things to consider that may help sort out the confusion much faster:

- Try as best you can to determine whether the anxiety symptoms you feel might be coming from restless legs, not just generalized anxiety.
- Find someone to sleep with you in your bed (the scientific method demands it!) for a few nights and ask them to notice whether you

are moving your legs.

- Ask your mother or father or siblings or any other blood relatives if they suffer from RLS or PLMD as the condition runs in families.
- Look carefully at your bed linens in the morning and attempt to quantify how messy they appear compared to when you first went to sleep.
- Pay attention to any leg or back soreness and pains you notice in the mornings because lower back problems may cause or contribute to RLS/PLMD.
- Any noticeable findings from these observations should raise suspicions for an underlying limb movement disorder as a disrupting variable in your sleep experience.
- Regardless of how you go about figuring out whether you suffer from limb movements—the waking (RLS) or the sleeping (PLMD) versions—it cannot be overstated how critical it may be to your mental health to find out the most accurate information in the timeliest fashion.
- Patients with either diagnosed or undiagnosed RLS and PLMD experience mental health symptoms severe enough to aggravate, if not cause, suicidal ideation. You do not want to take a couple years to figure out this potential sleep issue.

If you are reading this book, we know you are concerned about mental health issues or suicidal ideation or both in yourself or a loved one. If necessary, you must push your healthcare providers to send you to the right type of physicians (for example, sleep doctor, neurologist, or psychiatrist) with experience in diagnosing and treating leg movement disorders. It just might save your life.

Two final tips. First, both Appendix A on troubleshooting PAP and Appendix B on organizing your sleep treatment program provide more information on the value and steps in treating RLS and PLMD. Second, just like SDB though not as frequently, new innovations are coming to market to treat leg movements. The two most promising areas at the moment include pneumatic compression devices and electrical stimulation units. Most of this technology remains developmental, but I am hopeful it would hit the marketplace soon.

Parasomnias and Other Things That Go Bump in the Night

Mental health patients and trauma survivors in general, as well as PTSD patients in particular, experience a lot of extra movements in their sleep beyond RLS and PLMD. The term parasomnia covers this area and includes various conditions, each described under a subhead. Keep in mind two things about these disorders. First, nearly all are linked to assorted controversies, conundrums, or highly unusual physiological or neurological findings; thus, in every instance, your best strategy is to meet with an expert in the appropriate field such as a neurologist, psychiatrist, sleep specialist, or dentist. Second, and no surprise, if diagnosed with one of these conditions as well as OSA/UARS, you do not want to slack off in treating the sleep breathing problem as failing to treat usually aggravates the parasomnia.

Sleep Terrors

Sleep terrors used to be called night terrors, but as things don't spread far or wide from the field of sleep medicine, many healthcare professionals still speak of night terrors. This condition is not nearly as common as nightmares, yet many patients and providers confuse the two behaviors. The sleep terror looks and sounds a bit like a bad dream, but that's it for similarity. A sleep terror occurs from deep NREM sleep, whereas a nightmare occurs in all stages of sleep, though mostly in REM. When you wake from a nightmare, you know you had a bad dream and recall disturbing dream content.

During a sleep terror, you may not actually awaken to consciousness even though someone in the same bed or bedroom may perceive you as awake or crying out or screaming, or all the above. Very few sleep terror patients remember anything about the content of what they were thinking during the episode, and fewer still remember having the episode, that is they have no memory of waking up, crying out, or screaming. Last, because sleep terrors occur in deeper sleep, they mostly occur in the first third of the night when you generate delta sleep, whereas nightmares are more common in the final third of the night when you generate more REM.

Sleep terrors represent a kind of baseline for parasomnia conditions as all the other conditions described below share features with this phenomenon, in particular, the propensity to be moving or thrashing in your sleep without any memory of doing so.

Another relevant feature is the OSA/UARS connection. Some years ago, Dr. Guilleminault, the great sleep researcher and clinician who discovered UARS, wrote a few articles about parasomnias where he noted most cases were linked to sleep breathing problems and emphasized a huge proportion of cases resolved once the individual was successfully treated with PAP.[141;142] At our sleep center during a 20-year span, we helped several thousand patients with parasomnia complaints, and greater than 95% needed no further treatments for their nocturnal episodes once successfully using PAP therapy.

Those with sleep terrors, sleepwalking, and sleep-talking symptoms showed the greatest success following PAP use. Even patients with the more complex conditions listed below also responded well, including a surprisingly high proportion of trauma survivors with PTSD. Remarkably, in large numbers, the diagnoses were then changed as the PAP treatment completely eliminated the condition, which means the OSA/UARS was the real and invisible disorder causing the parasomnia. And, among those with persisting parasomnias, PAP provided clear-cut improvements in sleep quality, so patients continued their treatments for OSA/UARS along with other treatments for parasomnias.

Of course, some sleep terrors require their own treatment usually comprising one to three components: a medication; psychotherapy; and, attempts to regularize the sleep schedule. Psychotropic medications like antidepressants and antianxiety drugs may prove effective simply by decreasing the amount of deep sleep. Psychotherapy has been mentioned on the theory the episodes reflect unprocessed emotional distress, notably, anxiety or anger;[141-144] however, very little has ever been researched or written about this approach. Sleep schedules are important for these patients as a means to ensure adequate sleep, given sleep deprivation shows greater risk for sleep terrors. All three elements, however, carry their own caveats. Psychotropic meds may cause or aggravate sleep terrors, psychotherapy may take far too long to achieve clear-cut benefits, and creating a normal sleep routine often proves difficult for any sleep patient suffering complex sleep disorders.

REM Behavior Disorder (RBD)

RBD literally means acting out your dreams while dreaming in REM. As you recall, you are paralyzed in REM, so you shouldn't be acting out anything. Due to damage in a specific area of the brain, your paralysis goes away, and now muscles move too much during a dream. This condition is dangerous and leads to serious injuries to self or others in the same bed. In the discovery of RBD during the mid-1980s, we learned about individuals who had taken to tying themselves with rope to their bedposts to prevent injury while sleeping.[145] The good news about treatment of RBD is its outstanding response to the drug Clonazepam at low dosages (0.25 mg to 2.0 mg).

Beyond this simple formulation of RBD reside many more complicating factors that affect both attempts to diagnose and properly treat it. The first and very large concern about RBD in mental health patients is the likelihood of a medication side effect (typically antidepressants) or a disorder like PTSD causing the condition. The most compelling information to date is that the largest majority of mental health patients acting out their dreams are suffering from treatable OSA/UARS. Once treated, the behavior vanishes, so technically these individuals are no longer diagnosed with RBD. The good news on medication side effects is removal of medications in most cases also leads to no further symptoms, albeit one emerging theory asks whether the antidepressant is actually unmasking an RBD condition that would typically show up years later?[146] Things continue to get more complicated regarding three overlapping conditions known as posttraumatic nightmares, traumatic brain injury (TBI), and PTSD because each of them individually may signal a possible co-occurring RBD diagnosis.

In a nutshell, if you treat one of these three conditions and RBD disappears, then you never had RBD. But there's still another caveat: it is critically important to confirm no residual RBD due to its links to neurodegenerative diseases. RBD was originally discovered in middle-aged to older men who suffered from poorly controlled hypertension. Over time, RBD seemed to arise following a series of previously unrecognized mini-strokes inside the brain, after which the resulting damage led to acting out dream behavior. When these patients received follow-up 10 to 20 years later, far worse brain degeneration had developed since the original RBD diagnosis.[147] These neurodegenerative diseases are currently untreatable and eventually lead to extreme deteriorations in functioning and eventual death. Radiological scans of the brain are increasingly used in RBD patients to determine the type and progression of potential neurodegenerative diseases.

Overall, some patients suffer from RBD as well as one or more of the three conditions listed above (posttraumatic nightmares, TBI, and PTSD). These individuals experience a much more difficult treatment course that must include multimodal therapy, which in commonsense language means trying every conceivable intervention with at least partial evidence to support its use. In the military there are entire centers of excellence faced with such cases, and these individuals could be receiving as many as five to 10 therapies, including multiple medications, multiple psychotherapies, physical therapy, occupational therapy, yoga, acupuncture, massage, exercise regimens, and then all the appropriate sleep treatments, including PAP, medications for RLS/PLMD, insomnia therapies, nightmare therapies, and bright light or melatonin for circadian rhythm abnormalities.

Trauma-Associated Sleep Disorder (TASD)

TASD is a newly defined disorder overlapping with many parasomnias.[148] It includes disruptive nocturnal behaviors like sleep terrors, acting out dreams like RBD, nightmares with specific content related to past traumatic events, and specific and pronounced hyperarousal symptoms like sweating, fast heart rate, and rapid respiratory rate. Thus, TASD overlaps with patients who suffer from PTSD or TBI. As research data are sparse on TASD, it's possible the condition may turn out to be its own independent condition or perhaps a variant of PTSD or RBD. Of clinical sleep interest, the TASD patients also suffer very high rates of OSA.

Treatment research on TASD is sparse as well, but some patients have responded to combination therapies included the IRT method for nightmares (Chapter 16), PAP for OSA, and the drug prazosin for hyperarousal symptoms.

Nocturnal Eating Disorders

Sleep-related eating disorder (SRED) means you are eating while sleeping, but you still may experience various levels of awareness. The condition parallels aspects of sleepwalking as it occurs in NREM sleep and is triggered by co-occurring sleep disorders like OSA, PLMD, and other parasomnias. It also has been linked to sedative hypnotics, such as Ambien. SRED causes obesity in patients, which may be related to a desire for high caloric foods eaten during the episodes. Another disorder is known as night eating syndrome (NES), which occurs while you are awake and refers to a noticeable increase in appetite and ingestion of food late at night. The mainstay of treatment for these conditions is to aggressively treat underlying sleep disorders combined with pertinent pharmacotherapy and behavioral interventions as would be used with any eating disorder patients.

Traumatic Brain Injury (TBI)

A large and growing interest in TBI research will lead to promising interventions. One point to offer, because it seems routinely missed in those researching and treating TBI, is the higher prevalence of OSA/UARS as well as a greater than expected rate of CSA.[149] Damage to the brain appears to directly impact the respiratory drive centers, which is thought to explain the high incidence of CSA in these patients. So, if TBI is in your background or a loved one's, you want to seek a full-night sleep laboratory evaluation as the best procedure to test for CSA. If diagnosed with CSA, it is likely ASV therapy will provide the optimal treatment option.

Sleep Bruxism

Clenching or grinding your teeth while sleeping is very common and requires the use of dental guards bought at drug stores or manufactured by dentists and dental labs. These devices are not the same as OAT for sleep apnea, but if you use an OAT for OSA/UARS then it usually works as a dental guard too. The most interesting research finding on bruxism is its commonality in patients with sleep-disordered breathing. Of considerable research interest, it has been proven individuals must arouse or awaken first, and then they clench or grind. The question arises as to what is triggering these arousals? Could it be sleep respiratory events, leg movements, or some other arousal stimuli? No evidence currently demonstrates bruxism resolves by treating OSA/UARS, but it is clear whatever the cause of bruxism, the associated arousal activity is sufficient to disrupt sleep and produce daytime symptoms. Therefore, seeking evaluation with a dentist or a sleep center is advisable.

Sleep Seizure Disorders

Finally, a note here on the parasomnias—including seizure movements—caused by specific and irregular brain waves usually generated at specific sites in the brain. A host of these nocturnal seizure movement disorders range from the very benign to serious and harmful. Even a partial discussion of these more involved EEG patterns is beyond the scope of this book, but they are worth mentioning because some parasomnias require neurologic evaluations. While a fair number of sleep medicine specialists are also neurologists, most sleep doctors originate from internal medicine and pulmonary medicine. Therefore, if your parasomnias seem to be poorly understood, diagnosed, or treated, it could prove valuable to find a new sleep doctor with a background in neurology or a neurologist who specializes in parasomnias.

Closing Words

We would never want you to underestimate the impact of parasomnias or leg movement disorders on your sleep quality, and whenever you sense your treatment response is subpar or mediocre, it is very reasonable to ask yourself whether another condition is in play. Priority number one is often RLS/PLMD, and priority number two is another parasomnia. In a nutshell, if you toss and turn at night, and if this thrashing about fails to recede after treatment of OSA/UARS, then finding the cause of the tossing and turning could truly optimize your response, giving you a much higher sleep quality.

Sleep Research Pearl #9

Esmeralda participated in and gained much benefit from our research study on nasal dilator strips to treat insomnia when she was 65 years old and freshly retired from an occupational health specialist career at a major defense laboratory in New Mexico. A couple years later, she decided to look into PAP therapy because she developed morning headaches, as well as suffering migraines for years. Despite gaining relief from all her headaches with ABPAP, including the migraines, it took until age 71 and the repeated manifestation of leg jerks on her sleep studies before she chose to treat them.

Starting on Mirapex, she gained so much improvement she believed her sleep was noticeably better than with ABPAP alone. In a few months, augmentation triggered a round of upping the Mirapex dosage, which made her sleep worse, along with new RLS symptoms in the morning. We saw her in clinic and discussed the augmentation and the necessity to switch to another drug. We offered Neurontin, which was a nonstarter as she once used it unsuccessfully for headaches and developed a rash and stomach problems. That left opiates, as she had no interest in other GABA derivatives, and she understood another dopamine drug might rekindle the augmentation.

All these events occurred around the same time as the burgeoning opiate crisis was gaining coverage in the news media and in relevant medical practices. Esmeralda's husband was a family medicine physician and nearly blew a gasket when I recommended low-dose oxycodone. One consequence of the opiate epidemic caused many physicians to cower in their prescribing patterns, fearful of giving opiates to virtually any patient. I was fortunate to have trained in sleep medicine in the 1990s, and with my research background I had previously combed the literature and recognized opiates were the most tested and proven treatment for RLS/PLMD.[150] Being evidence-based, I had been prescribing codeine, oxycodone, and hydrocodone for years. Ever since 2010 onward, however, I needed to engage in many personal phone calls with other doctors and patients' spouses to explain why an opiate was an excellent therapy option. Oxycodone proved the most effective in my practice.

When the dialogue settled down into rational discourse, a low dosage of oxycodone was prescribed, starting at 5 mg pills to be broken in half or quarters and taken at bedtime. Esmeralda obtained fantastic relief on 2.5 mg and sometimes went as low as 1.25 mg of oxycodone. Several years later she discovered she could use low-dose Requip (one 0.25 mg pill) to provide additional relief for RLS without augmentation while continuing low-dose opiates.

Unfortunately, opiates get a bad rap regarding RLS/PLMD simply as a carryover effect from all the publicity surrounding opiate addiction, opiate deaths, and the ensuing opiate crisis. Nevertheless, using a personally tailored approach to medicine, opiates were the right choice for this patient, as they are for many with persistent symptoms. With hostile media coverage coupled with healthcare systems that now demand obedience to rules instead of encouragement to actually "follow science," sadly, many RLS/PLMD patients may never be offered the opportunity for low-dose opiates.

CHAPTER 10

Erasing Racing Thoughts the Natural Way

*How do advanced self-help mental skills conquer
insomnia and nightmares?*

The Proper Framework

Physical or physiological sleep disorders are the initial targets, because treating sleep breathing and sleep movement disorders leads to marked improvements in overall sleep quality. Enhanced sleep quality decreases insomnia and nightmares in many patients. Nonetheless, when repairing broken sleep in mental health patients, you must pay equal attention to the psychological aspects of sleep disorders.

Unfortunately, psychiatrists, psychologists, and other therapists often start off on the wrong foot by describing insomnia and nightmares as secondary symptoms of a primary mental health disorder without realizing nightmares and insomnia each operate as **independent sleep disorders.** Although the specific evaluation and treatment plan for your sleep disorders should include the physical side of restoring normal levels of REM and delta sleep as well as sleep consolidation, psychologically driven sleep therapies must also be considered for insomnia and nightmares. These approaches are especially relevant when physical treatments do not yield great results or if you defer physiological treatments.

Few healthcare professionals of every type elaborate on the co-occurrence of physical and mental components of sleep disorders. Most often, a mental health provider told you to address the mental problem (for example, PTSD, anxiety, or depression) and, supposedly, your sleep problems would vanish. Or your primary physician prescribed a medication that failed to cure any sleep problems or only partially treated them. In other words, insomnia or nightmares were minimized, and you never received encouragement to seek independent treatments for these sleep disorders.

The extraordinarily high failure rate using conventional strategies to treat sleep disorders (standard psychological or drug therapies) is compounded by literally millions of mental health providers who ignore effective, evidence-based, and direct treatments developed or utilized by sleep specialists for nightmares and insomnia.

These sleep psychological therapies have been researched and published in the scientific literature for more than three decades, and in this chapter and the ensuing five chapters, you will learn these "new" techniques to take control of insomnia and nightmares.

You have learned specific therapies target specific disorders like sleep apnea or leg jerks. This same point is true for nightmares and insomnia. These treatments are drug free, yet only take a few days or weeks to learn. Soon enough, you will be taking steps on your own and gaining superior results with surprisingly little effort. Here, truly, is an opportunity to take control of your own sleep problems.

For those already initiating treatment with PAP for OSA/UARS or medications/supplements for RLS/PLMD, all that follows remains applicable and may yield additional improvements in insomnia symptoms or disturbing dreams. Working on these mentally oriented treatments can also offer a break from PAP in particular and lets you alternate therapies. This alternation is highly advantageous for individuals who need to go slower with PAP adaptation.

Starting with Insomnia or Nightmares

Of the two conditions—insomnia and nightmares—mental health patients in general, and PTSD, anxiety, and depressed patients in particular, report insomnia as the most common sleep problem. By *insomnia*, we mean difficulty falling asleep or staying asleep. Perhaps, nightmare problems feel more intense, produce more distress, and worsen insomnia. Nonetheless, you must decide whether to treat one condition and then the other or to treat both simultaneously. In this format, we'll start with insomnia. And you will discover these two sleep disorders are closely related, so some steps for insomnia prove useful in treating nightmares.

TFI System (Thoughts, Feelings, Images)

We begin with a simple template depicting how the human mind operates, which offers a useful working theory on how and why insomnia and nightmares persist for so long. The model is called the *TFI system*,[15] standing for:

- T = thoughts
- F = feelings
- I = images or imagery (pictures) from your imagination

Thoughts and feelings are familiar terms, whereas imagery refers to the pictures illuminating your mind's eye. When somebody asks for directions to a location, you often see the streets or landmarks in your mind's eye, spontaneously creating a mental road map. Then you describe the roadmap to someone seeking directions.

This mental faculty is a highly advanced, precision instrument without which you would be at a great loss for operating in the real world, not to mention how sad you would feel in a world without daydreams and other satisfying mental images. Unfortunately, use of mental imagery appears to be a lost art frequently overlooked by healthcare professionals. Our goal is to reinvigorate your imagery skill as it possesses vast potential for enhancing mental health and sleep.

Thinking is something we do all the time, and sometimes the self-talk can be annoying, unpleasant, anxiety producing, and more. Your thinking can be focused or scattered; no matter, you are often aware of some thoughts. In contrast, feelings are a different story. People who suffer from nightmares or insomnia may intentionally or otherwise restrict awareness of feelings as well as limit the pictures in their mind's eye. These restrictions and limitations are typically attempted during *daytime or waking hours*.

Feelings represent a full range of sensations in your body, including pain and pleasure. But the feelings most relevant to nightmares and insomnia are the ones we call "emotions" because these feelings greatly influence your sleep. Very specific feelings to be discussed at length in the ensuing chapters often prove singularly relevant to insomniacs.

Two other very precise feelings are also relevant to treat your sleep problems. The first is "sleepiness or drowsiness," the sensation you feel when you are about to fall asleep or doze off in various circumstances. The second is "tiredness or fatigue," a sensation in your body more so than in your mind, when you feel low energy and would prefer to rest or relax instead of carrying on.

Take special note: tiredness and fatigue are not the preamble to falling asleep or dozing off. Before you fell asleep, you were feeling drowsy or sleepy. As you recall from our earlier discussion on sleepiness versus tiredness in sleep breathing problems, mental health patients often confuse these sensations and imagine they are one and the same. In learning to treat insomnia and nightmares, you will not only develop skills to recognize and experience the difference between sleepiness and tiredness, but this new insight will also prove therapeutic to your overall efforts.

TFI System and Insomnia

The TFI system is a potent way to observe the workings of your own mind, which is essential for insomniacs because they invariably report being unable to turn off their minds at bedtime. You probably call this problem racing thoughts, ruminations, worries, or feeling stressed. Nearly all insomniacs complain of this problem when they try to fall asleep at night or when they wake up in the middle of the night and cannot return to sleep. In both situations, the insomniac is suffering from an absence of sleepiness, and without sleepiness it is virtually impossible to fall asleep.

A common refrain is "If I could just turn off my mind at bedtime or the middle of the night, I'm sure I could fall or go back to sleep." This declaration is absolutely correct because it defines the problem yet begs for a not so obvious solution. For one, you cannot snap your fingers to make sleepiness wash away the racing thoughts.

By scrutinizing your own TFI system of thoughts, feelings, and imagery, the concept of thinking too much will be seen in a new light. Although it should be obvious thinking too much or sensing your mind racing along "out of control" disrupts your ability to fall asleep at bedtime or in the middle of the night, has any therapist or physician ever explained to you why you have racing thoughts?

Categorically, racing thoughts are not random or an accident or some genetic trait in most insomniacs. Clear and substantive reasons explain how or why you learned to use your mind in this way. Here's a big clue: if you look at what you are *not using* inside your own mind, you will find the main reasons your mental landscape is too "wordy." That is, instead of looking at what you are doing with your mind (racing thoughts, self-talk), we need to ask what are you *not doing*?

Of the three parts to TFI System, thinking too much readily stands out. Now, what about feelings and the pictures in your mind's eye? Are they hiding, suppressed, perhaps ignored?

Indeed, you have just learned the primary reason for your racing thoughts: **you have learned to think in order to avoid spending time with emotions and the images in your mind's eye**.

Said differently, the problem of racing thoughts does not fully explain your sleepless nights. Racing thoughts turn out to be the signal or marker of the problem. The real issue is your conscious or unconscious need to push away troubling emotions or problematic memories. But this effort fails miserably as racing thoughts emerge more or less as a replacement for the emotions and images you are trying to avoid.

If no one has ever explained this process to you, then you would naturally try to solve the problem of racing thoughts, say, by taking a pill. As you will learn, if you work just a little, and truly we mean just a little bit, on your feelings and the pictures in your mind, you will see the racing thoughts diminish, after which you will experience an easier time falling asleep.

It is crucial for the insomnia patient to learn how this lack of balance (excess thoughts, shortage of feelings or images) operates to cause insomnia.

To summarize, too much thinking means you are uncomfortable or unable or unwilling to spend more time in the realm of emotion or imagination. And the more one fears one's emotions or imagination, the more racing thoughts rule the night.

What you need to hear right now is that a natural human mind seeks to operate with a relative degree of equal time spent on thoughts, feelings, and images. Your mind was not designed to spend nearly all its time thinking by self-talking incessantly. The mind possesses a much richer capacity to operate in different realms simultaneously.

When you were young, you were blessed with the inclination to pay more attention to your feelings and the pictures in your mind's eye. As you grow older (and lose some of this innate wisdom) the tendency is to rely too much on the realm of thinking. Regaining natural access to your imagination and expanding your capacity to experience feelings often leads to an outright cure for insomnia. And this cure is powerful, because once you retrain your mind to regain balance you can usually reproduce this balance more than 95% of the time to overcome your struggle to fall asleep.

Letting the TFI System Rock You to Sleep the Natural Way

The TFI system naturally ramps up your capacity to solve insomnia because this system mirrors the actual way your mind falls asleep. When you get into bed, one of the first things to notice about the workings of the mind is a quick flurry of thoughts. These thoughts may arise because you are no longer engaging in your regular routine; you are not sitting or standing, and things are quiet around you. As a result, you might find yourself noticing more activity in your mind.

At this point, a normal sleeper finds it easy to let go of these thoughts and watch them drift into nothing in particular. This soon-to-be-fast asleep sleeper notices a degree of comfort in bed. It may be the pleasant feeling of lying down in bed or the temperature of the pillowcases or the softness or firmness of the mattress. One of the most important feelings sensed by the normal sleeper is the feeling of emotional closure, that is, whatever troubling thoughts or feelings that might arise from the day's activities, there is a strong sense this **day is done,** and tomorrow will provide plenty of opportunity to deal with life's fastballs, curve balls, and the occasional screwball.

In bed, we started with thoughts, moved to feelings, and now we finish with images in your mind's eye. Often, the very last thing occurring right before you fall asleep is the emergence of "dreamlets" in your mind's eye.[151;152] Among people who "watch" themselves fall asleep, most describe these little images or dreamlets arising in their mind's eye in the act of falling asleep.

Thus, the TFI system sequence of three letters (TFI) is no coincidence. TFI tends to be the order in which you naturally fall asleep. Clearly, at any step of the way, something can interfere with your thoughts (to make them too active), your feelings (to make you too aroused), or your imagery system (bringing unpleasant memories or provoking anxieties about what you might dream about).

There are many ways to work each part of the TFI system to improve your chances of eradicating insomnia or nightmares. As it is so common for nearly all insomnia patients to spend too much time thinking, we start in reverse order by explaining how to use the imagery system to rapidly solve insomnia, then move to the feeling component, an equally powerful approach to solving the problem, and finally, we move back to the thinking arena where some additional tools are available. These three elements will be explained in the next five chapters, and in each chapter, you will be trained to use specific and straightforward tools to put your sleep problems to bed.

Sleep Research Pearl #10

The *TFI system* was first introduced in my book *Sound Sleep, Sound Mind,* published in 2007. Leading up to the book's publication were nearly two decades of research and clinical work, reaching a pinnacle in our landmark study on the treatment of disaster survivors following the 2000 Cerro Grande

Fire on the perimeter of Los Alamos, New Mexico. At the time, we were formulating the program *Sleep Dynamic Therapy,* which is described in the *Sound Sleep, Sound Mind* book.[15] Moreover, we published the seminal paper on *Sleep Dynamic Therapy* in 2002 in the *Journal of Clinical Psychiatry* to spell out the necessity for a mind–body approach for the diagnosis and treatment of sleep disorders in PTSD patients and other trauma survivors.[23]

At the turn of the twenty-first century, most sleep and mental health professionals remained stuck in their silos, holding fast to the idea of focusing on their separate areas of expertise to treat PTSD patients. Our model, which was conceptualized and actively applied throughout the 1990s, described the essential requirement to aggressively treat sleep disorders as primary independent disorders co-occurring with mental illness.

This new model counters the prevailing wisdom (still current) that unapologetically declares sleep symptoms are secondary features of psychiatric disorders, and therefore the focus must remain on mental health treatment. Now, 20 years later, this inappropriate fixation remains the common practice among most mental health professionals, and, regrettably, many sleep professionals seem highly reluctant to involve themselves and their sleep centers in formal treatment of psychiatric patients with co-occurring sleep disorders.

We hoped the publication of our earlier works would have jumped over these hurdles, but we see there is still a long way to go. We trust *Life Saving Sleep* will continue the process of opening the eyes of those who seem unable to imagine the intricate, complex, and pivotal role of sleep disorders in mental health.

CHAPTER 11

Imagining Insomnia Out of the Picture

Is your mind's eye more powerful than a sleeping pill?

Imagine Falling Asleep

How easy is it to apply imagery steps to help you fall asleep at bedtime? Remarkably easy—so easy, you merely need to close your eyes and let the flow of images commence. But a problem arises here if you are reluctant to tap into your imagery system or if you experience difficulty doing so.

For these two reasons, we start imagery training with simple steps, and you are likely to appreciate almost immediately your imagery system is working well and safely. In a comfortable place (definitely not while driving a car or slicing tomatoes), sit in a relaxed position, close your eyes, and imagine your response to this question: "Please tell me how to drive or walk from your home to your favorite local restaurant." Okay, put down the book and watch what happens in your mind's eye when you reflect on this question.

Due to the global pandemic, you may not have been to this restaurant recently, so another scenario could be "Picture yourself walking in your own neighborhood on familiar streets and sidewalks."

Just spend a minute or two on this exercise.

Surprisingly or not, most people, including a large majority of very severe PTSD patients, show no difficulty with this form of imagery work.

Why are these results so predictable? These directions or walking paths are probably something you have repeated often. You have traveled the route or paths many times. In terms of imagery needed to reach this destination or follow the path, such as recalling the right landmarks, sidewalks, stoplights, street signs, potholes, curbsides, left and right turns, and so on, the whole thing is essentially over-memorized.

In picturing this journey, hopefully it's a safe trip, with no surprises and no worries about other images creeping into your mind's eye to distract or disturb you. Above all, virtually everyone notices they can and do see recognizable landmarks on this brief trip, because it is so familiar and accessible.

Compare this regularly traversed drive or neighborhood walk with any attempt to imagine a brand-new destination. Say you wish to travel to a beach or a meadow or a mountain you have not visited previously; or, suppose something traumatic occurred while at a location that shares similar features to a beach, meadow, or mountain. When you attempt to image your new destination, two problems arise. First, the lack of familiarity of the location yields vague imagery, or second, overt anxiety arises if these scenarios trigger other unpleasant scenes from past memories.

This anxiety erupts from the fear of flashbacks, daymares, or traumatic memories entering into and overwhelming the mind's eye, causing substantial emotional pain and bodily distress. When you initially practice imagery, we never want this problem to emerge, as you would then develop reluctance about trying imagery again.

We usually do not need to address this problem here because most people with even the smallest degree of imagery skill can use the mind's eye to fall asleep without these issues arising. Regardless, near the end of this chapter we'll help those individuals who are exceptions to the rule, that is, who experience unpleasant images during simple imagery steps. Also, as explained in Chapter 16, such individuals may need to work with a therapist to apply an exposure therapy technique before treating chronic nightmares. As you read on, you can determine the best approach for starting with imagery exercises, now or later.

Imagine That!

To fall asleep, you need to practice or rehearse a series of images with which you are very comfortable or simply respond to with limited reactions. When I first learned this technique 57 years ago, I pictured the furniture in my bedroom as soon as my head hit the pillow. Later, just for the sheer fun of it, I would revisit my most recent round of golf and would never make it past the fourth hole before nodding off. While the amount of variation in this exercise is limitless, the key is to avoid things too new or overstimulating. As I usually played golf at only one or two public courses, the terrain was well known to my visual system. If you regularly walk or hike a certain route, picturing the path or trail will ease you into this exercise. Whatever you select, your goal is to let yourself drift into your mind's eye. By spending time picturing things, you are literally slowing down the racing thoughts at bedtime.

Just to be clear, you could picture yourself cooking dinner, washing your car, viewing art or photos in a real or imaginary art gallery or album, painting a wall, gardening, drawing, or watching clouds drift across the sky. Again, choices are limitless, though pictures of your tax returns or anything else you find unpleasant are best ignored.

The imagery approach is your sure-fire step to triggering dreamlets that lead to the Land of Nod. Importantly, just because the technique capitalizes on your natural and innate capacity to see things in your mind's eye, do not imagine for a moment the technique is a weak tool. Imagery at bedtime for many insomniacs often proves more powerful than the most highly touted sleeping pills currently advertised on television or the Internet or in magazines as the latest and greatest cure for insomnia. In fact, it is rare for sleeping pills to produce a full cure for insomnia, whereas imagery may achieve this goal in short order.

Another potent feature of imagery is its impact on middle-of-the-night insomnia. Instead of popping another pill or drinking another beer, once you awaken and experience difficulty returning to sleep, how about letting a few images pop into your mind's eye? At 3 a.m. a few images can lead to a few dreamlets, and the next thing you know, the racing thoughts recede and the drowsiness returns.

Sleep is not somewhere far off on the horizon. Sleep is lying in bed right next to you, quietly waiting for you to melt into that glorious feeling of sleepiness and then sleep. Reminder—do not be surprised when imagery works so fast you do not even remember the sleepy feelings that emerged before you dozed off.

Wake on It

Some immediately access imagery at bedtime, whereas a more cautious approach requires daytime practice for certain mental health patients and trauma survivors. If the nighttime feels more vulnerable, daytime might offer greater safety and security. For example, sitting in front of your computer screen or taking a break from work or home routines, you only need to close your eyes and picture something pleasant for a few minutes. To start, you could practice just 10 or 15 seconds, but later, as you grow more comfortable with imagery, you can practice 10 to 15 minutes if you desire. After all, there are some insomniacs and nightmare sufferers whose imagery system is constrained, and they need more time to ramp up the flow of images.

Developing daytime imagery skills generates confidence in your efforts in using the mind's eye at bedtime. Let's do another exercise so you can embrace the simplicity of this refined and potent tool within your own mental capacity during waking hours.

As you sit quietly, look around your room or space and notice things. Let your eye wander over and under and around things. If you see a bookcase or shelves with assorted items, trace the outlines of the objects, see the various shades and colors, and, above all, notice how your mind might insist on continuing its self-talk even about these items. The very act of looking is a great way to prepare yourself for closing your eyes and conducting mental imagery.

This particular exercise can be repeated virtually any time. You simply look at things, then close your eyes and notice how easily you can generate images of what you had been looking at. I just looked up at a painting on the wall behind my computer screen. It's a sailboat in the ocean running parallel to a sandy promontory with a lighthouse in the background. I close then open then close my eyes again and see the difference between the blue water and sandy beach, wind billowing the sails outward toward me, and the lighthouse looking solid, white, and ready. This type of exercise a few times per day is a great "twofer." Not only does it build your confidence in gaining rapid access to your mind's eye, but also just 30 to 60 seconds spent in this mental space frequently relaxes you.

Another way to hone this skill is by looking at something that inspires you. Some will use a coffee table picture book of great architecture, landscapes, or artwork, turning through the pages and then closing the eyes to see what images can be recalled. One of the most natural scenarios is gazing at a sunset. Notice how sunset images are so beautiful and stimulating; you often feel awe or aesthetic pleasure in the mind and body.

Do not be surprised, though, when the self-chattering component of your mind insinuates itself into your viewing pleasure as the sun sinks in the west. Some self-talk may integrate well with the scene at hand: you make note of a new shade of orange or clouds drifting by or the dramatic change in light as the final ribbon of sunshine dissolves. Compare these self-talk remarks to a situation where watching a delightful sunset is coupled with thinking about how much is left in your health savings account, not forgetting to stop for milk and eggs, and the necessity of taking in your car for an oil change.

Why does the human mind work this way? Why are there so many different types of chatter in which we can engage—and some for no apparent reason? Can we gain more control over this chatter? In general, once you learn the link between how you feel and what you think, far greater control of self-talk is possible. When we pick up our discussion of emotions in the next chapter, you'll be able to learn, see, and test this theory, which proposes that we think about what we are feeling much more than we realize.

Practicing Imagery Could and Should Be Fun

Now back to the sunset or just your friendly home or work space. Our goal is not to completely eliminate the self-talk, because that's nearly impossible, but it is worth your time to do two things going forward. To reiterate, practice looking around at your environment every day a few times a day; just notice lots of things, and as you do so, notice whether the self-talk you engage in is of a type that's related to the thing you are looking at or the type that seems more random or chaotic, even pressured. Second, initiate eyes-closed mental imagery practices twice a day or more for very short periods, almost always less than 60 or 30 seconds—even 15 or just 10 seconds is fine. For this latter exercise, again pick familiar things: the furniture in the room; actual photographs or images of loved ones; a favorite painting, poster, or magazine cover; or, if feeling ambitious, go for big things like your last or best vacation spot and relive your favorite landscapes or scenery from this trip.

Finally, can you recall a lazy time when you were sitting somewhere doing nothing and just looking at stuff in front of you? At some point it almost feels like you are in a daze; you are not really thinking about anything obvious or particularly important, and your eyes are going in and out of focus on the objects in front of you. In this setting, you are defaulting to a system that lets your visual capacity nearly ignore your self-talk activity. When you achieve this sort of "just looking at nothing and everything" sensation, you'll realize you can achieve a similar sensation with your eyes shut when you practice mental imagery. By recognizing your natural visual skills with your eyes open, it yields confidence in producing similar results with your eyes closed.

Bedding Down with Imagery

Once you achieve a reasonable comfort level with imagery, which for most people requires a few days to a few weeks, you can use all your practice material at bedtime. Whatever the nature of your bedtime ritual, such as saying prayers or noting next-day reminders, literally within seconds of your head hitting the pillow you want to initiate imagery in the mind's eye. Of course, you can wait to feel more settled if you need more time adjusting pillows, assuming the most comfortable position, or confirming the temperature feels right, but immediately after doing so, initiate the imagery sequence.

Remember, an imagery session does not need your mind to be consumed only with images. Thoughts and feelings still emerge because the TFI system within your mind and body naturally generates all elements; however, unlike in the past where excess thinking was the norm, you want to create a new, more balanced system by linking your initial bedtime routine to imagery scenes.

In sum, you are not trying to stop yourself from thinking or feeling;

instead, you are infusing the almost magical element of imagery into your consciousness because doing so creates a strong potential to accomplish two relevant goals.

First, if you enjoy your imagery, it literally takes up space in your mind that would ordinarily be used to ruminate or worry with self-talk. Thus, consistent use of imagery at bedtime will decrease racing thoughts. Second, imagery will lead you toward those special dreamlets, technically known as *hypnagogic imagery*, that appear to be the very last thing you notice before falling asleep.

Plus, another somewhat artistic bonus to imagery occurs with a substantial number of individuals. As you are falling asleep, in addition to dreamlets, you may also see more abstract images, typically described as shapes, colors, geometric designs, and other unusual or not clearly definable components that shift or move or rapidly appear and disappear. An ordinary daytime practice of imagery usually does not go down this pathway, although abstract artists or similar personality types might describe such experiences.

These images may parallel experiences akin to "drug trips" where the shapes, colors, and designs seem to be highly random and often inexplicable. These images may be even closer to the state of sleep than dreamlets, so if you are fortunate enough to see such transcendent images, you are probably easily inclined to successfully use imagery to fall asleep, again with the possible exception of artists, who might find the imagery so stimulating it wakes them up.

There is one other caveat. In some individuals, distressing or disturbing images may burst forth from these abstractions. Mostly, this hypnagogic imagery is positive and pleasurable or neutral and boring, but for some individuals notably trauma survivors hypnagogic imagery leads to traumatic imagery that clearly blocks them from falling asleep, which brings us to our last section.

Dealing With Unpleasant Imagery

Unpleasant imagery is no small matter. In the context of PTSD, you might say imagery is everything, because it is the traumatic memories of awful events that can trigger a psychological cascade, essentially fixating the posttraumatic stress process into the mind and body.

Upon recall of a stressful life event, the mind and body jerk to full attention with a hyperarousal response, as would be expected when a highly charged memory instigates the "reliving" of the trauma. Once the hyperarousal is triggered, the mind and body seek to find solutions to avoid these triggers and prevent the onslaught of traumatic memories. The best example relates to our current effort to treat your insomnia. If you suffer from nightmares that relive traumatic events, why would you want to go to sleep? By avoiding sleep with your insomnia, you can theoretically prevent nightmares!

In fact, nightmares teach you not to go to sleep so you won't relive the traumatic events during the heightened vulnerability of dreaming.

In a nutshell, an entrenched PTSD cycle can start with a nightmare (a symptom called "reexperiencing"), which leads to a racing heart, sweating, and full awakening (a symptom called "arousal" or "hyperarousal"), and then over time the trauma survivor "learns" to not go to sleep to prevent the return of the nightmare (a symptom called "avoidance"). These symptom clusters (reexperiencing, hyperarousal, and avoidance) are one common way to define the PTSD process, and have been used to designate whether or not someone meets the diagnostic criteria for posttraumatic stress *disorder.*

You must determine whether your own imagery system is currently in a fragile state or whether you can proceed with the exercises detailed here. When imagery feels unpredictable, overwhelming, and ultimately out of control, then most likely we should assume posttraumatic stress symptoms or frank PTSD are in play, which means the above exercises should only be applied with the assistance of a skilled psychotherapist who is comfortable coaching you on imagery techniques.

When you find a therapist trained and experienced in the use of exposure type therapies, then the uncontrollable imagery from which you suffer can be worked through during a course of specific desensitization steps. With desensitization therapies, you learn to "expose" or recall past stressful events in a controlled and structured fashion; over time you learn to desensitize yourself from such memories. Exposure therapies are intimidating and certainly not easy, but in the hands of a trained professional these therapies are extremely potent and reliable and may lead to a complete cure of PTSD, albeit, to be sure, exposure therapies are not appropriate for all trauma survivors.

In Chapter 16 we will discuss treating nightmares using imagery techniques. As you will learn, the images in your mind's eye could be described as plastic or fluid in the sense they often are changing. For now, it's important for you to appreciate that as you develop more skill with the images in your mind's eye, you may notice you have the power to encourage, promote, or activate changes in the images that float across your visual landscape. In other words, there is a strong tendency for individuals who work with imagery to reach a stage where they can *acknowledge* the presence of an unpleasant image—even experience some bad feelings linked to the image—and then consciously *choose* to move to a new set of images to replace the distressing ones. I learned this concept from Dr. Joseph Neidhardt, and I must say at first it seemed far too simplistic. Nonetheless, if you practice it, you will see acknowledging and choosing is quite a powerful combo mental skill. You may want a therapist to coach you to gain confidence in this technique.

This control over your imagery system is possible, but it may require days, weeks, or months of practice for some to acquire this capacity and tap into it on a regular basis. The simple imagery steps described in this chapter are an excellent starting point for relearning what is actually a very natural skill you once regularly used in your early childhood, if not more recently.

Still, among those with more fragile imagery systems, keep in mind this fail-safe maneuver: **when suffering unpleasant imagery, *open your eyes*!** Some may need to use this step frequently in the early going, but hopefully over time you need to do so less and less. On the other hand, the more you find yourself needing to open your eyes, the more likely professional guidance is warranted, again most commonly a psychotherapist or a hypnotherapist skilled in imagery work.

Moving Forward with Imagery

To reiterate, although many individuals with posttraumatic stress symptoms suffer from unpleasant imagery, most of these disturbing images are not so regularly overwhelming as to make the individual feel completely out of control. Therefore, they can attempt brief mind's eye practices and eventually incorporate them into a bedtime routine. In going forward, we will make the assumption you have been using imagery during the daytime and at bedtime, or you have recognized the need to work with a trained professional in exposure therapy to help alleviate some or all of your uncontrollable images.

Now, to close this section on an uplifting note, I appreciate how imagery might seem incredibly simplistic and therefore not up to the task of treating insomnia. Yet, it is this very simplicity that marks the incredible powers within the human mind to solve exactly this sort of problem. At our sleep centers, we trained thousands of individuals in the use of imagery at bedtime, and virtually all these patients reported benefits from accessing their imagination in this tranquil manner when ready for sleep.

Moreover, as described in Chapter 7 in the *Pearl of All Pearls* section on imagery distraction, we have trained thousands of patients to perform imagery exercises to distract themselves from the pressurized air sensations of PAP or other sensations related to the mask or headgear in using PAP therapy. Creating beautiful scenery in the mind's eye, as one example of imagery distraction, has proven powerful in helping OSA/UARS patients overcome the newness or early discomforts with the PAP adaptation process.

As you continue reading, you will learn imagery is literally a multifunction tool you can employ on a daily and nightly basis to address many facets of your life's challenges.

Finally, at the end of Chapter 15 we'll return to imagery to offer another insomnia treatment that fits the category known as "cognitive-imagery" work. This technique blends thinking and imagery in a unique and unexpected way to combat insomnia. If for any reason you desire more steps in this realm now, please skip ahead to Chapter 15. As a cautionary note, Chapters 12 through 14 are the most intense portions of the book; some individuals require weeks or longer to digest and absorb the material on how emotional work can overcome insomnia. If you are not ready to pursue Chapters 12–14 just yet, Chapter 15 contains the next logical set of instructions to resolve persisting unwanted sleeplessness.

Sleep Research Pearl #11

Over the years, we have been astonished by the skepticism expressed by our patients, as well as by healthcare professionals, on the power of the human imagery system applied through the mind's eye.[153] At appointments, discussions, lectures, and workshops, an added dose of persuasion has been needed to convince people of the importance, value, and power of the imagery system. When confronted by this potential barrier, I almost always respond from the opposite perspective, requesting the person to "tell me what your life would be like without a mind's eye—go ahead, tell me, I'm listening."

This line of thinking proves invaluable when you reflect on the power or role of imagery in your daily life. As we learned from many of our early nightmare treatment patients, who applied the *imagery rehearsal therapy* described in Chapter 16, once individuals embrace imagery exercises, mind's eye imagery expands into other uses. Among those gaining benefits after decreasing nightmares, many started using imagery at bedtime to facilitate sleep onset. A few women applied daytime imagery to resolve difficult encounters with another person, the first such instance occurring in a woman who argued with her boss. She imagined a different type of conversation with him prior to their next encounter, and then was surprised by how easily the imaginative dialogue transferred over into the real encounter without any friction. Part of the change involved picturing different body language to arrive at the meeting with less tension.

What many of us may not realize or appreciate is how often imagery comes into play. Here's the simplest example of this phenomenon: you lose or misplace something in your house—keys, phone, hat, and so on. When on your way out the door, you can't find them. What do you do? Many will anxiously search everywhere in the home. Others begin by picturing where they had been inside the house before they start the search. And, finally, a smaller proportion searches each room in their mind's eye by picturing the activity they were doing in each room. If you had to guess which group finds the misplaced object fastest, you would be correct if you said the person who completes the detailed search first in the mind's eye.

Why would the mind's eye be so powerful and accurate? I believe the mind's eye is taking in a lot more data than you can actually think about in real time. I believe these numerous pictures of your activity, recent or otherwise, global or precise, are providing volumes of information you can choose to tap into as needed. And I would suggest you revisit the original question I would pose, "How exactly do you think you'd be operating in life without a mind's eye?"

Again, at a very simple level, and before we had GPS tools, how would you have traveled from one place to another? Only a map could guide you, and you would constantly be looking back and forth between the map lines and the road ahead displaying various signs. Moreover, if you needed to repeat a trip without the mind's eye, do you really think your thoughts could consistently tell you the names of the streets or where to turn? I'm doubtful. I believe it is the picture-memory that has solidified your capacity to drive over and over again to the same locale as needed.

Now, you could ask since your eyes are open, won't that permit memory of the trip? I would agree partially; yet, remember how often during a trip a person is actually reaching back into the mind's eye to recall some guidance, like "let's see, oh yeah, it's the second light after Bartholomew Street, and the huge car wash sign is on the left side of the road." You are not accomplishing the driving task only by looking ahead. Rather, before you get there, your mind's eye retrieved the old image because it knows the old image.

In day-to-day affairs, I encourage you to spend more time utilizing your mind's eye or paying attention to how your mind's eye operates. Most discover imagery is in play much more than they previously realized. Over time, I believe the dividends from the mind's eye will surprise you, especially when you learn how easy it is to bank on the human imagery system.

CHAPTER 12

SLEEP-RELATED EMOTION-FOCUSED THERAPY: GETTING YOUR FEET WET

How much emotional work can I attempt without a therapist?

Emotions Belong in the Foreground, Not the Background

Emotions are messengers that deliver "Emotional Intel" directly to your consciousness in order to serve and protect you. Despite this fact about emotional intelligence, more people are likely to view emotions as **messy**ngers because feelings and emotions frequently cause confusion and distress. Lamentably, some mental health providers view emotions as too messy for their patients and therefore may not challenge the individual to face his or her feelings.

As discussed above, exposure therapy—a form of emotion-focused therapy— is a powerful tool a mental health therapist can apply to help PTSD patients. Yet, many practitioners remain concerned about this style of therapy that desensitizes the patient's emotional reactions to traumatic events. The concern stems from the uncertainty and unpredictability involved in helping a patient manage the erupting emotions when reliving traumatic experiences. On balance, some research has postulated the "reliving" paradigm is not beneficial or even appropriate for certain trauma survivors if for no other reason than a fair number drop out before completing treatment.[154]

Another style of therapy in mental health offers patients the following instructions about emotions: "If you just learn to think about things differently, then your feelings would change too." Though this one sentence would likely be disputed as over-simplifying by some mental health professionals, it seems apparent to me as well as others that a fair proportion of therapists may discount and disrespect the intrinsic value of emotions and imply there is no need to work on emotions directly in therapy. Moreover, in having helped thousands of mental health patients at our sleep center, I am under the impression an astonishingly high proportion of mental health therapists are either inexperienced with or feel uncomfortable about aiding patients in addressing emotional turmoil at the core. This lack of emotional engagement leads to what is known disparagingly as "talking heads" encounters if and when this intellectualizing style limits the role of emotion.

Though "thinking influences feelings" is self-evident, the converse is true: "what you feel influences what you think." It is a distorted view of humanity to imagine feelings and emotions do not serve a valuable purpose. Moreover, it is inconceivable that working with emotions would provide only small benefit to your mental health.

Granted, it may be difficult to appreciate the role of emotions in mental health; yet it is a fact that learning to work with emotions in a forthright manner yields immediate gains by decreasing stress levels, reducing physical tension, and illuminating critical insights about the workings of your mind. Such techniques guide you down a unique pathway to understanding and conquering insomnia.

When an individual cannot digest an intense form of emotional work such as exposure therapy, there are newer approaches, known as *somatic therapies*,[155] derived from older techniques originally described as *bodywork*.[156] These somatic-oriented approaches deal with emotions by focusing on bodily sensations; for some, the experience is less daunting than the exposure form of therapy.

Emotions Always Win

An overwhelming majority of insomniacs—far greater than 90%—suffer from their inability to recognize, learn from, and process emotions during the daytime, which transforms this unprocessed energy into the very fuel that keeps them awake at night—racing thoughts. In short, unprocessed emotional energy arising from your waking hours gives birth to the great multitude of racing thoughts at bedtime. Here is the perfect example of "what we feel affects the way we think"—in this case, thinking too much or too fast! In this instance, we say, "emotions always win," meaning the feelings force the issue (racing thoughts) because the feelings never received the honest hearing they demanded.[15] Or, as my sagely friend and colleague Stephen Safer offers, "The mind repeats what the heart can't delete."

What is so maddening about this feeling-thinking connection is its near invisibility. Insomniacs frequently lose touch with this natural skill—otherwise known as healthy coping—to deal directly with emotions. Instead, as they go through the day unmindful of how to access and use emotions to their advantage, these feelings relentlessly transition into a great many worries and stressors. Thus, if one is not consciously monitoring these transitions, you only realize the outcome at the end of the day—racing thoughts or ruminations when you lie down to sleep, and alas, during bouts of sleeplessness throughout the night.

Without question, a huge proportion of insomniacs can cure insomnia if they learn to work directly with emotions during waking hours so no fuel is left to fan the flames of sleeplessness at bedtime. While this step seems like a tall order to those with mental health conditions, the good news is insomnia problems often respond to the most elementary emotional coping skills. Truly, just a spoonful of emotions may be all that's needed to make the medicine go down. And the great news is the medicine is drug free!

Basic Emotional Processing Steps

Technically, emotional processing comprises only three steps, which engage you to develop a capacity: (1) to **identify** (name) the actual feelings you experience; (2) to **feel** your feelings in your body and not just your mind as you go through your day; and, (3) to **process** or **work through** your emotions as best you can. This latter and most difficult step is termed **emotional processing**. However, to treat insomnia, you may only need to initially develop skills for steps one and two, identify and feel the feelings. Some individuals only need to identify their feelings to see substantial improvement in their insomnia.

Now, we're going to work on steps one and two (identify and feel) for the remainder of this chapter and a portion of Chapter 13. Then we'll zoom in on step three (emotional processing) in the remainder of Chapter 13 and dive even deeper for all of Chapter 14.

One Step at a Time: Identifying Feelings

You might think it straightforward to name what you feel, but in our culture emotions are frequently avoided, which leads to poor or simply inaccurate word choices in labeling them. This problem shows up consistently with the overuse of code words for emotions in daily communications. "Stress" is the ultimate and worst code word because "stress" reveals almost nothing about actual or precise emotions you are experiencing. When a person exclaims, "I'm stressed," a story is there that includes experiences involving very precise emotions. For insomniacs, the most commonly encountered precise emotions are frustration and anger. But if individuals limit vocabulary to "stress" terms, they do not drill down to the core or perhaps primary emotions of frustration or anger.

No volume of words written here will convey strongly enough how the wrong word degrades your ability to describe what you feel. Suffice to say, if you are unable or unwilling to accurately identify your feelings, you simply cannot apply emotional tools to rid yourself of insomnia, and you greatly increase your risk for depending on medication as the only "solution" to the problem. Words are powerful; using accurate words for what you feel gives you the power to know and work with your emotions. Using inaccurate terms dissolves your power.

If you find yourself uncomfortable giving up "stress" terms by replacing them with precise emotional terms, please consider a second reason "stress" is so problematic and, for that matter, why so many insomniacs are eager to use the phrase, "I'm stressed!"

If you pay attention to this phenomenon over the coming weeks, you will see it frequently serves as a "defense mechanism," which means a tool your mind activates when it does not want to be confronted by information predictably undesirable or unpleasant. Notice among your colleagues, peers, friends, and even loved ones how often the phrase "I'm stressed" is not voiced to initiate a healthy discussion about a recent dilemma or conflict; rather, the phrase is a big red stop sign, as in "*Stop*, I don't want to talk about this, now . . . or ever!"

When people consciously or unconsciously seek to avoid emotions, they adopt code phrases like "I'm stressed" because it relieves them of any necessity to delve deeper to discover the whole story about the core emotions in play. "I'm stressed" is used in conversation with another person, more often than not, as the unsubtle message "I don't want to go there." Whether you are "stressed" and actively reflecting on your own state of affairs or whether you are responding to another's question, this phrase is used to withhold information entirely or partially from yourself or from others.

The prime directive with emotional work is learning to use the proper language that does not cover up what you feel. If you feel angry, you need to call it anger; if you feel frustration, you need to call it frustration, and so on for sadness, fear, shame, embarrassment, guilt, not to mention happy, content, satisfied, and joyous.

Match the correct word to the feeling, and this single step immediately moves you in the right direction for decreasing sleepless nights.

Adding a Second Step: Feeling Feelings

Naming a feeling is much easier than feeling it, but naming or even guessing the type of feeling you are experiencing moves you closer to feeling the feeling in your body. And the body is exactly where you want to notice and experience your feelings, especially in the area of your chest surrounding your heart.

Most insomniacs and many patients with mental health disorders feel their feelings solely in their minds, that is, above the neck. When asked the question, "Where do you feel this stress or anxiety?" they literally point to their heads.

While your mind is perceived as operating inside your head (which accounts for 12% of your body weight), if you only notice feelings in your mind, you are probably "intellectualizing" these emotions and may not be experiencing them on a sensory level. That is, you are *thinking* about feelings without necessarily *feeling* them.

Recall how the problem of insomnia is largely due to racing thoughts. If racing thoughts are caused by not attending to your emotions, it stands to reason you must be distancing yourself from these feelings. This distancing leads to the habit just mentioned: "thinking about feelings" instead of feeling them. This common approach is known as *rationalizing* or *intellectualizing* your feelings because the emphasis is on analyzing the experience with more self-talk and mental manipulations.

Emotions, however, are designed to be experienced in the "heart," which is why the expression "listen to your heart" (or even "listen to your gut") means so much more than its metaphorical value. When you learn to work directly and comfortably with your emotions, you will feel things in your chest near your heart *before* you necessarily think about what you are feeling. Or, as suggested, you might feel it first in your gut.

Point to Where You Feel It

Let's start with the simplest feelings you are sure to feel and just as sure to locate in your body and not just your mind. Take one hand now and point to the location in the body where you would feel the following:

- need to urinate
- indigestion
- bumped knee
- stuffy nose
- hungry
- nauseated
- sore shoulder

I trust you get the idea, but please point your way through this whole list before continuing to read.

Now two more feelings, which are really two trick questions: point to where you feel sleepy and then point to where you feel tired.

It is axiomatic you feel the urge to urinate or defecate in your pelvis, or the pain in your knee or any other part of your body when you bumped it, or the sensation of a clogged nose or a tummy in need of a yummy. But where do you feel the feeling of sleepiness, that drowsy feeling that lets you know you are ready to doze off? Where do you feel the feeling of tiredness or fatigue, that worn out, low energy state where sleep does not beckon, but nonetheless you want to rest or stop what you are doing for a moment, a minute, or longer?

Here's a tip for bedtime. Sleepiness is felt exclusively in the head region almost as a mystical mental feeling inviting you to the reality we call sleep. Tiredness can be felt anywhere in the body, including the recognition of feeling tired in your mind. **It is of immense value to appreciate that insomniacs often fail to distinguish between tired and sleepy feelings and lose the game of slumber by hopping into bed when they are tired but not sleepy.**

More on this sleepy versus tired conundrum later.

For now, I would like you to generate some genuine curiosity about why it is so easy to feel many bodily feelings in the right spot—the place where it's happening? In contrast, why is it so easy to inappropriately transfer emotional awareness into the center of your mind (self-talk) and so difficult to appropriately feel emotions in the right spot (heart/chest)? The quick answer is you want to feel safe by distancing yourself from your emotions. By relocating them into your mind, you believe you can more easily control undesirable or unpleasant emotions.

How exactly does this sense of "control" operate in day-to-day practice? Usually, you will use self-talk to *talk* to yourself about your emotions so you can avoid *feeling* them directly.

Reverse Polarity

In some of the early sci-fi movies and TV shows, the protagonist would often shout "reverse polarity" to solve an impending doomsday scenario. This emergency action applied to whatever machine or weapon or other fantastic gizmo defused the destructive energy or directed it to an uninhabited realm. To my recollection, it worked every time.

Does the analogy hold for emotions? Can a person reverse the order of sensing emotion so your feelings first emerge from within the body, before or while simultaneously sensing them in your mind? If you reverse polarity, will your heart gain the first opportunity to feel what you are feeling, tamping down the tendency to overthink your feelings before you feel them?

The answers to these questions may surprise. Yes, it is relatively easy to feel your feelings in your heart first because you were not only born to do so, but also, you lived in this balanced realm during the initial years of your life. That is, you felt emotions originating from your heart and without any of the mental interference you engage in currently, which means you must have learned in childhood or adolescence, mostly involuntarily, to *not* notice your feelings in your body. Once you learned not to *listen to your heart*, you "matured" to believe in a new normal—the adult-like, thinking-about-feelings pattern.

The good news is you still know how to work directly with your feelings; you're just out of practice and may believe too much effort is needed. Certainly, changing any behavior strains your mind, and take note, this challenge is not even half the problem. You see, while feeling feelings ought to proceed naturally and easily, there's a huge caveat: feeling feelings brings pain! Pain, in fact, is why and how you "unlearned" this essential skill at a younger age when you were overexposed to emotional turmoil.

Think "broken heart" as the prime example, along with thousands of other troubling and upsetting encounters that trigger overwhelming, complex, and painful emotions. If you never enrolled in, let alone graduated, from the *Emotions 101* course offered by your parents, grandparents, older siblings, best friend, peers, or another adept person, there's a huge chance you learned to squeeze your feelings into a smaller and smaller space, compressing them to a point of near invisibility.

At such a time in your life, you no longer trusted emotions, so you thought it best to avoid them. You neither expressed emotion nor recognized emotions as a powerful and insightful human function. Instead, stuffing emotion became the new normal.

Despite all your history, you can regain some natural capacity to feel more complex feelings, known as emotions, as well as learn to let yourself receive the information delivered by these emotions. Reversing polarity is not far, far away in some distant galaxy. For example, you feel heartburn in your chest or stomach, which informs you of a current state of indigestion, therefore you already feel some feelings with specificity; you realize where you feel it and understand what it means. Why not make room in your body for other feelings and emotions?

Indeed, everything stated so far is in complete accord with your natural capacity to develop or redevelop self-awareness of your *TFI system.* To reiterate, you are not going to be learning something new; you are relearning something old and innate to your mind and body.

A Safe Place to Start

When was the last time you felt happy about something? The smallest thing counts for our efforts to move forward. Someone smiled at you, and you felt good. You opened a door for an elderly person and were pleased about being attentive to someone else's need. You finished a task at work and were satisfied with your effort before moving on to the next one. You remembered to stop at the store to pick up ingredients for a favorite meal you planned to cook, and you felt enthusiasm about its preparation and eventual consumption. You pulled out a beer, plopped down in front of the TV to watch the game, and enjoyed a sense of contentment.

All these events promote positive feelings: happiness, satisfaction, enthusiasm, contentedness, and so on.

Where did you feel these feelings?

I guarantee no matter where you imagine or think you felt them, these feelings emerged in your body in assorted ways. The feeling may start with something relatively subtle, where your breathing releases a sigh; a sense of relief ensues as you let go of pent-up physical tension in your chest or abdomen. It may also hit you all at once, like a bolt of energy, when your team scores a touchdown, or you finally meet a deadline at the last minute, or you relish the exquisite first bite or sip of a favorite dish or beverage. These positive, pleasant, and desirable feelings emanate from places *in your body* that enable you to feel these emotions instantaneously instead of merely thinking you are happy, satisfied, or content.

For starters, many insomniacs and other mental health patients must accentuate the positive, though not because of a secret plan to turn them into optimists. No, this positivity is very technical.

For just a couple moments in a day, please reflect on a few experiences that yield happiness, joy, satisfaction, or contentedness. Learning to clearly feel these positive feelings in your body prepares you for the more difficult tasks ahead when you must ultimately turn your attention to the negative emotions.

Indeed, before we go negative, pause right now to think, to do, or to imagine something that brings a smile to your face and notice how your body feels. As needed, repeat as many times as you like, or at least enough to gain a minimum of confidence in how to feel your body's response when dealing with the good things in life. Again, this exercise is neither about the power of positive thinking nor about tricking yourself into changing your current mood. This work is a not-so-subtle introductory step to prove to yourself how your body actually functions when experiencing feelings and emotions—in this case the positive ones.

Approaching the Crossroads

The difficulty in learning to appreciate bodily sensations for so-called "negative" emotions is all about the *pain*! Each of the more unpleasant emotions (anger, fear, sadness, embarrassment, shame, or guilt) feels unpleasant and downright painful at times. It would seem natural to avoid such pain, and the easiest way to do so is to "think about your feelings" instead of feeling them, which at least decreases some intensity, or which may squeeze these sensations into extremely small if not invisible spaces.

When someone undergoes an emotionally charged life event such as a death in the family or of a dear friend or colleague or comrade-in-arms, pain is guaranteed. The same holds for other such traumatic events, like victimization during an assault. In other instances, a person may engage in aggressive behavior as part of their work in the police force or fire department or military. Such actions may lead to the injury or death of another individual, which may prove difficult to process over the long run, leading to feelings of deep remorse or guilt.

Once a person experiences intense negative emotions, generally two paths emerge. One is to work with these emotions directly, learning to process them in ways to promote broader, deeper, and healthier perspectives about life. Unfortunately, this approach appears less natural or common, arguably because the second path teaches us to do whatever it takes to ignore or repress emotional experiences to avoid the pain.

The avoidance of emotional experiences is epitomized by the insomniac who suffers from racing thoughts. The racing thoughts are the most straightforward way to occupy the mind so emotional sensations can be vanquished both in the short and long run. Thinking is a classic way to numb the body, making it insensitive to feelings by using general or imprecise words to describe emotion instead of using the body to experience the feelings.

Thus, we arrive at a crossroad for many insomniacs. Do you actually want to relearn to feel your emotions or not? What are your options? Continued racing thoughts? Sleeping pills? Stronger sleeping pills? How about adding stronger psychotropic medications, antidepressants, antipsychotics, mood stabilizers, and let's not forget antianxiety drugs? These are the pathways doctors and mental health professionals frequently recommend to their patients for the specific goal of shutting down the racing thoughts.

Do these medications work? Do they turn off your mind?

If you are reading this book, chances are the drugs have not turned off your mind at bedtime, and now you know the reason why. Your mind is dealing with a volume of emotion you had the opportunity to fully experience during the daytime, but which your body was not permitted to sense, recognize, and explore.

You now need to ask yourself, what are these medications doing to aid your efforts in working with your emotions? Or, as is commonly reported by many individuals, are these medications merely numbing the body and the emotions along with it? Perhaps, this numbing is a very appropriate step in the short run if someone is acutely suicidal.

What about the long term? Is there a more effective way to work with emotions in conjunction with the medications? Are there techniques focusing directly on emotional work to engage you more meaningfully with your feelings instead of simply numbing them? "Yes" to both questions, and you are already learning the initial two steps of a sleep-related, emotion-focused therapy program.

When you learn to name your feelings and feel them in your body, you are fundamentally transforming how you feel. As you continue reading, likewise continue with additional support from your own therapist or counselor, as well as friends and family. Use the time to gain clarity on how your mind and body can actively and successfully engage your entire emotional network. Doing so just might save your life, and resolve your insomnia as well, not a bad two-for-one!

Sleep Research Pearl #12

Avoidance behavior is a key component to mental illness and leads directly to struggles with coping in general and in working with emotions specifically. At one point or another, nearly all individuals with mental health issues reckon with the problem of avoidance. In fact, avoidance usually turns out to be the largest barrier to effective emotional processing. If you refuse to enter the arena of emotion, not only do you lose out on the opportunity to gain considerable insight about your difficulties, but you also may forfeit your chances for regaining a healthy and satisfying life.

Avoidance may start out looking like a minor thing. A trauma survivor, as a clear example, may choose to avoid certain people, places, and circumstances that provoke memories of past traumatic events. Sounds logical and rational, to be sure, yet over time the avoidance if unchecked often expands to more and more people, places, and circumstances. Such an individual may not go to movie theaters to see violent movies, and then over time stop going to movie theaters at all. Then, it might expand to no longer watching movies at home, and it may eventually include being unable to listen to people talking about scenes from movies. In extreme cases of PTSD, this progression of avoidance leads to a very restrictive lifestyle where the individual may no longer be capable of working, let alone functioning normally in family or community life. All such restrictions are based on the fear that emotional tidal waves would drown the individual in feelings and sensations too painful to bear.

At heart, avoidance means you are engaging in a behavior to thwart or otherwise prevent you from feeling emotions you don't want to feel. In a common circumstance, avoidance is seen among mental health patients who choose not to enter into therapy despite suffering from conditions interfering with their daily life and relationships. This point is not to suggest psychotherapy or medications are the only way to address mental health issues. However, when a person has shown no interest in or desire to address impairing issues, or if they have attempted and failed to gain improvement with less "invasive" means (for example, using exercise to treat depression), the question of why the individual avoids considering professional help should immediately come to the forefront. The answer most often offered out of the mouths of such individuals is "I don't want to go there" because they are at least minimally aware of the anxieties and fears sure to be "there."

The next two chapters on emotion-focused therapy (EFT) are the most intense of the book. The information offered should prove insightful for someone who is looking to understand the powerful role of emotions in mental health. As a bonus, working on your emotions may lead to more rapid resolution of vexing problems like nightmares and insomnia, and it can help you manage various hassles when attempting PAP therapy.

The more you engage with the ideas in these next two chapters, the less you are likely to avoid working with your emotions.

Still, the chapters only serve as a framework for EFT. While several practical steps and examples are offered, ultimately you must decide whether you wish to pursue this pathway in depth, with or without a therapist, or whether other factors stand in your way in your efforts to get to the heart of the matter.

CHAPTER 13

SLEEP-RELATED EMOTION-FOCUSED THERAPY: BEYOND THE SHALLOW END

The way you experience your feelings could prove the greatest factor in how well you cope with mental health problems—true or false?

Where You Feel Is Where It's At!

One of the most difficult components of emotional processing is learning how to feel your feelings and how to feel them in their natural home—the area of your chest and, not infrequently, your gut. Even if it hurts your ear, let me repeat: most people struggle to feel emotions in the core of their bodies because they prefer to think about feelings in their minds.

While sensing something in your mind seems like a reasonable starting point, in truth, most patients resorting to this intellectual style often spend years before embracing the notion that feelings emerge in the core of the body. Many believe emotions descend from the mind into the body. However, we want you to learn a reverse pathway where the heart sends the message to the brain to yield the *Emotional Intel*, which we'll explore in depth in Chapter 14.

For now, other common sites for feeling your feelings outside your head include neck, shoulders, and hands. Some emotions may be experienced in unusual places such as the anus, perineum, or certain muscles or joints of the body. With one exception, the farther away from the core you feel your emotions, the greater the distance you must travel to discover the "heart of the matter." The exception is your head, whose "density" could make the distance that much farther. As the goal of the first two steps is to identify and precisely feel what you are feeling, there is no greater system for success than your natural capability to let emotions spring from your heart.

How Not to Process Emotions

It sounds odd, but emotional processing is easier to comprehend by looking at examples of the opposite behavior, that is, avoiding the "heart of the matter." You probably know the term *psychosomatic*, which refers to psycho (in the mind) somatic (in the body). Unfortunately, a lot of people, including many healthcare professionals, use the term incorrectly and in unflattering ways, as if to suggest you are making it all up. Allegedly, you report a symptom that's not really there.

The most accurate starting point to define psychosomatics is "you are unable to feel things in a normal way, so your mind redistributes very real feelings to another part of your body." However, you usually do not recognize this sensation as an emotion. Instead, it feels like some type of symptom, the most common being pain. In sum, there is nothing unreal or made up when you suffer psychosomatic pain; you really do feel what you say you are feeling! Virtually everyone in childhood, adolescence, or as an adult has experienced psychosomatic symptoms.

The tummy ache is the classic psychosomatic response experienced by a child who is suffering fear or anxiety. In one scenario, a child does not complete a homework assignment and fears the consequences. Similarly, a child bullied at school wants to avoid the next encounter. The child may or may not immediately reveal these details, but with gentle probing, a child—in ways more skilled than an adolescent or adult—can not only bring this knowledge into the foreground, but also, and most remarkably, his or her coping capacity is so naturally advanced, the tummy ache almost always disappears within seconds or minutes after an honest discussion about current events.

Also, notice the tummy ache feelings rest in the gut, which therefore aligns with one of the two locations in the body most conducive to sensing emotion. In this sequence, the child starts with a tummy ache; and, as the parent-child discussion proceeds, the anxiety and fear quickly replace the tummy ache, meaning anxiety and fear are now felt in the abdomen. Finally, the emotions disappear altogether after the candid conversation leads to a well devised plan for solving the initial concerns (that is, homework, bullying).

As a clue to what's ahead in Chapter 14, compare this straightforward example to an adult developing psychosomatic depression where several symptoms emerge early on. Can you imagine how much more complex the exploration would be to search for the cause, if not causes?

As we age, another common psychosomatic response, or what's called an emotional "holding area," is a tension headache, often emerging in the latter part of the afternoon when fear, anxiety, or anger develops regarding an earlier conflict at work or in personal affairs. In this situation, you might realize something is bugging you, although you are not able to connect the stressors to your headache. You may receive relevant advice from friends or family about troubling issues in your life, but unless the deeper connection is made to the emotional components of your problem, the headache persists. Worse, you may have friends and family who prefer to avoid feelings and invite you to drink alcohol or to ingest/inhale some other mood altering substance. Bottom line, in these very common circumstances, the individual's "adult personality" has erected sufficient barriers to prevent emotions from breaking out, so the headache prevails as the substitute experience.

This headache undoubtedly grabs your attention, but your first, second, and third thoughts are not directed toward a deep dive to uncover the sources of the emotional tension. Moreover, a conundrum arises because this classic headache response might have prevented you from blowing up at your boss or someone else in a personal relationship. The mind-body possesses a great deal of wisdom, does it not?

Ultimately, however, if the real problem is anger, and you do not spot your anger or what you are angry about, then you are operating like a craftsman missing key tools. Emotions are instruments you learn to use with great precision, and you can often find them handy in your emotional toolbox when you understand where to locate and apply them. Which means circling back to steps one and two to identify and feel the feelings before you react or overreact.

In time, you will spot plenty of cues beyond tummy aches and headaches. As adults we are prone toward clenching teeth, tight jaws, chest tightness, rigid, crumpled, or tense posture while sitting or standing, hunched, rounded, or raised shoulders, or blood pressure elevations, to name a few. Once you gain awareness of these physical changes occurring in your body, you've positioned yourself to ask, "Is this physical feeling or change actually driven by a previously undetected emotion?"

Responding to the Response

Responding to psychosomatic reactions in general and emotions specifically is much easier for children than adults. In a child with a tummy ache, any number of questions can be asked by a parent, then the child pours forth information about troubling issues, and this venting process releases emotional residue. Make no mistake, while venting, this child is feeling stuff in the chest or gut, which facilitates the release of these emotions, leaving a healthy tummy in their wake.

Once the tummy ache evaporates, a clever parent educates the child with an insightful comment, "Hey that's pretty interesting; just by talking about problems you have with the teacher, your tummy ache is gone. I wonder, if you talk more about things bothering you, would you have fewer tummy aches?"

Oh, to be a kid again!

To restate, please do not think for a second the kid is simply engaged in a talk therapy variation. At a young age, when a child talks about troubling things, the words and emotions are closely linked, so much so there is a clear opportunity for feeling and releasing feelings through venting. For a child, it's as easy as taking off the bonnet to release the bee.

For adults, it requires accessing your emotional history to see more clearly the origins of your adult defense mechanisms. With practice (and/or help from a well-trained therapist), you learn how to feel emotions routinely without blocking them. Ultimately, you gain the capacity to feel things so clearly, you develop a satisfying sense of "control" instead of being controlled by hidden and unprocessed feelings.

Pause, and think about this paradoxical point. Most people never view those who are overly emotional as being in control of their feelings. These people seem out of control—some reach heights of hysteria. Correct, hysteria is neither the type of emotional expressiveness to learn here nor is it the pathway to gaining the insights you need. Hysteria is unhealthy, and technically called *maladaptive emotional processing*.

We are describing a highly adaptive form of emotional processing that will serve you well and make you considerably healthier. And one of the first ways to start this new approach is to address the frustration and anger so common to those suffering insomnia. Unfortunately, many insomniacs do not see these strong emotions staring them in the face. Instead, they suffer from a range of psychosomatic responses, including racing thoughts, tension headaches, neck strains, digestive issues, chronic pain, and frequent upper respiratory tract infections. Yes, failing to work with emotions directly can cause or contribute to any of these types of symptoms or illnesses.

Would you like to consider a different approach to resolving these unpleasant and disturbing emotions? Chances are extraordinarily high that direct targeting of frustration and anger will dramatically improve several health issues. Or do you believe you are destined to lock up the frustration and anger, presuming they are too dangerous to uncage?

Where we are headed is the place where you could learn to feel the anger and frustration and yet not react or respond to it. Sounds difficult, doesn't it? Of course, many imagine it's impossible not to respond. They think once you feel anger, you must unleash or vent it in some way, perhaps verbally or physically. The million-dollar question is, why do people believe these actions are the only responses to anger? In fact, anyone who outwardly expresses anger usually learned to respond in this way because they are reacting to an underlying threat or fear. By now, you must have heard on TV, radio, movies, or the Internet that anger is an extremely common response when feeling threatened. For once, the media got something right; this concept is an entirely accurate description of the human condition. After all, who wouldn't expect to react overtly if your security or safety were threatened?

In day-to-day life, most with anger problems have not trained themselves to reach for that singularly invaluable pause to reflect on the degree of threat, and then let the anger pass when there is no immediate or urgent sense of danger. This literal pause means before you open your mouth or launch a fist, you learn to take a split second to feel the anger in your body and then interpret whether a response is needed. This reflective pause, or what I describe as a "SOLO" moment in my *Sound Sleep, Sound Mind* book, could just as easily reveal no response was necessary. The SOLO technique stands for:

- *Stop* doing anything.
- *Observe* yourself: know your mind.
- *Let* yourself be: just breathe.
- *Observe* yourself: know your body.

When you apply a SOLO moment just prior to an imminent emotional discharge, you greatly increase your opportunities to "listen to your heart" to discover the "heart of the matter." This is the exact content of the message the anger is airmailing.

In time, you could learn to express nearly all your emotions to your inner self even if you're not aiming to become the world's greatest poker player. In this early stage of recovering your emotional processing skills, self-expression of emotions could soon feel like the most straightforward and natural way to deal with emotions.

Permit me to remind you there is no natural or healthy reason to use anger to commit an act of road rage or punch someone in the nose or kick your dog. There is nothing natural about this behavior; you must have learned at some point it was an acceptable or perhaps the only way to release anger.

With healthier emotional processing techniques, you learn to choose **no response** to an emotion—just feel it instead and let it go. Seriously, you can learn to feel the emotion and let it slip away, as it will nine times out of 10, if not 95 times out of 100.

Yes, there are many difficult situations where emotions linger longer and therefore cannot resolve quickly; this issue will be taken up in the next chapter.

Connecting Emotional Intel to Real-Time Emotions

Now let's go down a different pathway to show how the body naturally wants to experience its feelings and emotions and thereby allow them to pass through without much commotion most of the time.

Consider this thought experiment. Imagine a dream vacation and bring up images and feelings of what you want to see and experience. While sitting at home with this picture in your mind's eye, you are not "reacting" to it other than enjoying the imaginative pleasure of wading in the ocean waves or climbing to the top of a mountain. It's an experience that creates happy and pleasant feelings during which your mind and body are more than capable of letting you feel something in a natural way without any outward reaction. Moreover, there's no attempt to block what you feel; you'd like to feel more, right?

Most people with poorly adaptive emotional problem-solving skills do not realize they can learn to use their minds and bodies exactly the same way with an unpleasant or negative emotional experience. Yes, it's more difficult, but the overwhelming majority of adults utilize this system every day. Truly, you can learn to feel anger course through many places in your body, and as long as you remain motionless and inactive with this feeling in your body, the anger will literally disappear on its own or transform into another emotion that might really expose the "heart of the matter." More to come on this transformation process.

Grab another image for a moment. Picture a scene of something that makes you angry. Briefly relive something frustrating or something that angers you. Notice how different places in your body react to these images. Do you feel tightening in your jaw, hands, or chest? Whatever scene you choose, try as hard as you can to build the intention *not* to react to it; instead, focus everything on what you are feeling anywhere in your body.

If you pictured an angry encounter with your boss, your anger is likely fueled by some concern about how well you are doing your job or how well your boss measures your performance. Such questions would lead to more questions: will you get a promotion, when is the next raise, does the boss recognize your worth, and so on?

If you carefully review the possibilities, you may notice similarities to the point made earlier about the element of fear underlying at least some portion of each question. Which means the heart of the matter for anger is *fear*. And this explains the earlier statement about transformation. If you sit with the anger, you might quickly spot the Emotional Intel and recognize fear is the actual driving force. When this step occurs, you will be pleasantly or unpleasantly surprised to see anger vanishing as it is replaced by fear.

These kinds of workplace circumstances plague nearly everyone because everyone in some way or another must complete tasks to be evaluated by another person, whether it is a boss, a consultant, or a colleague. Even those not working still must bear responsibilities and meet obligations around their homes or for friends and family. In the real world, someone else eventually, if not regularly, rates you with approval or disapproval about activities in your life.

The anger directed toward your boss is actually a good thing because it is offering you a chance to become aware of emotional insights previously under the radar. Now, as an anger builds, your mind and body are literally declaring you must pay attention to these insights and deal with them. From this vantage point, anger is the messenger of valuable information, revealing certain fears you can address directly instead of responding to the anger. If you stuff the anger, you miss out on the Intel. In most cases, lashing out in anger usually means you misinterpreted the message.

In the next and final chapter on emotional processing, we'll go through specific examples of how individuals experience and process emotions in the healthiest of ways, even though initially they struggle to do so.

Sleep Research Pearl #13

Formal research in the field of psychosomatics seems limited compared to its vast potential. Frequently, relationships are drawn between a physical illness like diabetes or hypertension and an individual's stress levels. Often, bidirectional relationships demonstrate how hypertension or diabetes makes anxiety and depression worse, and how anxiety or depression makes diabetes and hypertension worse. Don't get me wrong. It's great this research is conducted; however, there are two follow-through areas that rarely get coverage in the research studies or in popular media.

First and foremost, the information about psychosomatic medicine does not spread into most medical practices where internists, family medicine doctors, general practitioners, and other primary care professionals should be watching for these connections, every single day, arguably with all patients. Many more mental health professionals are aware of the links and will discuss them with their patients. Nonetheless, if medical professionals, including nurse practitioners and physician assistants, learned more about psychosomatic medicine, it would greatly heighten a patient's confidence in moving forward with steps to address the psychological aspects of their physical illnesses.

Second, and more problematic on the mental health side, the essential tool of emotion-focused therapy is ignored by a substantial proportion of professionals, including therapists of all types. I hope you are starting to see how the theories and workings of emotion-focused therapy are essential to high quality psychotherapy. Specifically, those who practice emotion-focused therapy realize anxiety and depression are frequently secondary emotions covering up primary feelings like anger, fear, or sadness. These experts are not anti-medication, but they are very skilled, for example, in helping depressed patients explore deeper emotional states, which often prove to be the real cause of the depression.

In Leslie Greenberg's research[157-163] and in his more than 40 authored or co-authored books, he describes cases detailing exactly this phenomenon. Often, the individual had been or was currently using antidepressant medication. Over time, the individual was guided to tap into the deeper emotional states and arrived at an epiphany where he or she realized the depression was covering up other more painful emotions like anger, fear, or sadness, not to mention shame, embarrassment, or guilt.

Although EFT requires time, it takes less time than standard talk therapy because the focus is on getting to the heart of the matter. For this reason, questions should always arise when a patient reports working with one therapist for years. Obviously, exceptional cases occur where an individual may need such support for a long time, but this lengthy period should usually bring up the "elephant in the room" metaphor. Namely, how much progress is the patient actually making? How much have emotional and coping skills improved? Is the individual in fact learning how to manage his or her own therapy issues, or is the individual now therapist-dependent?

These points are a very big deal in the field of mental health because they harken back to key historical junctures in psychiatry and psychology where controversies have arisen about what works, how well it works, and who is capable of delivering an effective therapy. We'll pick up this history in the *Sleep Research Pearl #14* in the next chapter after you've had the opportunity to read about practical cases of emotion-focused therapy in action.

CHAPTER 14

SLEEP-RELATED EMOTION-FOCUSED THERAPY: DIVING IN!

*How can I apply EFT steps to overcome insomnia on
my own or with a therapist?*

Diving Into the Deep End of the Pool

We continue discussing anger as well as other emotions—especially so-called negative ones of fear, sadness, embarrassment, guilt, and shame—that can also be managed in similar ways: identified and felt, then processed in a healthy manner.

Nevertheless, when mental health patients are asked to actively dive into the deep end of the pool, the benefits do not seem readily apparent. Will your landing be a painful belly flop or a nifty slice into the water with barely a splash on the surface?

What if past experiences led you to believe emotions are harmful? Many suffer trauma and believe their emotional responses are unequivocally harmful. And many children are told by their parents in the strongest ways that emotions must be avoided, indicating something is bad about feelings. Regrettably, lots of people in childhood, adolescence, or adulthood have accustomed themselves to spending as little time as possible in dealing with their feelings.

In extreme circumstances, among individuals who suffer lingering guilt or shame throughout the day (discussed further in Chapter 18), we understand how they would find emotions dangerous and damaging. No surprise, they would prefer to squeeze these emotions into a very small space or find ways for total avoidance.

One final point for anyone choosing to work more regularly with emotions—you may be wondering how much skill you can develop with or without the assistance of a therapist? On this point, please read carefully the *Cautionary Note* at the end of this chapter, either now or later.

All the above requires reflection on your part, and in no way are we suggesting emotional processing is a smooth, simplistic, or short-lived experience. Still, the majority of strong emotional responses you experience in life often prove much briefer when faced head-on. It may shock you to hear, but many intense emotional responses may turn out to be measured in seconds or minutes.

That emotional intensity can die down quickly is actually common sense, but not the common sense of fixing something quickly with a simple solution. No, this common sense refers to the true nature or purpose of emotion. **To repeat and in bold: emotion is nearly always if not always trying to serve you, protect you, and in some way help you grow into a person more capable and more resilient in dealing with life's challenges.**

Emotions are not designed to plague or torture you, though circumstances arise where it may feel as if that's the way things are unfolding before your eyes. And when such episodes occur acutely, urgently, and with great intensity, it is understandable the net result in the moment might be a very unstable set of symptoms. In some cases, a person needs urgent help if he or she is suffering what may be called a nervous breakdown or other terms indicating mental decompensation.

More urgently, if someone is contemplating or engaging in self-harm, mental health professionals and psychotropic medication are likely the best tools available in the twenty-first century.

What About All the Other Episodes?

Few people live in crisis mode all the time, and those going down such paths, voluntarily or involuntarily, may require hospitalization.

For all the remaining individuals and for most of everyday life, nearly everyone has some capacity to develop new ways to cope to pull themselves through difficult encounters.

Emotion-focused therapy in general and our sleep-related emphasis are worthy of your attention because you could gain healthy opportunities to turn reactivity into reflectivity. This reflection allows you to hit the pause button, though not because you are trying to tamp down or avoid emotions. Just the opposite—you want the emotions to course through your body in order to feel with great certainty and accuracy exactly what you are feeling. Doing so will confirm how the penultimate step in emotional processing is almost invariably transformative. One emotion will truly turn into something entirely different than what was experienced at the outset of the emotional reflection.

As mentioned in the previous chapter, anger frequently turns to fear. And fear may then turn to sadness. And then maybe you discover sadness is really what's going on, not really so much anger or fear.

Do you see yourself never letting the anger transform into another feeling and then believing you could never let go of this anger? In fact, you might be very concerned the anger will lead to something harmful to you or others. That's possible. However, 90% of the time or greater, when someone feels anger there will be another deeper layer of emotion fueling his or her wrath.

When you discover anger is covering up fear or sadness, it is quite an eye-opener; a new way to relate to your emotions is just around the corner. Surely, you can appreciate your behavior or actions would be different when you feel anger compared to feeling fear or feeling sad.

A big question might arise at this point: do you want to know the deepest layers of your feelings? Are you actually more attuned to feeling anger or even feeling angry much of the time? How much would your life or lifestyle feel disrupted if you realized all along you needed to contend with your fears or your sadness? What if anger has been a long-held disguise to prevent you from feeling the fear or sadness?

As a side note, recall that fear was brought up in Chapter 8 to discuss how sleep apnea patients become apprehensive about thinking too much about their breathing. It's certainly scary not to breathe, and therefore you could scare yourself by spending too much time imagining what it's like to suffer abnormal breathing episodes in your sleep in the middle of the night.

One part of this fear comes from the awful feeling of not breathing, but the second part of the fear is usually greater; it is hating the awful feeling of fear itself. Fear is paralyzing to many, both heroes and cowards. The greatest progress is made when you no longer fear the feeling of fear; and the same is true for any other emotion. You may hate to feel shame and guilt because it is so horrible to feel shame and guilt. Nonetheless, fear is usually the biggie, which is why the TV show was called *Fear Factor*, not *Some Other Emotion Factor*.

This point is not insignificant, because an enormous number of mental health patients find it "easier" to maintain a current state of avoidance for whatever reasons or circumstances. If you know your emotions in one certain way—for example, you choose to think about your feelings instead of feeling them—you are more likely to continue down this overly analytical path.

In contrast, emotion-focused therapy declares, "Bring it on!" Not because of a confrontational style or thrill seeking, but from the honest awareness and recognition your emotions are attempting to deliver important messages, the *Emotional Intel*. Once the information is delivered, 90% of the time most of what you have been feeling begins to subside or begins to transform into the next layer of emotion.

Delivery of the Intel, though, does not always mean your work is done. It may mean you are just getting started. Or, just by feeling the feeling and knowing its source provides sufficient information to continue with the rest of your day and improve your sleep at night.

Let's examine how various situations move forward toward full emotional processing.

Albert the School Teacher

The first example describes what I call *self-contained* emotional processing, which means it's all about the individual, and no matter how many other people or factors seem to be involved, it's really all about one person's emotional work.

Albert is a 32-year-old middle school science teacher, engaged to be married and eager to settle down and raise a family with Miriam, a special ed teacher at a different school. While they both enjoy aspects of teaching, Albert developed insomnia over the past two years that he attributes to his work. It's noticeably better when school is out in the summer but returns with a vengeance the week before the new fall session. Occasionally, he takes OTC sleep aids, tries to keep a regular sleep schedule, and routinely searches the Internet for new sleep cures.

In the past six months, Albert noticed the loss of sleep made him irritable in ways he previously would have not thought possible. He's had to bite his tongue on several occasions in dealing with his school principal. At home in their small apartment, Albert spends quality time at the dinner table complaining about school while Miriam coaxes him to see the brighter side and stop focusing on the negative. Turns out, the brighter side for Albert is the few kids in school who take their science studies seriously.

As much as Albert appreciates his fiancé's perspective, he senses a frequent feeling of something bugging him. When he gains a moment of clarity, he vents to Miriam about so many kids being uninterested in learning and not completing their assignments. Despite his best efforts to come up with real-world science topics to spark interest in middle schoolers, he sees few gains for his efforts. Adding insult to injury, he feels there is scant support from the principal and has grown frustrated and angry almost every time they meet.

At this point, when Albert visits our clinic, we start with the tools involving much of the material covered in these past four chapters on the *TFI system*, mind's eye imagery, SOLO reflections, and basic steps of sleep-related emotional processing. Though he enjoys the imagery technique and gained some benefits, he notices intrusive thoughts interrupting his efforts during more severe insomnia episodes. For these reasons, we suggest further work on emotional processing, and Albert is comfortable with a plan to further investigate his frustration and anger. To be clear, what he will learn could also be applied before bedtime or virtually any other time of day during a few uninterrupted minutes.

As we discuss his use of the steps that follow, bear in mind this process could be occurring during a period of a few days, weeks, or months in an insomnia patient. In Albert's case, the steps unfolded over a period of 4 to

6 weeks, though condensed here for the sake of brevity.

As he had already identified two strong emotions, frustration and anger (completing Step 1), he next found a place in his home to sit and relax and attempted to pay attention to where in his body he feels the anger and frustration (Step 2). In a short time frame, he notices tension in how tightly he holds his hands and the stiffness in the back of his neck. Even though these are not ideal locations, it's a healthy start because he isn't just intellectually aware of the feelings; he actually feels them in some part of his body.

Now comes a challenging phase. Can he let himself feel the anger and frustration at its source, that is, his chest/torso/heart regions? When Albert reflects more about things at school that make him angry, he conjures up a picture of the principal, which then spurs a new level of anger. In the context of Albert's self-observing mode (SOLO), some anger creeps into his chest, which yields a clearer sense of how upset he is about the whole school experience, particularly his lack of support from the principal. At this point, Albert is making good progress with Step 2.

So, how does this example play out as entirely self-contained? Doesn't Albert need to do something to process his clearly recognized anger? Doesn't he need to find ways to gain more control over the classroom? Doesn't he need to confront the school principal to help find ways to enhance the classroom experience?

All these questions would be reasonable and demand answers if Albert were someone else in similar circumstances needing this type of resolution. But Albert's story is not such a one.

Albert's breakthrough moment occurs while seated by himself in a chair in his apartment. He starts out feeling parts of the frustration and anger in his chest and makes no effort to block these emotions. As the anger builds, it reaches a crescendo and now starts to subside. Though this declining intensity surprises Albert, what surprises him more is the next feeling creeping into his chest as it replaces the anger—the feeling of fear. Albert wonders what he is afraid of and senses he has worries about getting married, raising children, and finding a new place to live.

But these fears fade away quickly as he notices his mind going back to the school environment, and he now wonders whether he is afraid of losing his job.

In another instant, he finds himself welling up as if to cry. Indeed, his eyes moisten, but then suddenly he bursts out laughing. Why? Because he discovered the source of all these emotions led back to one thing, just one thing. He was the source of the anger because he had failed to keep the promise he made to himself seven years earlier when he said he would commit only five years to teaching and then reevaluate his position and career intentions.

Having gotten caught up in the negativity of the school environment, he turned his anger outward at the students and the principal even though he knew seven years ago teaching might not be the best profession for him. Now, with the clearest of observations, he felt the real problem was the need to make a decision on his future and stop using the external factors as an excuse to avoid his truth.

Thus, he completed Step 3 by using real-time emotional processing through layers of increasing complexity to gain a clear message about his current status and his possible future. This pattern is exactly how emotional processing works, and in Albert's circumstances real time could mean an hour or a day or a couple weeks' worth of effort on Step 3. And pay special attention to how Albert was able to reverse polarity, that is, he certainly attempted to use his intellect throughout the steps to find answers, but the ultimate solution arrived in Step 3 when he first welled up as if to cry and then burst out laughing.

Once he acknowledged fear as the deeper emotion, he let his body continue to transform his emotions. This transformation is subtle, and some would argue Albert must have had a thought or something else to cry about before he welled up. Correct, he had awareness he may have missed the boat by ignoring his promise to reevaluate his job status, and he literally and painfully forgot to do so. Nonetheless, the time interval here for this epiphany or breakthrough is a matter of seconds or nanoseconds.

Within a moment of putting these insights and feelings together, he wells up as if to cry out. This interval is very different than the person who takes several months or longer ruminating about why he is still working as a teacher and finally becomes tearful at some later point down the road when the emotions are allowed to break through. Nonetheless, emotional processing can still be achieved over a longer period, but Albert's efforts were expedited once he sought care at our sleep center and chose to pursue deeper emotional processing steps.

Another clarifying point might ask whether this scenario lends itself to a chicken and egg analysis, that is, which came first for Albert, the emotion or insight? While it's a fair question, I submit it may be overthinking the point. Clear emotional experiences trigger clear *Emotional Intel* (insights) in the blink of an eye, which is to be distinguished from taking weeks, months, or years of ruminating and sorting out emotional turmoil only with your intellect and potentially never permitting oneself to feel the emotions.

Going forward, Albert might choose to select a different career path. He has always been good at reading about and dissecting scientific investigations and could enroll in a master's program to formalize his skills as a researcher, a job often allowing more latitude in day-to-day tasks and clearly offering a different people dynamic compared to teaching young students.

Albert's laughter was provoked by his realization that for the past two years he would not admit his own anger to himself and instead wasted a lot of time and energy venting about the school system. Laughing at himself was a very healthy response instead of getting caught up in more frustration and anger.

Finally, no action outside of Albert's domain was needed to address anything in the school environment, and Albert's insomnia receded very quickly because he now had the action plan to move forward—whether he chooses to do so immediately, over the coming months, or longer—having clearly received the message from his emotions he had been blocking for a few years.

In sum, Albert was initially aware of frustration and anger and soon appreciated these feelings were what some experts call "secondary emotions," that is, a layer covering a deeper primary set of feelings, which in this case was fear. While the initial fear response was about losing a job, the actual fear response was related to the fear of never achieving a new career milestone.

Instead, he might be stuck in a work environment that felt like a dead end.

Once he worked with the fear, he knew a decision was forthcoming, but the decision was self-contained by Albert's personal choice of lifestyle. Clearly, it is not self-contained in so far as his future wife's input, but the frustration, anger, and fear no longer needed to be communicated to anyone but himself and his fiancé. No interaction with any school official was needed other than establishing the right timetable for leaving the profession.

Self-Talk to Self

Surprisingly or not, a majority, and some would say an overwhelming majority of emotional processing experiences are self-to-self communication. Oftentimes, when people hear about emotion work in general or emotional expressiveness in particular, they are persuaded the whole thing is about messy communication with other people "to express your feelings."

Nothing could be farther from the truth because in the greatest number of circumstances, you are the person who needs to know what you are feeling, and you are likely to discover you are the only one who needs to know. When you consider the vast number of emotional experiences anyone feels in one day, how could any of us possibly function if we needed to constantly inform others in our inner circle about our inner feelings?

When you know what you feel, you possess new information and insights to work with and arrive at decisions on how to proceed. As alluded to previously, a skilled poker player is a prime example of someone in specific circumstances who is acutely aware of his or her emotions and works effortlessly or otherwise to prevent anyone else from knowing. Your goal is not attempting to hide emotions from others; you simply must recognize the importance of your candid conversations with yourself.

The next example is quite complex, so much so, it entails more history about the patient long before she sought care for her sleep problems. Moreover, the process unfolds over several months, and for some patients would take even longer. Some readers will find parallels to these more severe challenges. If Albert's story proves sufficient to propel you toward action steps to use sleep-related emotion-focused therapy, you may want to skim through the next case or start in with cognitive-behavioral therapy for insomnia (CBT-I), discussed in Chapter 15.

Janet, Part I: The Dangers of Sleep Obsessions and Fixations

Janet is 55, a regional manager of a local supermarket chain and married to a veteran and current pharmaceutical salesman, Gabriel; they have five children, the youngest 17. Janet endured insomnia sporadically for several decades and avoided seeking help as she never had time to consider she suffered from a sleep disorder, let alone treat it. The past five years had taken a turn for the worse; sleeplessness was occurring in one form or another most nights. The problem deteriorated so much she no longer sleeps in the same bed or bedroom with her husband, both because she does not want to disturb his sleep, and because she experiences too much anxiety "trying" to fall asleep there. In the other bedroom, she experiences less anxiety but still suffers severe insomnia that flares up as hours-long difficulty returning to sleep after an awakening. During this five-year period, her primary care physician prescribed various sedatives, and she added OTC sleep aids. Though she is dependent on both agents, her results are so-so. Also, antidepressants, antianxiety pills, and psychotherapy entered the therapy regimen off and on during these years.

As best she recalls, this five-year battle began around the same time as a protracted dispute with her husband about fixing the electric garage door. The gist of several heated exchanges was his desire to keep tinkering with the motor, chains, and pulley system to keep it running, while she wanted to buy a new, less noisy, and more reliable door. After several arguments during the span of a year they agreed to buy the new one, but Gabriel insisted he could install it. Now when the garage door operates, she's convinced the job was substandard; and though it works reliably, the noise is aggravating every time she hears it.

A key component of her insomnia was an intensifying fixation on all things sleep, which in turn led to a crisis-like atmosphere in the home. Janet's obsessions were further fueled by chronic clock watching and time monitoring calculations so she could determine whether to plan for a good day, a fair day, a bad day, or a truly horrible, no-good, rotten day. In her mind, observations about each night of sleep or lack thereof yielded predictions about the next day's affairs, and she was obsessed with letting these predictions govern her daily and nightly lifestyles.

This type of obsession is very common in mental health patients with severe sleep problems, and if you have experienced these severe symptoms and the severe anxiety that goes along for this very bumpy ride, you may be aware that deeper emotional turmoil is the most common underlying factor fueling such episodes.

Identifying the Core Emotional Turmoil

Deeper emotional turmoil often spans a protracted period of years, often decades. Janet's original events, all traumatizing to various degrees, precipitated her bouts of insomnia as well as chronic nightmares, including the first and worst event when her mother divorced her father, a veteran unwilling to pursue any treatment for intractable alcoholism. The divorce itself was surprisingly amicable, but being a young adolescent girl, Janet was devastated by the turn of events and often broke down in tears repeatedly over the next year. Both insomnia and nightmares emerged within weeks and continued sporadically depending on her life circumstances. No one discussed the potential for psychotherapy during this period.

Roughly three years later, she and her mother grew more distant, but only due to her mom's increasing workload as she was hoping to put her daughter through college. Her 12-hour night shifts as an LPN plus overtime at the hospital led to a mostly unsupervised adolescence for Janet, and by age 17 she began experimenting with marijuana and fantasized about experimenting with sex.

Despite protestations from her high school girlfriends, she accepted a date from a sophomore in college whom she met at a local college function. She had socialized with the young man for all of one hour and impulsively agreed to a date the coming weekend. When her girlfriends heard the date was dinner and a movie, they collectively shook their heads and cautioned her on what to expect. Naively, as it turned out, she looked at the whole thing as a "first date," and therefore insisted there would be no expectations. On the other hand, to herself she admitted having fantasies of a sexual encounter as she was physically attracted to this older man.

The dinner and movie, as well as the conversations, all went well. When he drove her home but parked his car in a more secluded section of her neighborhood, she immediately tensed up. "Relax," he said. "Just thought we could talk some more and listen to some music. I've got a joint if you're interested in smoking."

The next hour was exhilarating for Janet, who thought she was connecting well with her date, though she wondered in the back of her mind whether it was the marijuana or the increasing physical attractiveness. One thing led to another, and the canoodling began. They were making out for a while when he made several highly intrusive advances, which she gingerly pushed aside.

At this crucial point in the escapade, the young man lost his cool and began shouting at Janet, attempting to shame her with the usual epithet of being a tease. He became so infuriated, he raised his hand as if to slap her, at which point she started crying horribly into her hands. He backed off, started the car, drove her to her house, never apologized and Janet jumped out and ran inside her home.

She never told anyone about the episode, not even her girlfriends, and certainly not her mother. Within a matter of days her nightmares worsened; and after awakenings, sleep was elusive. She stayed up later and later, hoping to avoid bad dreams, which generated a new sleep cycle of late morning wakeup times without respite from the nightmares. As no one else knew about the events of the disturbing date, and since her mother was rarely present for her daughter's evening and nighttime schedules, no one was available to suggest therapy or anything else. The problems persisted at moderate to severe intensity for about two years, but once community college started, things settled down to more manageable levels, though the sleep loss affected her schoolwork.

Janet was not enamored with college with the exception of math. She did exceptionally well in all math classes compared to average or below average in everything else. Business accounting caught her eye, and she excelled in it so much, an instructor recommended she find a part-time job; he provided several leads for apprenticeship bookkeeping jobs at local accounting firms.

Things were looking up for Janet as she saw a career option in accounting, giving her motivation to tough it out at college. Then, everything turned sour in one week when two incidents rocked her life and lifestyle. The first was a worse replay of her bad high school dating experience. She went to a party of college students, drank beer like everyone else, and was dancing away and enjoying the night when an older college student with a very impressive physical presence somehow guided her into a room with a bed, slammed her onto the mattress and began groping her. No amount of screaming reached above the din of the loud music, so no one came to her rescue. She struggled mightily to push him off, more because of his weight and drunkenness, and these factors allowed her to finally win out as she literally curled up in a ball and kept rolling around underneath him until she slipped out and fell on the floor, hitting her head. Nevertheless, she ran out of the bedroom and outside into the cold air and felt her heart pounding. She was angry, and then more angry, and wanted to break something, anything, into a lot of pieces.

Her girlfriends found her just as she started vomiting, and they took her home.

That same week her mother injured her hip during a transfer of a morbidly obese patient at the hospital. It was the recurrence of an old injury, and the very bad news was the likelihood of immediate hip replacement surgery, the same surgery recommended five years earlier. Though her mom did not expect to go on disability, she finally realized she could no longer maintain her rigorous work schedule, not to mention suffering the financial hit from the surgery.

Janet, despite new rounds of nightmares and insomnia, experienced a real-life wake-up moment and knew she must rethink her finances and education. Aside from math and accounting, college offered nothing of special value. The harder decision-making emerged when she recalled past advice from her father with whom she still spoke a few times per year. He had encouraged her way back in her early teens to think about a military career to get a solid and fully paid education.

The National Guard was a perfect fit, and at the age of 21 she signed up for a lengthy stint to make sure she received the full educational benefits, which she used not only to graduate from college with a major in accounting but also to complete a master's program in Business Administration. Topping it all off, she eventually met her future husband, Gabriel, who had recently finished a tour of duty in Iraq. Though battered and bruised from his efforts, his mild PTSD and newly developed pain issues were manageable. Only later did chronic pain factor into their quality of life and relationship.

Janet's experiences of entering the reserves, completing her education, working her way up in various job positions, and, most importantly, birthing four children and adopting one more kept her so busy in her twenties, thirties, and forties, she was able to cope with her insomnia and nightmares, by and large, by ignoring the problems and maintaining an exhausting schedule. The nightmares were increasingly sporadic and more like chronic bad dreams, with fewer awakenings. The insomnia, though ever present, was dealt with, as is often seen in a large majority of patients, by simply sleeping fewer hours and finding a way to maintain fair to great functioning depending on the needs of the day and proper dosing of caffeine.

Now, in her fifties, she realized the sleep loss was affecting her mental health, particularly through anxiety and depression symptoms, and at the encouragement of her husband she sought help, which led to an on-again, off-again relationship with antidepressants or antianxiety pills or both. Prescription sleeping pills were also used nightly along with the sleep aids, and throughout this period she heard of no other treatment options save drugs. No one recommended therapy, so she sought counseling on her own.

She found no benefit from weekly sessions over the next six months and felt all that occurred was talking and re-talking about things in the past, the present, and what might happen in the future. The therapist mentioned she was suffering from mild PTSD based on how her nightmares persisted for so long after her two sexual assaults and her mother's divorce, but this professional opinion seemed like an afterthought to Janet as she recalls no details or discussions about dealing with PTSD. To top it off, she went through menopause, and it aggravated all of her sleep issues and mental health symptoms. Finally, Gabriel's chronic pain added another major pressure point in their family life.

When Janet finally got around to seeing a sleep specialist, the sleep obsession had taken full hold of her, and a question always arises at this stage regarding what pathway the patient will pursue. We often see two pathways, one in which the patient acknowledges and addresses the sleep obsession, and the other where there is no escaping the obsession.

Sleep Fixation Pathway 1

The first pathway develops into a firm and incontestable belief all things revolve around sleep, even to the point all mental illness is caused by the lack of sleep or bad and broken sleep. In other words, Janet and patients just like her believe that if their sleep problems were fixed, anxiety and depression would disappear. Although you won't get an argument from me on the strong potential for sleep gains to generate mental health gains, I have not seen on any regular basis how a complete eradication of sleep disorders cures all mental health disorders. Rather, much gains, few cures.

For those who insist 100% resolution of all mental health problems will occur with successful sleep disorders treatment, this sleep fixation may serve as a defense or avoidance mechanism to divert attention from the stigma of the mental disease. The first objective is to help patients realize no one solves their sleep problems by obsessing about perfect sleep. As much as I encourage every mental health patient to do everything imaginable to "perfect" their sleep, eventually the individual must establish reasonable and accurate expectations and goals.

Sleep Fixation Pathway 2

The second scenario is alarmingly worse than clear-cut fixation because it starts out along the same path obsessing about sleep and then degrades further into a demoralizing and debilitating attitude, which then leads to deteriorating waking functioning. In scenario number one, a person fixated on sleep while suffering all the related impairment may still hold down a job, raise children, socialize with friends, and maintain a household environment, just as Janet did. It may be stressful, overwhelming, draining, and painful, but the individual carries on for several years, specific to his or her constitution, personality, and upbringing. In contrast, in this second scenario, the burdens are too great for various reasons, and the individual no longer operates in anything close to normal fashion on a day-to-day basis.

Many of these second scenario individuals go through a panic mode where they suffer fears about going to sleep, fears about what goes on during sleep, and fears about not sleeping, all rolled up into very challenging levels of anxiety and, ultimately, desperation. Some individuals are at the highest risk for suicidal thoughts or behaviors. Others may end up hospitalized in order to be heavily sedated with large dosages of "knock-out" drugs to temporarily break the cycle.

Ultimately, once "stabilized," these folks are usually maintained for lengthy periods on multiple psychotropic medications, yet their functioning gradually declines to almost a bare minimum of survivability. They no longer work, struggle mightily with household chores, avoid most social relationships, and check out much of the time in raising their children. In their own minds, they may believe they are doing the best they can, and there is no reason to believe they are not trying to do the best they can. Yet, effort and motivation are in short supply.

The ultimate explanation in many of these cases, though not necessarily all extreme cases, is the sleep factor provides cover against the deeper emotional turmoil too difficult for individuals to confront. By expending all their energy in the conquest of sleep, there is a sincere albeit misguided belief, most if not all other health troubles will change for the better when sleep solutions are discovered and treated. It's great that so much benefit can be gained by treating sleep disorders, but some unfortunate souls choose to put all their eggs into one basket.

Again, I endorse the theory sleep gains yield mental health gains, but in these two scenarios, which we would label as high- and low-functioning sleep fixators, these individuals eventually must reckon with the unprocessed emotional turmoil they have avoided.

Here's how Janet's story continued, and please keep in mind some of the following occurred in our clinic space, while other activities occurred with Janet taking her own initiative at home.

Janet, Part II: How to Stop Losing Sleep over Losing Sleep

Janet fits the high-functioning model. As she begins work on basic emotional processing skills to identify and feel her feelings, she is faced with the conundrum of needing to simultaneously deal with her fixations on sleep.

Questions then arise: How likely is she to recognize the sleep obsession as a major part of her problems? Would she be able to acknowledge the sleep obsession actually worsens her sleep problems? And what kind of intervention would help address this obsession?

Before we track down the answers, let's briefly follow up on Albert, the science teacher, who suffered no sleep obsessions. His sleep improved dramatically as he recognized the full scope of his previously dormant emotions (frustration, anger, fear, sadness) and received new emotional insights regarding his job. He no longer needed any therapy of any kind to deal with his insomnia because he was at peace with his decision to move beyond the teaching profession. It's true he might be at risk for future episodes of insomnia, but because he was never fixated on sleep, he was very capable of trying out the emotional processing pathway and getting to the heart of the matter quickly.

Janet's attempts at emotional processing are much more likely to be thwarted by her huge sleep fixations. If nothing else, just the sheer amount of time and energy dedicated to the sleep obsession subtracts from the time and energy needed to work through emotions. Making it more complicated, sleep obsessions themselves are emotionally driven and easily overlap and interfere with any other emotional work. Finally, the intensity of the sleep obsession is so strong it literally distorts cognitive processes and leads to poor judgments and decisions on how to proceed in treatment.

Even among high-functioning individuals, the trance of the sleep obsession is beyond their immediate grasp. Some might acknowledge, "Yeah, I'm pretty focused on my sleep stuff." Such perspectives are almost always a superficial or intellectual statement, not one with sincere depth like, "Holy Guacamole, this whole time I'm losing sleep by wasting a ghastly amount of time worrying about losing sleep." For short, we call this LSOLS, *losing sleep over losing sleep*.

Almost none of the above information and insights are available to someone like Janet until she starts working with a sleep specialist who understands how to engage a patient to realize all her attention directed at sleep is actually making things worse, and not in a superficial way. The mind's trance causes everything to revolve around sleep and is truly a harmful and sometimes dangerous mental state that must be confronted. Unfortunately, many prescribing providers and other mental health providers know almost nothing about the intricacies of LSOLS and too quickly either jump to a prescription pad or simply miss the whole point of the problem and move on to another area of therapy.

In No Time at All

In my work with Janet, she learned to confront the sleep obsession and was willing to forgo certain behaviors to stop the fixation. In part, she achieved these results by assiduously taking steps to eliminate clock-watching and time monitoring behavior (TMB).[164] In virtually any severity level of insomnia, cessation of TMB is guaranteed to improve insomnia from a little to a lot. Some people need to remove the clock from the bedroom or turn it around. All need to realize that listening to the sounds of traffic or birds outside or noting the changes in outside light are still forms of TMB and must be eliminated.

Solving TMB problems is a great step forward, but the ability to do so requires a capacity to confront LSOLS directly. Because TMB is a microcosm of LSOLS, successful reduction in TMB augurs a greater chance to stop the LSOLS as well. Nevertheless, just because a sleep doctor possesses a lot of experience managing this special problem and can repeatedly demonstrate to the patient how spending time *worrying* about sleep *kills* your sleep, the individual must at some point break down her own resistance, that is, figuratively or literally look in the mirror and finally accept responsibility for making a choice to stop the obsession. This step will only occur when the individual carefully looks at her own behavior and realizes with absolute clarity her sleep obsession is unequivocally wrecking her sleep.

Once this step is achieved, there remains the question of what mental content will be floating around in the mind of the individual who has ceased both LSOLS and TMB?

Imagery to the Rescue

At bedtime or in the middle of the night, for most individuals the use of imagery distracts them from looking at the clock or listening to the environment to make time calculations. Over time (no pun intended), the vast majority re-discover their innate feelings of sleepiness and appreciate how sleep is even closer than just around the corner.

As discussed, imagery is extremely powerful and exceptionally reliable in helping insomnia patients fall asleep. Once patients loosen their grip on LSOLS and TMB, they become more flexible and open-minded about trying different techniques. Using imagery at bedtime and during the night after awakenings is an invaluable tool to regularly pull out of your toolbox to meet the challenges of sleepless nights. Once imagery work proves satisfying and successful, it may prevent lapses back into sleep obsession behaviors.

Janet, Part III: Searching for the Core Emotional Issues That Fuel Insomnia

Once Janet has broken through the trance of the sleep fixation and attempted imagery exercises, there's more opportunity for improvement. For the first time in years, Janet openly speculated about her potential to sleep without drugs. Nevertheless, the deeper emotional turmoil remains unresolved as she's never dealt with her three traumatic experiences and never concretely connected them to her insomnia or nightmares. Now she becomes more willing to consider the general paradigm of sleep-related emotion-focused therapy because all her focus is no longer fueling the sleep obsession.

From the historical narrative above, Janet's past trauma would be an obvious target in connecting the dots. But, in practice, a sleep doctor may use sleep-related emotion-focused therapy based on how the patient is currently identifying her own problems. In this case, Janet had quickly pointed out some difficulties in communication with her husband, and therefore common sense dictates looking at this potential area of emotional turmoil before delving into the trauma history, whereas a skilled psychotherapist might target trauma and PTSD initially.

Janet finds herself in a place outside a self-contained environment, as described earlier. Whatever she learns from her deeper emotions, it appears she will need to communicate something to her husband about a problem she perceives in the relationship. These emotional issues are not isolated to her own growth and development.

What then is the problem?

To start, we could imagine how the communication about the garage door suggested mixed qualities, that is, information was exchanged, but one wonders about the friendliness or courtesy in the dialogue, a strong indicator of respect or disrespect felt for the other person. Then again, such analysis is only rationally describing a conflictual behavior. The meat (or vegan burger if you prefer) of the issue is the nature and intensity of the emotions Janet experiences. Sooner than later, it will also involve her husband's emotions.

When Janet sits in a chair and lets these feelings come into awareness in her body without trying to overthink them, she starts with obvious irritation about her husband's behavior. No matter what words she uses to describe his behavior (obstinate, procrastinator, know-it-all), the irritation is the key because it is a superficial emotion covering up the deeper stuff. To be clear, the irritation is real, very real, but when Janet lets things flow, she realizes she's angry at her husband, a feeling much stronger than irritation.

As individuals become aware of anger, originally thought of as simply irritation, this single experience is an eye-opener. People do not like to experience anger for many reasons; one in particular is it makes the person question whether or not they are a mean-spirited individual. After all, who gets angry about such petty things like a garage door and its noise?

This recognition, coupled with the bodily sensations of anger, may feel over the top at the outset, so the person becomes perplexed about such strong emotions. In these circumstances, if you were experiencing this insight, you might immediately try to suppress the whole experience, waving away the emotion as if to say, "that's not me."

An emotionally attuned individual recognizes anger also may prove to be a superficial emotion, and when Janet sits with the anger for just a short interval, it would usually wash away. In this case, when the anger dissolves, it is replaced by the next layer of emotions that have been fueling the anger. These feelings are the deeper more meaningful emotions yielding the most important insights and information.

In Janet's world, much like the hidden emotional world for most of us, her anger is a combination of feelings involving portions of embarrassment, sadness, and fear, which swept over her once the anger subsided.

Cascading Emotions

In actual experience, when the individual sincerely settles into this process, it's true all the emotions may flood the person in a decidedly overwhelming way. This type of experience is very difficult, challenging, and disturbing and may serve as a pivotal factor in how the individual seeks medications or, preferably, is managed properly by a compassionate therapist.

On the other hand, the more we fear emotions, the more likely they will push back with much greater intensity as they seek to be expressed, that is, expressed to you.

In Janet's circumstance, she notices how her anger turned into embarrassment as the next layer of emotion. Her embarrassment is a form of excessive self-consciousness, as if to say, "How did I get into the mess I'm in?" but she may also be embarrassed with herself just for having felt so much anger. Further, she might be embarrassed about her own nagging or nit-picking behavior directed at her husband.

If the emotional processing were complete at this point, she might look at the experience as an epiphany and directly apologize to her husband. But embarrassment was only the next layer. When she sits with the embarrassment and learns its primary message, most commonly the embarrassment subsides, and in its wake, the next layer appears on the scene; in this instance, the next feeling is sadness.

When Janet sits with the sadness, it would be very common for her to not just feel sad but actually tear up, if not start crying, without necessarily any immediate clarity whatsoever on the insights or information being delivered by this strong emotion.

Rather, while she is actually crying—and again, not necessarily before—various insights or information reveal themselves as the crystal clear fuel behind the crying. Let's repeat, Janet is not sitting thinking that she's sad about something and then starts crying. The sadness took over and precipitated the tears, and this equates to "listening to your heart," where the emotions traveled north from the chest, not south from the brain.

This healthier sequence is less intellectual and more experiential. It often provides a predictably common way of initially feeling an emotion and then sitting with this feeling until it starts to subside. During this transformation, Janet experienced images in her mind's eye while various thoughts streamed across her awareness of her own annoying behavior in communicating with her husband, realizing again she was feeling embarrassed only because she saw herself as a nag.

To repeat for clarity's sake, as the embarrassment ebbs but before she becomes aware of any new thoughts, she suddenly starts feeling sad and may or may not have a brief insight about what's making her sad. Once the tears are flowing, the individual is more inclined to *listen to her heart*, after which the insights rise into her consciousness. Again, in this example of reverse polarity in which the heart is thrusting information upward, Janet quickly realizes she is extremely disappointed, unhappy, and sad about the state of her relationship with her husband.

She is looking back (picturing) over several years and sees and feels a deterioration that includes a great deal of disrespect between the two of them, which is so different than what transpired in the nearly first three decades of their marriage, leading up to the garage door incident five years ago. She knows full well it takes two to tango, and her crying persists and intensifies as *she continues to listen to her heart*, revealing the poor state of affairs and the obvious questions about how things turned so sour.

At this key moment, resistance could be at its highest to prevent uncovering further depth to her feelings, because the next emotion, which is actually fueling or accompanying the sadness, is likely to be fear.

When You Fear the Message, Remember the Artichoke

Before proceeding further, it is crucial to hear why a person has so much resistance throughout the processing of emotion as well as resistance toward dealing with deeper emotions. The short answer—individuals realize, ultimately, emotions do carry messages, but the prediction that swirls around in our heads is almost always emotions have something to tell us that will prove unpleasant, bad, damaging, or disturbing, and it's going to cause lots of problems, so we don't want to hear any of it.

In this circumstance, I sincerely explain to my patients that emotional processing is not at all like peeling layers of an onion, though at first it might seem analogous since tears and crying are extremely common in deeper emotional processing attempts. The better analogy is peeling an artichoke, where at the end you get to the *heart of the matter*. Moreover, the analogy holds because the heart of the matter invariably provides you with much greater clarity and, many times, a greater sense of the truth about yourself and those around you. Truth ultimately tastes best even though it may taste bitter at first.

In other words, despite some pain involved, gaining truthful knowledge about yourself and your relationships is one of the most liberating and thus satisfying experiences an individual can go through. And when the person comes through to the other side, there is much greater motivation coupled with clearer insights on making the best decisions going forward.

How did this play out for Janet?

Janet, Part IV: The Heart of the Matter

Janet soon realized she was experiencing a great deal of fear along with her sadness, and it wasn't, strictly speaking, about her marriage. Rather, she identified her real sadness as the feeling of losing a best friend. The beauty of her relationship with her husband had been the early and steady belief they were soulmates; they had gone through thick and thin and always seemed attuned to each other during trials and tribulations, while also finding so much joy and satisfaction in each other's company during the good times as well. It popped into her mind to ask not whether she and her husband were still friends, but were they still best friends?

Her feelings of sadness and fear indicated something was wrong, and she realized this downhill slide could not have just happened overnight, when suddenly the image of the garage door popped into her head. She briefly relived the episode in her mind, and two very unpleasant feelings coupled with insights emerged. The first was just the sheer oddity of the encounters that transpired involving so much back and forth bickering, a style of conversation that brought up the second realization of how alienated she felt during that time. In reliving the episodes, she reexperienced the feelings of alienation and started shaking and then broke down with tears streaming out.

She let sink in the horribly unhealthy character of the episodes and suddenly felt shame and embarrassment for not having identified how unnatural the occurrence had been. She posed to herself a series of guilt-ridden questions: Where the hell was I when all this was happening? What was I thinking? How could I possibly let things slide into this mud pit? How could we let things slide into this unfriendly mess?

Janet became increasingly angry with herself and went downstairs into the basement and let out a scream. Her husband, Gabriel, rushed down the steps and blurted out, "What's wrong?"

She looked at him for several agonizing seconds, then walked over to him, wrapped her arms around him, and chokingly whispered, "We're wrong!" And started crying again.

The next several hours of heart-to-heart discussion were a catharsis for both husband and wife. Each recognized the past five years was like living in a kind of trance. As Janet's insomnia had worsened, Gabriel saw her as more distant, thin-skinned, and easily irritated. He remembered "backing off" a bit, thinking breathing room was a time-tested palliative, but now realized five weeks had turned into five years.

Janet learned for the first time the garage was largely a budget issue. Gabriel had been embarrassed to reveal his increasing reliance on and increasing dosage of OTC pain meds for chronic knee pain. He was convinced the only solution, per his consulting physicians, was knee replacement surgery, but the insurance co-pay and deductible were beyond their means. He had a plan to save more funds, but it was slow going. His doctors insisted he switch to opiate painkillers, but he wisely refused given a prior history of alcohol abuse in the early years of his marriage.

As they went back and forth, honestly discussing their problems and honestly expressing what they were feeling, they both experienced a beautiful meeting of the minds moment, where each person literally sees the other person in a new and more positive, not to mention more loving, human light.

216

The realness of each person's appearance is so powerful, it overwhelms the other with good feelings and a strong sense of the moment as well as the love shared between the two.

That night, Janet actually slept like a baby—not the kicking and screaming kind—but the peaceful, dreaming away in the Land of Nod kind.

Janet, Part V: Tying up Loose Ends

This level of emotional processing has a dramatic capacity to cure a person's sleeplessness when the underlying emotional tension from all the unaddressed emotional turmoil is finally and coherently brought forward into consciousness. When there is no fear to feel fear or any other feeling, emotional expressiveness and insight can release an enormous amount of emotional tension that had been stored unwittingly in the body and in the mind.

Still, not every individual achieves a complete cure with emotional processing. The more likely outcome is how the release of emotional tension frees up the mind to be more receptive to any and all new ideas on dealing with sleep problems. Said another way, emotional tension functions like ill-suited body armor, a concept described by several early psychologists and psychiatrists. This armor carries a reflexive response to avoid things that would cause chinks in the armor, which might let emotions in or out. As long as the armor holds firm, a person can continue to "think about his or her feelings" instead of feeling them.

When the armor is abandoned, the individual has a grand new opportunity to boldly go where he or she had previously been too timid to venture. Nevertheless, each person who goes through such an epiphany does not solve all life's problems and still must deal with life's pressing challenges and conflicts.

We know Janet still needed additional evidence-based psychotherapy for her PTSD, which ultimately was one of the most influential mental health conditions that caused her emotional processing skills to deteriorate over the years, starting as a young teen. A hallmark of PTSD is *avoidance*, and this avoidance leads people away from thinking about both their past history and their emotional responsiveness such that over long stretches a person can enter a trancelike state. This "trance" describes exactly how Janet ended up eventually developing a five-year period of deteriorating mental health and sleep, during which she was unable to recognize the superficial character of the standard options offered to her, namely, talk therapy and lots of medication.

With evidence-based treatment of PTSD and more sessions of emotion-focused therapy, Janet enhanced and entrenched her emotional processing skills. In so doing, Janet now gained a deeper appreciation and understanding of how the early traumatic episodes actually colored all the difficulties she was having in communicating with her husband. For this key reason, Janet could have been rightfully frustrated and angry for never having been offered therapy for her PTSD in the first place because such therapy might have led to far less problems with insomnia and nightmares and far better communication with her husband. Or she might choose a path of gratitude for having found greater meaning in her life.

Finally, on the sleep front, it turned out menopause led to her developing a moderate case of obstructive sleep apnea that required the use of the OAT device. For persisting insomnia, she actively pursued strategies to taper off all sleep aids. Her success included the practice of a mild form of sleep restriction therapy, which in her case simply meant going to sleep at night when she began to yawn outside the bedroom. And, she noticed her emotional reactions to the tapering and restrictions were much milder due to her enhanced emotional processing skill. That she easily tapered off both a prescription sedative and an OTC sleep aid was a testament to how EFT makes insomniacs much more receptive to CBT-I steps. Sleep restriction could be attempted early in many insomniacs while some fare better, like Janet, by adopting CBT-I only after learning to cope more effectively with her emotions.

In the next chapter, we will delve into this area known as cognitive-behavioral therapy for insomnia. Finally, her improving but persisting nightmares were treated with the IRT method described in Chapter 16, but it should be noted that just by improving her sleep breathing she quickly saw some improvement in her disturbing dreams.

Concluding Thoughts about Emotions

With all the intensity we've delved into for this specific chapter and the emotions therapy chapters in general (Chapters 12–14), please appreciate how much benefit there is to be gained from sleep-related EFT. As your skill at identifying (Step 1), feeling (Step 2), and processing emotions (Step 3) improves, you have the chance to capitalize on two distinct areas to help you sleep better. First and foremost, recall how we described sleepiness as a kind of feeling or sensation that is not exactly an emotion, but certainly fits into the category of things you feel or sense. Most importantly, you want to feel sleepiness at bedtime or in the middle of the night if awakened and seeking to return to sleep.

With advances in emotional processing skill, you are now going to spot, more often than not, how sleepiness hides beneath other layers of emotions. Think about it: if you are anxious or angry, how or why would you notice the feeling of being sleepy? You would not notice any drowsiness because, for all practical purposes, the sleepiness is nowhere to be felt. Instead, it's hiding in plain sight. Thus, if emotional processing resolves previously neglected unpleasant feelings, you should start noticing how racing thoughts are replaced with sleepiness, a feeling that eases into the foreground of your mental landscape.

You can experiment practically with processing right at bedtime. A firsthand experience might identify a feeling of frustration, and then you let yourself feel the frustration in your body, and finally in processing the insights from the message delivered by the frustration you feel satisfied some closure was achieved. All of which may lead to genuine sleepiness. In such circumstances, you drop off to sleep without even remembering the last of your efforts. That's how rapidly emotional processing steps may work.

The second area involves PAP therapy. You may need to pick up these pointers again when you delve into Appendix A, but for now let's note emotions, feelings, and sensations frequently interfere with PAP adaptation because your awareness kicks in regarding the heightened stimulation of placing a bulky, cumbersome, and annoying mask on your face, along with the unnatural fluctuations of the pressurized airflow.

Again, as healthy emotional processing allows you to directly confront experiences without worrying about the feeling itself, in short order you often discover PAP-related sensations are nowhere near as bothersome as initially experienced. What changed? Simply, you changed, and now you no longer amplify your attention and make these sensations worse. Instead, you learn to pay less attention to these sensations because you don't want to suffer the irritations or vexations from the mask or the pressurized air as long as you accept they are a normal part of the adaptation process. You learned to adapt and cope with them, just as you learned to adapt and cope better with your emotions.

A Final Cautionary Note

Sometimes, problematic emotions and emotional turmoil linger for the most obvious of reasons, such as a recent traumatic event, or ongoing abuse, or chronic conflictual relationships. We would not expect sleep-related EFT to be effective in such circumstances, which need more regular interventions like exposure therapy, counseling, advanced psychotherapy techniques, 12-step programs, or even medications. Ongoing psychotherapy may be the most relevant thing and should be strongly considered when no obvious solutions to emotional turmoil are available. And, most importantly, if suicidal thinking or behaviors are involved, it is most imperative to work regularly with trained and experienced mental health professionals.

Other times, however, there are scenarios where the emotions linger more so because the individual has developed a pattern of ruminating on life's problems in unhealthy ways. In this situation, the individual spends so much time thinking or talking about troubling issues, there is little time left over for actually working on emotional growth. The end result is somewhat obvious: by continuing a pattern of thinking about problems, the individual is ultimately thinking about feelings instead of feeling feelings.

This point cannot be overemphasized because if you suffer from the habit of talking or thinking too much about emotions instead of actually trying to address these feelings with healthier coping mechanisms, then indeed your emotional residue is going to linger indefinitely.

The problems described in this cautionary note are sometimes very difficult for the individual to sort out and almost always require a skilled intervention from a professional who has the best training and experience in emotion-focused therapies or its variations.

Keep these points in mind going forward if you feel stuck trying to regain your natural sleepiness using sleep-related EFT. Your situation may prove too complex for the instructions provided in these chapters. And there is no reason to keep banging your head against the wall if SR-EFT does not work for you. It works for many, but others also require the assistance of a therapist to gain more benefit. If success is not emerging as you would like, seek additional help. The added education, coaching, or therapy might be what you need to reach your goals.

And to reiterate, while many aspects of suicidal thinking or behavior appear to decrease once your sleep improves, it cannot be overemphasized that the persistence of such thinking or behavior warrants immediate professional attention.

Sleep Research Pearl #14

An undeniably brief history of the formal mental health profession starts with the psychoanalytic revolution at the end of the nineteenth century when Dr. Sigmund Freud and the Vienna Circle got patients taking a very deep dive into all sorts of experiences in their background, upbringing, and current thinking and feeling patterns. Though the movement has lived on in many ways and achieved considerable success for many, the earliest criticism was psychoanalysis was too long, too expensive, and just plain too much to ask of most people. That said, the key element of the program was *catharsis*, the ability to reflect on past events and feel a deep emotional connection to what occurred in the past and then process the information to gain valuable insights about how your emotional responses in the past have affected your current state of being. As you can see, it should already remind you of both exposure therapy and EFT.

The mid-twentieth century saw the birth of cognitive-behavioral programs where the emphasis was far less on the deep penetration of the past. Instead, there was a notable shift away from emotions and toward thinking (cognitive) and action (behavior). The result was a huge growth in various forms of CBT pioneered by Dr. Aaron Beck and Dr. Albert Ellis, which challenged the patient to spend more time "thinking about what they are thinking about" as well as taking action steps in the mind or in one's lifestyle to improve mental health. A very simplistic example would be the patient with mild depression whose lifestyle unwittingly became more sedentary after marriage and children. With CBT, the individual might rapidly discover just by adopting a regular exercise regimen the depression all but disappears. In this instance, the chief determinant of long-term success is whether the patient maintains the commitment to the exercise program. That is, was the depression a simple psychosomatic process where the shift away from physical activity led to a decline in mental functioning that resolves with exercise, or will it turn out the depression has other and potentially deeper causes?

By the 1970s, if not earlier, a niche of researchers and clinicians recognized CBT often missed out on the emotional content of their patients' psychological turmoil. And here's where things got really interesting, because by this time and certainly earlier, the term "talking cure" was in wide use, which ultimately led to a great deal of confusion in clinical practice.

You see, "talking cure" originated with Freud and others who were promoting talking to lead to deep emotional catharsis. Somewhere along the way, many in the profession or in the media or both started using the term "talk therapy" either to replace "talking cure" or redefine it. The redefined version clearly left out the emotional content.

Now, very recently, perhaps in just the past decade, there is a new trend in the world of CBT called "third wave CBT,"[165] which—you'll never guess—seeks to bring certain aspects of emotions back into the therapy equation.

Bottom line is psychosomatic medicine in general and psychotherapy in particular typically must include emotional content, sensations, and insights as an essential, if not the essential, component of treatment. That said, it is still true psychoanalysis remains prolonged and expensive for many people, and it's equally true traditional CBT fails many patients for its lack of attention to core emotional principles. In this regard, we know emotion-driven therapies like exposure or desensitization are wildly successful, with the caveat they may be poorly implemented in ways that overwhelm some proportion of patients. EFT, on the other hand, tends to be a longer (though not long) therapy providing the patient with plenty of homework to test out new approaches to experiencing emotions and gaining new, life-changing insights (Emotional Intel) through the process.

Eventually, nearly all psychosomatic oriented therapists as well as most other mental health professionals must revisit the works of the early psychoanalysts and realize emotion-focused therapy (including what are known as the "newer" somatic therapies) represent the most natural and likely most relevant underlying principle of psycotherapy in the twenty-first century.

———•———

A final clarification on EFT is necessary due to the tumultuous times in which we live. Regrettably, many adults express very adolescent, egocentric opinions about the role of emotions in human life. Their view is epitomized by the phrase: "if it feels good, do it!" Healthy emotional processing stands in opposition. To repeat, emotions serve and protect you; using feelings as an excuse to satisfy selfish desires or to stew in your grievances, is a sure sign of *unintelligent* emotional processing. From the incredible gifts and insights we may receive from the depths of our emotions, it remains our duty to responsibly work through the Emotional Intel to make healthy choices and decisions. Reason rules!

CHAPTER 15

ADVANCED COGNITIVE-BEHAVIORAL THERAPY FOR INSOMNIA

How can I use CBT-I to effectively treat chronic insomnia problems?

Thoughts to Change Behavior

Instructions so far engaged the imagery and emotional, or feeling, systems of the human mind/body. Both approaches are extremely powerful, and in many ways are the most powerful in solving the universal problem of racing thoughts. It's worth taking a moment to reiterate why this point is so relevant to your long-term resolution of chronic insomnia.

Chronic insomnia is, well, chronic because individuals who develop the disorder almost always suffer from a chronic imbalance in the TFI system. The most common imbalance is too much thinking. And, you can take it to the sleep bank, racing thoughts are predominantly caused by unprocessed emotional turmoil or blockages in the imagery system. Notwithstanding, many folks decrease or eliminate racing thoughts soon after initiating PAP for OSA/UARS. This physiological intervention is described in more detail as the "Respiratory Threat Matrix Model of Chronic Insomnia" in my *Sound Sleep, Sound Mind* book.

Returning to the *TFI system,* when you work directly on daytime emotional residue to identify, feel, and process the cascade of emotional insights layered into the various feelings you uncover, it is most satisfying when you attain closure on the day. Closure at the end of the day is a hallmark of successful emotional processing.

Regarding imagery, it is equally satisfying when you discover your racing thoughts aren't as powerful as they seemed once self-talk vanishes following regular use of guided daydreaming at bedtime.

Still, there are individuals who may feel uncomfortable or awkward attempting manipulation of either the imagery or feeling systems. Or they simply prefer something more cognitive (thinking strategies) or behavioral (action strategies), which leads to an equally tried and true method, cognitive-behavioral therapy for insomnia (CBT-I).

You Don't Need to Sleep on It

The standard way to teach insomniacs how to overcome their sleeplessness is through cognitive restructuring, a technique in which you learn specific facts and information about insomnia, which in short order guide you to change the ways you think about and behave toward the problem. Cognitive restructuring is at the core of CBT-I.

CBT-I is a potent therapy that works for many insomniacs, but it lacks completeness because it offers no specific strategy to treat racing thoughts. Nonetheless, CBT-I instructions are definitely worth knowing and applying because this framework may prove initially easier for understanding and addressing insomnia. Moreover, it is plausible CBT-I indirectly decreases racing thoughts in some.

After establishing a CBT-I routine, you could also revisit techniques such as self-guided imagery or sleep-related emotional processing, which often leads to more sustainable results.

Revisiting Tiredness Versus Sleepiness

A basic premise of CBT-I contends the insomniac has lost the feeling of sleepiness or has become confused about what it means to feel sleepy and how to regain this sensation at the right time. As discussed, sleepiness can be generated by using your mind's eye to drift toward pleasant images, or sleepiness is induced by using your feelings to process emotions to dissipate racing thoughts. CBT-I offers a different behavioral opportunity to infuse sleepiness into your system when needed.

The first part of CBT-I requires paying close attention to the distinctions between feelings of sleepiness and feelings of tiredness, which leads to a very strict rule to never get into bed and attempt sleep if you only feel *tired*. Instead, you must wait until you feel *sleepy*.

You can see how "force" enters this equation because at first you must force yourself not to go to bed if not sleepy. If you only feel tired, do not "try" to go to sleep. When you force yourself to stay awake, eventually your body generates feelings of sleepiness, after which you hop into bed and drop off to the Land of Nod.

Undoubtedly, this system may prove painful at the outset because you are so tired you just want to get into bed and sleep. But this point illustrates one of the most illuminating ideas behind CBT-I: never try to make yourself go to sleep! Sleep is a natural process; you merely need to relearn to let it happen. By staying awake for longer periods of time during the first week of treatment, you will discern with far greater precision the distinctions between feelings of sleepiness or drowsiness and feelings of fatigue or tiredness.

As you relearn to experience drowsiness, two critical insights emerge. First, you realize there were times in the past where you had been jumping into bed when not sleepy. Second, once you start feeling the sublime if not seductive sensation of genuine sleepiness, you will also realize you were previously able to recruit this feeling, if inconsistently. With these insights, you build more confidence and momentum to generate sleepiness when needed. Finally, by paying close attention to these different sensations during the day, you tend to observe more accurately the feelings of tiredness during the daytime, while hopefully experiencing more sleepiness closer to bedtime.

These concepts might seem impractical at first. Notwithstanding, once you actually start to feel the differences between tiredness and sleepiness, it is almost natural to redirect these feelings to the proper time of day or night and naturally fall into synchrony with your 24-hour sleep–wake cycle.

Sleep Restriction Is Not Torture

Sleep restriction therapy (SRT) is a cardinal principle of CBT-I and works well because the absolute fastest way to ever go to sleep is to stay awake until you cannot stay awake any longer. Warning—this is true for nearly everyone, but patients suffering from bipolar disorder may discover a reverse effect (mania), so SRT is not typically advised.

The exciting thing about SRT is it frequently works without going to extremes. Consider this common example at a sleep clinic. The patient reports she sleeps five hours per night but lies in bed for nine hours; tossing and turning makes up the other four hours. In classic CBT-I instructions, the rule dictates a reduction in time in bed down to about six hours.

Six hours is not some magical figure. If you slept for five hours yet spent only six hours in bed, the sleep efficiency (time asleep/time in bed) approaches 85%. Among strict behavioral sleep specialists, the recommendation might be 5.5 hours in bed to sleep five hours to gain sleep efficiency > 90%. While these rigid instructions work for select patients, many individuals find these adjustments extreme and downright scary. As they have grown so attached to their bed and bedrooms, they cannot resonate with the idea of giving up all these "hours of opportunity" to sleep.

Targeting high sleep efficiency at the outset of treatment as a fixed rule often proves counterproductive for the obvious reason it puts far too much pressure on someone who has been under the "spell" of seeking more time in bed to procure more time asleep.

Even after the insomniac hears a fundamental principle of CBT—"more time spent in bed not sleeping leads to more time not sleeping in bed"— the individual still may not embrace strict SRT. And even though it's true someone who radically restricts time in bed would likely achieve a large benefit, the vast majority of patients cannot employ these instructions when they first hear them.

The good news is an insomniac may only need a small taste of sleep restriction to start gaining benefits. In the above example, we would suggest reducing the number of hours in bed from nine down to eight instead of from nine down to 5.5. Happily, just this little drop produces its own domino effect, causing many insomniacs to suddenly start sleeping more hours.

This positive change probably occurs because it gently breaks the harmful habit of prolonged time in bed. It would not be unusual for this patient to return a week later and exclaim, "Sleep restriction really seemed to move things in the right direction, so I decided to cut another 30 minutes off my time in bed."

Can you see how empowering it would be to observe and determine the right amount of sleep restriction for yourself instead of being ruled over by some data points that may not immediately make sense to you regardless of how well the math was explained?

These data points usually derive from a sleep diary in which the person tracks time in bed and time asleep for a week or two beforehand. Even though sleep diaries are invaluable for specific patients, most insomniacs can reasonably estimate useful time components, that is, the amount of time spent in bed and the amount of time spent asleep while in bed. Even if these estimates are way off quantitatively, it rarely matters. The nature of the problem is a qualitative one: lying in bed awake breeds more time awake in bed. To break this cycle, even the smallest change, say 30 or 60 minutes less time in bed, works wonders among those individuals committed and motivated to try.

Yeah, but What Do I Do When I'm Awake in the Middle of the Night?

The nighttime post-awakening routine is the single greatest concern among insomniacs who attempt CBT-I. They do not just balk at the request to spend less time in bed; they also develop fears and anxieties when the instructions demand, "When you are not sleeping, you must get up out of bed and return only when you are sleepy." To which the patient replies, "WTF am I supposed to do when I am awake in the middle of the night?"

As straightforward as CBT-I specialists may approach this dilemma, this problem requires a personally tailored solution based on the complexity of the individual case. In fact, it may be necessary for the patient to hear that a multilevel plan of options is available, so if the first or basic step does not work, the patient ascends to the next level to attempt another idea on the list.

At the first level, the individual receives the classic CBT-I instruction,

"Do something boring or non-stimulating until you feel sleepy again." It does not need to be something as annoying as "read the telephone book—backwards," but the gist is to not overstimulate yourself. Instead of reading a fast-paced novel, how about nonfiction on a dry subject where you would never read more than two to ten pages. Some of my favorites include *Safe Mopping Practices for Home and Office*, *Dietary Restrictions of Religious Heretics in the 16th Century*, and *An Annotated History of Shoelaces*. Hint: If the title makes you sleepy, it might be the right book.

Will this technique work? It works for some, but not necessarily those with severe insomnia because it really does not address their fears or anxieties when faced with the challenge of getting up out of bed in the middle of the night. If they could simply sit up in bed and read the book for a while it might suffice. But if reading does not do the trick, then the question arises whether the bed and bedroom must be vacated temporarily until the sleepiness returns?

Many patients with severe insomnia do not succeed by sitting up to read in bed in the middle of the night (even though it may work at bedtime) and so would now be confronted by the daunting task of leaving the bed and bedroom for some other place in the house—to do what? Read there instead?

What If Getting Up Out of Bed Doesn't Appear to Make Sense?

Unfortunately, these seemingly simplistic tips only work for a small proportion of very severe insomniacs, and there are complex reasons why they do not work when applied simplistically. Nonetheless, it's worth a shot to consider getting up out of bed for now so you have more of a fighting chance to beat insomnia with CBT-I.

Bear in mind, I'm just asking you to consider getting up out of bed.

Over time, I also want to remind you to consider circling back to strategies involving imagery or emotional processing, which afford you the opportunity to solve insomnia right there in bed without ever having to employ this unpleasant strategy that goes by the technical term *stimulus control*.

Stimulus control means you linked your bed and your bedroom with *not* sleeping; therefore, you must take control of the stimulus causing this problem, namely, your habit of suffering insomnia where else but in your bed. By moving yourself to a new place, you hope to regain the sensation of sleepiness and then return to your bed and fall asleep without any effort—at least that's the plan. Indeed many insomniacs will fall asleep if they move to a different bed in their own homes, just as many sleep better for at least the first or second night in a hotel.

Stimulus control is a stronger way of redirecting your energy so you do not feel the pressure to fall asleep in your bed at those times when you cannot fall asleep in your bed!

By leaving the bed and bedroom, your mind-body soon forgets this nasty habit of walking into the bedroom and suddenly feeling wide awake—a habit you of course had little to no control over. After all, if you are not sleeping, a person's natural tendency would believe it makes sense to hang around the bedroom and lie in bed to see if at least you eventually get more hours of sleep.

Makes perfect sense except it doesn't work. But it does present the perfect opportunity to appreciate how the "less is more" approach in the short term is the path forward. After all, the less time you spend in bed, the more likely you are to tap into your natural sleepiness, as we described above using the concept of sleep restriction.

But here's the big problem: if you do not know what to do in the middle of the night, that is, what to think, or feel, or picture—or what behavior you are supposed to engage in and why—if you do not know all these fine points of strategy, then stimulus control usually would not and will not work for you. If so, we need to go to the next level to clarify the core reason you are not sleeping and to tease apart the related reasons for struggling with stimulus control rules.

If You Can't Get No Satisfaction, You Probably Can't Get No Sleep Either

When discussing the role of emotions in fueling racing thoughts, we mentioned that anger and frustration are leading indicators, complaints, or symptoms experienced by insomnia patients. Some insomniacs need more time to resolve this emotional distress and understand how to use this processing to decrease racing thoughts. Notwithstanding, you may want to ask, "If I am frustrated about something, can I do something to become un-frustrated?"

The answer usually is a simple "yes." Most insomniacs are frustrated during the day because they are not satisfied with the way their day is going or the way their day went. Discontent or dissatisfaction could take many forms of emotional symptoms (bodily tension leading to a backache) or behavioral acting out (slamming a door, kicking a trash can). These signs are fairly reliable in demonstrating to the individual he or she is feeling keyed up about something. I am not suggesting it is imperative you identify and work through the cause of this frustration at this point in the timeline because it may be too difficult to do so. Moreover, there may be more subtle signs of dissatisfaction that would only be discovered with a more vigorous personal inventory.

Our goal for now is to learn to "reverse polarity" in a new way by focusing on the positive potential you have in front of your eyes to gain satisfaction. This step may not fully solve the insomnia problem, but it may sufficiently reduce bodily tension formed during waking hours and thus pave the way to recruiting ample sleepiness to lead you back to slumber town.

This approach is simple on the surface but complex at the core because you must find something that yields satisfaction but does not trigger a desire to stay up for hours on end. If you know that reading a racy novel or nail-biting suspense thriller will be overflowing with fun, then it solves the problem of dissatisfaction but causes another problem of too much alertness and no return to sleep.

What works in this situation?

Like I said, it can be quite a chore to sort it out. For example, some people get out of bed and clean their homes and do laundry, and they report satisfaction from completing these tasks, which not only made them feel better, but in fact led to a new round of sleepiness. Someone else might make repairs to small problems in the kitchen or rearrange furniture while clearing out house clutter. Again, I know individuals who perform these tasks in the middle of the night and report satisfaction plus newfound sleepiness.

Others go for more intellectual activities, like writing letters, memos, papers, or short stories or books. The irony is not lost on me; in 1999, I wrote one-third of my second book, *Insomnia Cures,* in the middle of the night. Some people record shows they have wanted to watch for months or years and view a couple episodes at 3 a.m.

In these examples, notice how the individual takes control of his or her life at this dark and dreary moment of sleeplessness in the loneliest part of any night and turns it into something productive or pleasurable for a long enough period of time to gain satisfaction without being overstimulated. Sleepiness returns, which to reiterate was always lurking, hidden from immediate view; and, it resurfaces in a reasonable amount of time, permitting the person to head back to the bedroom and gain some shut-eye.

In my clinical experience, helping people in this manner has proven much more effective than the traditional model of stimulus control that mandates boring or non-stimulating techniques. Our model asks you to face the fact you are not satisfied with some aspect of your day. While it would be great if you could immediately recognize what caused this problem and fix it, most people cannot identify and resolve such problems so quickly.

In our method, we want you to accept that enlisting your own efforts to feel satisfied about *something*, without overstimulating yourself, may prove adequate to reduce or erase some of the day's frustrations. Gaining satisfaction also makes you feel *in control* and gives you new ways to look at the problem. Instead of seeing it as a period of lost sleep, you now view it as a time of found opportunity. In the short term, you gain the advantage and fight back against insomnia episodes. This change of attitude is crucial in attempting to use the satisfaction-seeking approach.

But What If All I Do Is Worry About Not Sleeping When I'm Not Sleeping?

Now we arrive at the very heart of this recurring question: what to do at night when you are awakened? The answer may surprise you and may even cause some consternation even though you heard it in earlier chapters. You must . . .

Never lose sleep over losing sleep!

Which means, when you think hard and deep about it, no matter how you choose to occupy your time during the night, never let sleep issues occupy your mind. Never think about sleep. Literally, do not care about sleep! Go so far as to laugh at sleep and declare open hostilities toward it, telling it to leave you alone while you are awake gaining satisfaction from the thing you are playing with or working on.

Seems like an extraordinary recommendation for someone feeling so miserable about lost sleep. But again, the truth is this simple: the degree to which you adopt this frame of mind predicts the degree to which you will succeed in resolving your insomnia. Indeed, with this single instruction to *never* lose sleep over losing sleep, we see insomniacs gain marked improvement over the problem in a matter of days—sometimes the very first night.

Usually, it does not matter what you are doing at night unless you pick the "wrong" thing that triggers a cycle of overstimulation and excess alertness. What really matters is occupying your mind with its own current reality of solving a crossword puzzle, ironing shirts, framing a picture, watching a sitcom, or, if in a safe neighborhood, taking a walk. Such actions should promote only a mild degree of alertness, and eventually the sleepiness will creep back into your consciousness; you'll start yawning, your eyelids will grow heavy, and you'll recognize it is time to journey back to the bedroom and slide into bed and fall fast asleep.

This huge Sleep Pearl can never be repeated enough times: changing your attitude about your loss of sleep will lead you in a positive direction faster than you can say, "Sweet dreams and good night." This mindset is unbelievably powerful among a huge proportion of insomniacs where their fears of losing sleep are the greatest cause of their insomnia. To repeat, losing sleep over losing sleep is so diabolical it leads to suicidal ideation, and it will induce some insomniacs to demand more and more medications to solve their sleep problems. That's how dangerous things become if you do not adopt a new mindset to "stop caring about your lost sleep."

For patients on the brink, it is a critical intervention to teach them how this unique mindset may relieve so much of their suffering; and although there is no research on this specific point, I would wager that teaching insomniacs to stop losing sleep over losing sleep might save some lives. That's how seriously we take this imperative.

There is an important caveat for psychiatric patients with manic depression because the loss of sleep might provoke a manic episode. These folks must pay special attention to their sleep schedules, and sometimes the only way to achieve a regular pattern is with specific sleep aids. For the rest of us, learning to honestly give up the quest for sleep at this vulnerable moment in the middle of the night while gaining the feeling in your heart you do not care whether you sleep, can truly turn into a lifesaver for many insomniacs.

As difficult as it may be to swallow and digest this special Sleep Pearl, it is one of the most remarkable strategies of all as it teaches the individual to stop imbibing the awful and virulent poison of losing sleep over losing sleep (LSOLS).

Clock-Watching Is Just Another Form of LSOLS

In the emotion section, we briefly touched on time monitoring behavior (TMB), and here we'll elaborate because one of the fastest ways to overcome losing sleep over losing sleep is the immediate recognition that watching the clock or otherwise monitoring time is just another way of expressing your frustration about lost sleep. Even though you look at the clock and believe you are earnestly making calculations to sort out how much more sleep you might gain that night or perhaps how to rearrange your schedule accordingly for the next day, the underlying reason you look at the clock is your worry about lost slumber. Thus, clock-watching is a disguised version of losing sleep over losing sleep.

Clock-watching makes insomnia worse in another way because you are spending conscious time not sleeping while calculating how much sleep you lost, how long it might take to fall back asleep, and how much sleep you might still gain. In other words, you are engaging in waking activities that indirectly teach your mind-body to believe the bed and bedroom are the place to engage in waking behavior, which clearly is the opposite of sleeping behavior.

There are two ways to gauge the intensity of your clock-watching, a behavior engaged in by the majority of chronic insomniacs. First and foremost, when time monitoring is deeply entrenched, you will be surprised at the difficulty in relinquishing the power the clock has over your thoughts and feelings in the middle of the night. In fact, among insomnia patients who eventually refuse to stop time monitoring, a huge proportion end up using sleep medication(s) chronically.

The second gauge is the potential relief gained by simply removing the clock from the bedroom (or turning it to face the wall) compared to your renewed efforts to search the environment for gross clues to substitute for time monitoring. Classically, checking the outside light, hoping and praying for dawn's early light, is the dead giveaway you really have not ceased time monitoring behavior. Other clues would be listening for the sounds of dogs, roosters, traffic, or hustle and bustle in your neighborhood. Some will even go to the limit of internal evaluation, declaring a certain number of hours must have been slept based on the current feelings while awake.

Surprisingly or not, among those who accept the principle that time monitoring worsens insomnia and then proceed to eliminate the behavior in a robust fashion, chances are extraordinarily high for pronounced benefit. Some people take longer to process these ideas and want to experiment slowly for a few weeks, whereas others embrace most of the instructions in no time at all when they quickly connect their clock-watching with their frustration about losing sleep over losing sleep.

If you are among the time clock diehards, let me be perfectly clear: you may not realize it yet, but time monitoring is a very big psychological issue for you. For some, it's actually terrifying to give up the clock, and some long-term insomniacs will express these fears straight up. In such cases, I would never push for the change in clock-watching behavior until individuals gain greater command and control over emotional processing skills. Such skills unequivocally help someone work through the anxiety and fear over the potential loss of time information during the night.

Those who cannot cease TMB, unfortunately, are at much greater risk for starting or continuing to use sleep medication(s), but candidly, ceasing TMB just does not sit well for these individuals under various circumstances. Knowing when to alter TMB is crucial, and for those hesitant to do so it is essential to work on the problem with a sleep or mental health professional to come to a reasonable temporizing solution, certainly in the short term and likely the long term.

Finally, the question often arises as to what to do if you are not looking at the clock or not otherwise engaging in arithmetic gymnastics to determine how much sleep time is left in the night? The answer goes back to what you discovered to be the right things to do in the middle of the night after an awakening. These same strategies are equally designed to replace clock-watching, and at the top of the list, most insomniacs eventually discover imagery distraction techniques are the best remedy, short- and long-term.

Newer Advanced Strategy and Some Old Fallback Maneuvers

As promised, we now discuss a newer cognitive approach to insomnia that recently sprung up to directly target racing thoughts. It certainly sounds hokey at first, kind of like fighting fire with fire, but truly has some potential. Moreover, I am developing a variant of the technique by combining it with imagery distraction.

The basic principle is known as "nonlinear thinking," which stands in opposition to how racing thoughts run their course when you cannot fall asleep. When you ruminate, worry, or otherwise experience a motor that won't turn off, your thoughts may go all over the map; but if you carefully scrutinize the pattern, you will see how the "sentences" in this unbearable discourse make perfect sense. In other words (literally), racing thoughts are usually not bizarre, psychotic, random, chaotic, or inexplicable sequences of thoughts. Rather, they are about something, often work, relationships, family, vacations, stressors, food, hobbies, deadlines, and so on. Judged separately, you would have no confusion about the content of each thought or worry.

Now, as you recall from our earlier discussion of the *TFI system,* thoughts are the first thing sleepers notice when they lie down to go to sleep, and for nearly everyone these thoughts begin with a linear pattern, something like, "Oh yeah, I need to remember to get gas tomorrow when I stop at the supermarket for the groceries." But then something magical happens; the thinking grows increasingly less linear to the point where it starts making no sense. Indeed, among individuals who pay too much attention to such thought processes (like researchers obsessed with sleep), you could actually come to full alertness and blurt out, "That was ridiculous." What thought sparked such a reaction? Maybe something like, "the cheese barn times slowly."

As the words make no sense, the thought is nonlinear, and therefore you could attempt to replicate this style by consciously attempting to create nonlinear thought; for example, you speak in your mind "elbow . . . rain . . . cake . . . calm." Each word could be thought for a second or several seconds apart from the previous word, and your consciousness might drift closer toward sleepiness and then sleep.

Revisiting the progression of TFI as you drift toward sleep, the nonlinear words could prove more powerful than imagery distraction in that you would be falling asleep before you ever knowingly encountered the third and final phase of imagery. On the other hand, if nonlinear words do not initiate the drift toward sleep, you might never arrive at your natural imagery to open the final doorway to the Land of Nod. Instead, what if the nonlinear thoughts just trigger a new round of racing thoughts?

Therefore, why not combine the two approaches—nonlinear thoughts with imagery? That is, pick the word, then see its image, then pick another word and see its image, and so on, keeping in mind (pun intended) each new word should usually emerge with relative spontaneity, if possible, but regardless needs to be at least somewhat disconnected from the past word.

So, your word sequence would *not* be "car . . . boat . . . train . . . plane." Rather, it could be "book . . . pebble . . . cauliflower . . . harmony." Each of these words offers possible images, so after the word is said in your mind, try to picture a book . . . and then a rock . . . and so on. Using a more abstract concept like "harmony" may also yield interesting images. The beauty of adding imagery here is while some folks strain to conduct imagery, now you are only asked to try to image one thing and then another thing, so there's very little work involved in completing the task. Personally, I have attempted both systems, just the words and word-pictures, with some success. I also find the process humorous, which adds to its relaxation qualities.

Regarding the combo, if the imagery takes off, you might discover you see the book, then the book opens, and then pages are turning. Maybe there's something on the pages or maybe they're blank. By the time you finish with the book, you might already be asleep, but if not, you see a pebble. Do you pick it up and feel the smooth surface? Do you throw it sidearm and skip it along a lake? Do you toss it into a pond and watch the ripples flow outward?

Notice everything so far involves nouns, that is, tangible things. What about something more unconventional where you start thinking about adjectives and adverbs, like "gently . . . smooth . . . green . . . cool"? Using imagery here requires more creativity, and by expanding your imagination you would conceivably have more success. Perhaps "gently" evokes images of rocking a baby, "smooth" images of comfy pajamas, "green" images of a meadow, and "cool" images of a refreshing breeze while walking on a beach.

The sky's the limit, so I would encourage use of this cognitive–imagery combination as another tool for resolving any difficulties falling asleep or going back to sleep if awakened.

Still, with all you've learned in Chapters 10–15, not every technique works for every individual every time. Occasionally, and hopefully rarely, you may get stuck and frustrated over a particularly vexing sleepless night. Gravitating toward a few old fallback maneuvers in the heat of the battle may provide at least some relief. Distraction of the mind is the key to all these strategies, which can be used at bedtime or in the middle of the night. I'll list a few with a brief comment:

- Colorku is puzzle game, a colorized version of Sudoku. Instead of nine numbers, you are sorting nine round colored balls, and each of the nine squares on the board must be filled with all nine colors. The beauty of the game is it can be as challenging as you like, and if you look carefully at the color of each ball, soon you'll notice it's very difficult to maintain a rapid mental chatter.

- "Aural imagery" is the principle of turning off self-talk by listening to another sound. The most common sound is music. If you have a favorite lullaby or ballad-style artist (think Nat King Cole at the top of the list), the tune, the lyrics, and the style are so overwhelmingly pleasant, a person falls asleep to such input without ever realizing he or she is getting sleepy. Personal tastes dictate the choice.

- "Aural imagery technologically-derived" fits into the category of artificial white noise or natural white noise. These artificial devices act to mask out other noises and leave in their wake a steady hum or sound that hopefully is loud enough to block out the sound of your mind but not loud enough to stimulate you. I find the natural version more pleasing, something like rain on a roof with occasional distant thunder. An Internet search on your phone brings up hundreds of videos that often run for 10 straight hours of rain pouring down on a tin roof. On the rare occasion I've attempted this approach, the sound is remarkably soothing.

- Never underestimate advances in technology as new devices of distraction are frequently coming to the marketplace

- Also, as the emphasis in my *Sound Sleep, Sound Mind* book using the *Sleep Dynamic Therapy* model involves additional psychological approaches, it's another resource to consider for those seeking additional coverage in this area of sleep disorders.

- Finally, breathing "tricks" to induce sleepiness are widely offered. Buteyko, 4-7-8, and diaphragmatic breathing are popular modes that temporarily raise or lower carbon dioxide levels. This change promotes relaxation or sleepiness.

> ### Sleep Research Pearl #15

Sleep restriction remains controversial as it may cause an increase in daytime sleepiness by having "robbed" the individual of extra time asleep at night. The concern has merit but has received limited research attention, showing mixed results.[166;167] This theory also reflects biased perspectives among two factions of sleep physicians and researchers. One group favors the use of sleeping pills and often includes researchers who received funding from the pharmaceutical industry. A second group might include those who insist CBT-I is the be-all, end-all in the treatment of chronic insomnia.

The problem needs mentioning because specific patients are susceptible to this side effect of unintended daytime sleepiness. Traditionally, a very large proportion of chronic insomniacs report little or no sleepiness during the daytime. Harken back, please, to our discussions on tiredness versus sleepiness. These patients complain about tiredness and rarely if ever fall asleep during the daytime. Among this group, it is possible yet unlikely the loss of 30 or 60 minutes of sleep would cause this issue given these patients are usually very uncertain how many hours of sleep they are currently gaining. Such cases are usually the most difficult as the patients frequently draw cloudy pictures about when they go to bed, when they wake up, and how much sleep they are really receiving.

Another insomnia group, however, with a noticeable degree of daytime sleepiness, is more susceptible to this sleep restriction side effect, leading to a question about trade-offs. In the early phase of SRT, these individuals are ecstatic when they sleep more continuously through the night. The psychological respite of a "full" night of sleep does wonders for their mental outlook. However, there's an added cost if these individuals now suffer increased daytime sleepiness. This point is confusing and confounding because an individual might have slept fewer yet deeper hours, and therefore the expectation is no further daytime sleepiness whatsoever should have emerged.

Based on the principles in this book, you must also consider another underlying confound should the daytime sleepiness be triggered by untreated sleep-disordered breathing. In other words, by promoting continuous sleep during the night, perhaps an untreated SDB patient is exposed to more breathing events, leading to worse sleep fragmentation and thereby a cause for worse daytime sleepiness.

Regardless of the cause, the alternative approach of using sleeping pills is fraught with potholes, many of which you cannot easily drive through or around. First and foremost, based on our experience in the sleep lab, the majority of sleeping pill users do not obtain improvement in sleep architecture despite the pervasive advertising claims of deeper sleep and better quality sleep. Individuals may gain more continuous sleep, though if lighter it's a setup for worse sleep breathing events.[168] This side-effect may contribute to some sleeping pill users reporting more daytime sleepiness. Second, sleeping pills almost never cure insomnia, so you are going down a path treating a symptom and not addressing its cause. Third, benefits from sleeping pills wax and, more commonly, wane in far too many individuals, which lead them to switch to the next pill until the results wane again, leading to yet another pill. Fourth, sleeping pills cause side effects, particularly cognitive issues that worsen the longer you use the drugs.

Bottom line, SRT should be used vigorously in certain insomnia emergencies with proper guidance from a sleep specialist or other knowledgeable therapist. Once the emergency is over, sleep restriction may be employed over a long period of time if needed, but usually the restriction is a shorter interval, less likely to cause residual daytime sleepiness. Even so, anyone using SRT must be made aware of this potential side effect, especially as it would relate to morning commutes, driving commercial vehicles of any type, shift work, and engaging in any type of manual labor or physical activity where safety issues are present.

In my opinion, SRT is the much preferred pathway compared to drugs in the largest proportion of insomnia scenarios.

CHAPTER 16

Nightmares: A Very Treatable Condition

*Why do so few healthcare professionals realize nightmares or
disturbing dreams are a treatable sleep disorder?*

Direct Nightmare Treatment

Chronic nightmare patients are best treated with direct nightmare therapies, if only they knew such interventions existed! If this book were written in 1980, very little could be offered, but several historical developments have demonstrated chronic nightmares can be successfully eradicated with a cognitive-imagery technique known as *imagery rehearsal therapy* (IRT), the use of PAP therapy, the drug Prazosin, psychodynamic psychotherapy, several types of dream therapy, and emotion-focused therapies.

This knowledge remains largely obscure because chronic nightmares are still most commonly defined as a secondary symptom of an underlying mental health problem even though they only surface during sleep. In this circular view, anxiety dreams mean you suffer from daytime anxiety, which then triggers anxiety dreams when you sleep. Up until recently, the mental health scientific literature never spelled out the converse point of view— nightmares cause anxiety, so if you treat nightmares, anxiety will decrease.

These new and paradoxical theories cause confusion, because the individual nightmare sufferer does not really understand the nature of bad dreams despite feeling the psychological distress at night, as well as the aftershocks from bad dreams during the day. They are more than familiar with waking up at night sweating, short of breath, or heart pounding; and, they connect some of the dots between what happens at night with daytime residue like daymares, flashbacks, and other traumatic memories and images that feel very similar to the nightmare experience.

While wishing to fend off this 24/7 onslaught, a chronic nightmare sufferer usually doesn't know where or how to find relief while suffering from the problem for years or decades. The concept of direct nightmare treatment sounds odd because it implies placing nightmares at the top of a list of conditions to treat. And rarely would any therapist or other mental health professional recommend nightmare treatment as a first step.

Finally, making matters more confusing, how could so many different treatment pathways solve this particular condition that for centuries has always been perceived as an uncontrollable, unconscious behavior? Though it seems reasonable multiple types of psychotherapy or drugs might work, how do we explain the effectiveness of such diverse treatment approaches as mind's eye mental imagery or PAP therapy?

Let's tackle this conundrum by taking a step back, asking what causes nightmares and why they persist for so long?

The Key: Nightmares Are an Independent Disorder, Mental or Sleep—Take Your Pick

People develop nightmares for many reasons, most due to psychological or mental health factors. Our understanding of human nature makes clear that a stressful or traumatizing experience could lead to disturbing dreams or nightmares about these events. Most mental health professionals believe nightmares are natural, if not healthy, in the early going after trauma or other difficult life events. The nightmares serve the purpose of "forcing" the person to confront, work through (emotional processing), and overcome painful emotions and troubling memories from a traumatic event the individual survived.

The theory of nightmares serving a purpose is well established and valid, but in the long run many patients with chronic nightmares do not accept this viewpoint after suffering disturbing dreams years on end. As the very best example, consider patients seeking treatment for PTSD. After completing successful specialized psychotherapy, nightmares often persist. Then the patient rightfully asks, "My PTSD was treated with excellent results, so why do the disturbing dreams persist?"

Exposure therapy, the highly effective PTSD treatment discussed previously,

243

reduces or eliminates posttraumatic stress symptoms; yet scant evidence suggests this therapy consistently resolves posttraumatic nightmares. In fact, mounting evidence reveals nightmares persist after various mental health treatments for other psychological disorders, such as anxiety or depression.

The unexpected findings from PTSD studies conducted all over the world, combined with our research studies on nightmare treatment, stimulated new theories, chief of which states: **nightmares take on a life of their own after the trauma and require a specific treatment distinct from PTSD therapies.** Our view is nightmares or "nightmaring behavior" (a term developed by my friend and colleague Dr. Michael Hollifield)[20] becomes entrenched in the brain, leading the mind to develop a learned behavior—the habit of experiencing nightmares. The nightmare experience repeats over time in susceptible PTSD patients or other psychiatric patients.

We recognize trauma itself triggered the nightmares, but it seems as if this learned behavior sustains the nightmares in the long term.

Can You Unlearn to Suffer from Nightmares?

The learned behavior theory of nightmares is difficult to digest and absorb among nightmare sufferers. Resistance to this theory arises within nightmare patients who were repeatedly counseled over the years the only way to treat nightmares is to treat PTSD. "Treat PTSD, and nightmares should disappear." If you heard only this perspective for several years and from several mental health professionals, a conflict emerges when we offer this newer theory of nightmares as a learned behavior.

Perhaps, you need to pause, take a deep breath, and ask whether you are ready to consider this new idea of the learned behavior theory. This thought-provoking theory creates an intriguing opportunity for self-empowerment. Specifically, if a behavior is learned, there is potential to unlearn it, which suggests nightmare patients possess a capacity to directly influence their own bad dreams. This direct influence may arise outside the traditional spheres of psychotherapy or psychotropic medications.

Rather, it may exist inside your own mind.

Have I got your attention?

Our first glimpse of this theory emerged by gaining insights from the vast majority of individuals who report nightmares soon after traumatic exposure. Contrary to what you might have heard elsewhere, an extremely large proportion of trauma survivors develop nightmares early on, yet the bad dreams disappear within a few days to a couple weeks. Eight out of 10 people suffer events in their lifetime that trigger posttraumatic stress symptoms or PTSD, yet fewer than one out of 10 continue to experience a chronic nightmare problem.

Clearly, some individuals manifest greater risks for persisting bad dreams and nightmares lasting years or decades, after which it seems disturbing dreams no longer serve a purpose other than making life and sleep miserable. The percentage of those suffering chronic nightmares or other disturbing dreams may be as low as 4% to as high as 8% of adults in Western civilization. That's a lot of people.

The big question is "Why do nightmares disappear in so many people who have suffered trauma?" If we could explain this spontaneous improvement, then we could probably find ways to help those patients where nightmares persist.

Setting the Stage for New Treatments for Chronic Nightmares

The oldest treatment theory involved dream interpretation. More recently, the idea developed that specific mental health treatments (drugs or psychotherapy) of mental disorders would yield a decrease in bad dreams. And most recently, there is a medication known as Prazosin that works to treat nightmares in certain patients.[169] Finally, on the cutting edge, we and others have published scientific articles on treating sleep breathing problems as a way to decrease nightmares, though this research is in the early stages.

This array of treatment options unequivocally informs us how the very logical and simple explanation linking trauma to nightmares is no longer a satisfactory or complete theory on the nature of disturbing dreams. While this unexpected insight on nightmares is great news, it is imperative to recognize how many medical and mental health providers know almost nothing about this research and related clinical studies.

Which brings us to the learned behavior theory, a thought-provoking approach in light of its success rate using treatment based on an "unlearning" method. Again, paradoxically, this approach as well as some mentioned previously, do not place attention on the cause of the nightmares. The learned behavior theory of nightmares never discounts the fact trauma gives birth to nightmares. Instead, newer approaches do not address what caused the nightmares because nightmares may decrease or disappear without ever having to explore or discuss the cause of the bad dreams.

Sounds very counterintuitive, doesn't it?

These findings laid the foundation of the learned behavior theory of nightmares and raised related questions, such as:

- How can you tell when your nightmares are a learned behavior?
- Does the original trauma still influence nightmares even after suffering from bad dreams for months or years or decades?
- When nightmares are a learned behavior, what works to unlearn them?

In your efforts going forward, keep in mind you are likely to experience resistance when you broach this topic with mental health providers who are wedded to the belief treating your primary mental health disorder (PTSD, depression, anxiety) is the only sure way to treat your nightmares. This exclusive mental health perspective is questionable, and after you hear more evidence about all the other options, I believe and hope you will welcome the various methods from which to choose.

We start with the treatment that is arguably the most powerful nightmare treatment ever developed, and it utilizes the same system we described in the treatment of insomnia—the human imagery system.

Imagery Rehearsal Therapy

In our work with nightmare treatment dating back more than three decades, we developed *imagery rehearsal therapy* where you learn to work directly with nightmares while awake. The technique is simple and straightforward: ask the nightmare sufferer to **select** a disturbing dream, **change** it while awake into something different, and then **picture** the changed version of the dream (we call it the "new dream") using mind's eye imagery.

Even though these steps are not applied while sleeping, the effort apparently influences what you will or will not dream about at night. You may not necessarily dream about the "new dream" you created, but the process of actively working with your daytime imagery seems to deliver a lingering and favorable influence on your dream imagery while sleeping.

This technique, originally described as "auto-suggested" dreams dates in the scientific literature to 1934,[170] but our research team was fortunate in 1992 to have published the first randomized controlled trials proving the efficacy (it works) of imagery rehearsal therapy,[22;27] or IRT as it is now called (coined by Dr. Hollifield).[20] Since then we published other randomized controlled trials on many different types of nightmare patients, and our hallmark study involved sexual assault survivors with PTSD and chronic nightmares, which was the lead article in *JAMA* in August 2001.

This study showed IRT worked successfully in PTSD patients, but more noteworthy, it showed treatment of nightmares decreased our patients' PTSD symptoms as well. We conducted long-term follow-ups of 18 and 30 months on other patients who applied IRT, and they also sustained their improvements. Numerous other researchers and therapists throughout the world have either completed their own research investigations into IRT or have integrated IRT into their clinical practices, all with resounding success. In fact, in July 2016, the first Nightmare Treatment Summit was held in Düsseldorf, Germany, which gathered 20 of the leading nightmare treatment experts from around the globe. Unquestionably, IRT and its variations received the most attention at the conference.[32]

In our experience with IRT, disturbing dreams start decreasing within a few weeks or a few months following just a few minutes of practice each or every other day. As a point of context, bear in mind we are describing trauma survivors who have suffered from posttraumatic stress symptoms, including nightmares, for years or decades, and after only a few weeks of using IRT, they reported changes in their dreams for the better. Initially, the change might be a decrease in frequency or change in intensity, but as weeks become months among people who actively used the IRT method, greater than 90% reported clear and satisfactory reductions in their nightmares. A fair number reported a cure.

Tips on IRT Use

The simplicity of IRT steps may confuse first-time users because so little effort is required to achieve results. The first step, selecting a nightmare or bad dream, seems obvious enough; still, remember this caveat: do **not** start with the worst nightmare you ever experienced, and do **not** use nightmares that feel like a replay of an actual event you have lived through.

Make things easier on yourself by selecting a bad dream that does not vividly replay real-life events and does not produce the most severe distress levels when you recall it. In other words, you will be targeting more severe nightmares later, once you feel comfortable applying the IRT steps.

Upon selecting this bad dream, there is absolutely no objective to spend time reflecting on the dream's content; as soon as you choose a disturbing dream, go to step two and immediately engage your imagination (the mind's eye) to change the images to something different than the original nightmare.

Got it? You are awake, so do not let the nightmare play in your mind like a broken record. Instead, just make the decision, often coming from instinct or from your gut or directly from the mind's eye, to change certain aspects of the nightmare, changing content of any type to make it a "new dream."

What should you change? We follow the original instructions of Dr. Joseph Neidhardt, one of my three main mentors on nightmare treatment. Dr. Neidhardt's exact words were "change the nightmare any way you wish."[22;27] Which literally means change the beginning, or the middle, or the ending. Change one scene in the dream out of 10 scenes, or change all 10 scenes. Change a color in the dream, change a smell, change the lighting—or change the whole thing to create a brand-new location and dialogue—everything different or just a little different. It does not seem to matter.

Now take your new creation, the new dream, and close your eyes, and for the next few minutes—anywhere from two to 20 minutes—rehearse the new dream you have created. Rehearsing for longer periods is not typically needed. Some only rehearse a couple minutes or less.

If you would like an additional resource, my wife, Jessica, and I created the *Turning Nightmares into Dreams* audio workbook manual, and it remains a very popular tool for both patients and therapists who desire more coaching on the use of IRT for nightmare treatment. The workbook contains 20 lessons, and each lesson includes a brief audio section, usually five to 10 minutes, and few workbook pages. The workbook runs 100 pages and includes graphics, charts, fill-in-the-blank exercises, and tips on skills development, all of which are easy to use.

You can find *Turning Nightmares into Dreams* on our three main websites, www.nightmaretreatment.com and www.barrykrakowmd.com and www.sleeptreatment.com.

Refining the Learned Behavior Theory of Chronic Nightmares

Since 1988, we tried making sense of these remarkable findings. It has certainly been a fortunate experience, for which I feel blessed, being among those able to pioneer and spread the word on a treatment that provides so much relief to so many people who suffered for so long from vexing dreams.

As I learned more by encountering so many patients with problematic nightmares and treating so many, I attempted to refine the learned behavior theory. In so doing, my approach has transitioned into a more precise theory about the human imagery system.

Simply stated, we all accept the development of nightmares after trauma as a natural response. However, most of us forget, as mentioned earlier, that the largest proportion of those traumatized see their nightmares disappear within days or weeks or months. And to reiterate, spontaneously!

If the natural experience of most patients is "nightmares come and go" over short periods of time, what is the crucial distinction revealed by this acute natural healing tendency compared to those whose nightmares persist for months or years? Is there something in the human imagery system that explains why or how disturbing dreams do or do not diminish early on after trauma? Finally, does the mind innately possess its own capacity toward an IRT mechanism to jump-start this naturally occurring healing process, so common to many traumatized individuals?

We can turn to the field of dream research for some answers. When a dream therapist works with a trauma survivor, the patient undergoes a dream metamorphosis during which the patient's nightmares are gradually changing over a relatively short period of time depending on the success of the dream therapy.[171]

In *dream therapy*, the patient and the therapist emphasize the salient content of the dreams and the precise emotions within the dreams at the very first appointment. Engaged in this emotional processing technique, the patient often returns at the next appointment and is already reporting changes in his or her nightmare images or other dream content. And after several weeks or months, such a patient may report the dreams have changed so much, they are no longer disturbing or nightmarish. Or, the frequency of bad dreams is lessened so much, coping is easier.

From this known evidence from the field of dream research, we could hypothesize the exact or nearly identical process must be underway in those who develop nightmares but for whom no formal therapy was provided. That is, they are receiving "self-therapy," the mind's natural tendency to change the images in the dreams. Within the brief span of weeks or months after the trauma, we know most people do not seek counseling, and yet most report nightmares disappear.

The parsimonious explanation for these results would be a natural tendency of the human mind to work through the nightmare images using mental imagery, which causes them to change into non-nightmare dreams. From the outside looking in, we might call this process spontaneous, but I think it more useful to give due credit to the mind's natural capacity to heal.

Because of its survival value, I cannot think of a good reason to counter this idea. Perhaps, in the short run, it makes sense to dream about the trauma to remind you to be safe or safer in similar situations encountered in the future. Then, once you "get the message," why would you need to keep dreaming the same disturbing images?

Said another way, if this pathway is what occurs in dream therapy, most likely the same metamorphosis is occurring naturally in the human mind. Therefore, among chronic nightmare patients, perhaps IRT inserts itself into this metamorphosis to catalyze the necessary transformations. If so, we speculate those with chronic nightmares are suffering some blockage in this natural transformation, or perhaps the mind got stuck. Had this barrier never been present, the argument would be the patient's nightmares would have receded in a short time, as they in fact do for so many more people who don't develop chronic nightmare conditions after traumatic events.

Digging Still Deeper into the Mind's Eye

Assuming IRT encourages or influences this changing process within the dreams, we further speculate on a very specific mechanism regarding how images are formed in the mind's eye and how they could be affected by waking imagery. Let's take an example of a patient seeking help through dream therapy a few months after a trauma or a few years after unresolved posttraumatic stress symptoms.

A successful timeline might go as follows. The individual first describes a dream to the dream therapist that feels like a replay of the traumatic event. The dream may be something very close to an exact replay or replay-like, wherein the patient describes scenes, feelings, and sensations that convince the individual this particular nightmare is clearly linked to the traumatic event due to the degree of similarity.

The patient then discusses his or her emotions experienced during the dream, and the therapist instructs the patient to attempt to "work through" these emotions. *Working through* refers to the idea of experiencing difficult emotions, including painful aspects of these feelings, with the goal of coming out on the other end having accepted these feelings and, ideally, having learned something from the emotions. (Note the similarity in this description to the concepts of "emotional processing" discussed in Chapters 12–14). Within just a few sessions, it would be common for the metamorphosis to commence, and soon the individual returns to clinic and reports the disturbing dreams feel less replay-like and appear more symbolic.

What's the difference between replay and symbolic? If a person were traumatized by a physical assault in a parking lot, then a replay or replay-like set of images would feel or look or seem like an attack in a parking lot, whereas a symbolic representation of such events re-creates very similar feelings of being under attack or being hurt, but now the dream image might convey the sense of being overwhelmed, for example, by dreaming you are swept away by a tidal wave or unable to stand your ground against fierce hurricane winds. Such dreams are common and may symbolize the original assault, and if so, this transformation suggests the dream therapy is working because the images moved from actual event images to symbolic pictures.

In this example, another possibility for the change in dream content might look like an open area or open space that's not exactly a parking lot, and the attack might be less precise, as if someone were going to attack or there was a concern of an imminent attack, but the attack actually does not occur in the dream. This variation again suggests a transformation is underway as the dream is no longer a replay or replay-like; if the person reported this variation early in dream therapy, it would be a fairly obvious change and likely indicator of the images shifting into a symbolic form.

Over time, with more dream therapy, the images continue to transform or metamorphosize until eventually the nightmares are gone or the dreams are considerably less disturbing, if at all.

Summing up, these types of experiences with dream therapists reconfirm the human mind is naturally geared to solve the problem of nightmares and probably does so rather easily through the system described above. For those nightmare patients where this system does not appear to function well, IRT is probably jump-starting this natural process. In some ways, you could argue IRT is not a therapy at all; rather, it is a technique to teach you how to pay attention to your mind's eye in a way that will eventually yield the desired natural transformation of dream imagery to make bad dreams less disturbing, and eventually no longer bad dreams at all.

Why Do Other Nightmare Treatment Options Also Work?

The changing views on chronic nightmare disorders are further confirmed by the evidence of so many different successful therapies, and yet it appears confusing why nightmares would respond to so much variation in treatment. Usually, the more we know about how something works, such as with any specific therapeutic technique, the more confidence it generates among professionals providing the treatment, as well as among patients seeking help for the condition. Both patients and healthcare professionals are more willing to try out a therapy when a valid explanation indicates how or why the treatment should work. Penicillin is time and evidence tested for treating strep throat and, more importantly, preventing rheumatic fever. Antibiotics kill bacteria and thereby dissipate their toxic by-products as well—pretty simple.

Above, we described theories on how the human imagery system may naturally resolve nightmares through a process where dream images either change over time on their own or are stimulated to change by the treatment known as IRT. Is there something similar we can describe about Prazosin, now considered an option by some mental health professionals for the treatment of nightmares? Likewise, why would PAP therapy used to treat sleep apnea patients cause nightmares to decrease?

The short answer is we do not know the mechanisms to explain these results, but working theories may provide some understanding and give you more confidence if you wish to consider these options.

Prazosin most likely works by reducing a PTSD patient's reactivity to certain stimuli. PTSD patients suffer symptoms of hypervigilance and hyperarousal during waking hours; therefore, nightmares and insomnia surely reflect a continuation of this hyper state, which in medical terms is called *high noradrenergic activity*, meaning the neurotransmitter norepinephrine fuels the rush of energy that makes one's mind and body feel overly activated (that is, fright, flight, or fight response).

In this scenario, if there were a drug to block the effects of noradrenergic activity, it would make sense the severity level of the hyperarousal would be lessened. In fact, Prazosin is a drug that blocks the actions of the "α_1(alpha-1) adrenergic receptor" in the brain's prefrontal cortex, which leads to decreases in various PTSD symptoms, including nightmares. Thus, Prazosin receives the pharmacologic label "α_1 adrenergic receptor antagonist."

To my knowledge, nothing about this theory suggests Prazosin is directly targeting the human imagery system. Instead, the drug is decreasing the reactivity accompanying nightmares. Conceivably, a person on Prazosin still might suffer nightmares, but the intensity of the dreaming experience decreases so much the individual no longer perceives the dreams as nightmarish.

Dovetailing with this idea is the telltale clinical experience described by many patients who stopped using Prazosin altogether (for whatever reasons) after months or years of successful eradication of their disturbing dreams; namely, a noticeable return of the nightmares to levels as painful as originally experienced.

This issue raises questions on how long someone can safely use Prazosin, and the good news is the medication may be used by many people for months or years. Furthermore, the side effects seem to be mild and rare in general, the most common one being dizziness, lightheadedness, or fainting when moving too quickly from a lying position to sitting or standing. In other words, don't get out of bed quickly when using Prazosin until you clarify whether the drug affects you in this way. Like many other drugs that act on the central nervous system, other symptoms, though less common, include drowsiness, headache, low energy, nausea, and nervousness. A prescribing physician will alert you to other relevant side effects that might be specific to your case.

Finally, it may also turn out that knowledge will expand to show a connection to noradrenergic activity in the human imagery system. Available evidence already shows how noradrenergic activity is linked to emotional memory consolidation, which explains in part how Prazosin could thwart the intensity of the emotions triggered by nightmare activation.

While this change in reactivity would appear to be a downstream influence on the disturbing feelings occurring during bad dreams, we could speculate the brain, with so many millions of synaptic connections, might then transmit a feedback signal to the visualization centers of the brain that influence the dream imagery. I could not find any research supporting this hypothesis, but dream researchers and other neuroscientists are likely groups to investigate such links.

Treating Sleep Apnea Treats Nightmares

The working theory on sleep apnea is you awaken more frequently, so you remember more dreams, good or bad. The overarching problem of sleep disruption and fragmentation caused by sleep apnea certainly could occur prior to a nightmare. However, we don't know if sleep apnea simply makes you more aware of your nightmares or whether sleep apnea actually causes or worsens nightmares. When using PAP therapy, we could speculate that improved sleep consolidation decreases awakenings, thereby making you less aware of bad dreams.

Although this theory has some validity, it's paradoxical because using a PAP machine effectively leads to an uptick in well-consolidated REM sleep such that the average patient reports more awareness of dreaming. Thus, nightmare awareness reduction appears too simplistic.

Many clinical psychologists, dream therapists, and dream and nightmare researchers strongly believe REM sleep has numerous higher-level functions that transcend the act of sleeping. Numerous studies suggest REM facilitates remembering things, learning things, and more effectively processing emotional experiences in one's life. If all these functions were factually proven, then REM really is a therapist-in-residence because in any good therapy session you must remember events that affected you and then try to learn something from these experiences, and throughout the session you must work on emotionally processing (again, working through) both your memories and what you have learned. REM sounds like a pretty powerful medicine, don't you think?

Therefore, a more potent working theory regarding nightmares and sleep apnea might relate to the specific sleep fragmentation of REM sleep stage. As might be obvious, REM sleep must be connected directly to your imagery system because you are picturing things in your dreams, and your most vivid dreams seem to occur in REM. Therefore, when sleep apnea disrupts REM, which it appears to do quite easily, it must be having an impact on the links between REM and your imagery system. Simply by treating sleep apnea, this linkage is now restored to its normal functioning. Conceivably, the explanation may be as simple as treating OSA/CSA/UARS leads to decreases in nightmares, because REM is again permitted to work in its normal state and function.

In trauma survivors who suffer from both PTSD and SDB, we would expect a great deal of overall sleep fragmentation; and, depending on personal sensitivities, we would expect varying degrees of REM sleep fragmentation. As discussed in the earlier chapters, we focus a great deal of attention on consolidation of REM sleep when titrating patients on their PAP devices. We anticipate future research will demonstrate connections between the consolidation of REM sleep and more normalized functioning of the human imagery system, all of which would contribute to the theory of how a breathing device decreases disturbing dreams and nightmares.

As a footnote, we should never discount the possibility that difficulty in breathing during sleep is likely to induce an unconscious fear response of varying degrees of intensity. Perhaps, this fear provokes bad dreams. If so, normalization of breathing should eliminate the fear and thus the nightmares.

Finally, although high quality randomized controlled trials have not been conducted as yet on the impact of PAP on nightmares, there are roughly 10 studies strongly pointing to the likelihood PAP decreases nightmares.[172;173] Therefore, please keep this pathway available as a reasonable option in light of the strong probability you may be suffering from a sleep breathing disorder.

Additional Psychotherapies

We've mentioned four methods. The last two involved psychodynamic psychotherapy and exposure therapy, including EMDR (eye movement desensitization and reprocessing). All these psychotherapies invest considerable focus and energy on resolving emotional conflicts or otherwise helping the individual process difficult emotional experiences. Thus, when these therapies are successful, and they are highly effective when applied by well-trained and experienced mental health professionals, they lead to marked reductions in emotional tension.

Any drop-off in emotional tension usually leads to decreases in other symptoms. For example, suppose an individual were treated with psychodynamic therapy for anxiety and chronic headaches. It's a distinct possibility both the anxiety and the headaches (if related to tension) would improve markedly after a successful course of therapy.

This same pattern holds when someone is treated for PTSD and nightmares. An exposure therapy such as EMDR might prove very successful in decreasing posttraumatic stress symptoms, of which nightmares are a common one. Therefore, in some cases, the nightmares will dissipate to a large extent.

Earlier, I mentioned these emotion-based therapies may not work to reduce nightmares, so to reiterate, while these therapies are highly effective in the right hands, some patients respond accordingly and nightmares diminish, whereas some patients improve their PTSD, yet nightmares persist.

Because so many people with PTSD are offered exposure therapies, and other mental health patients may be offered psychodynamic psychotherapies, I want to be clear that substantial benefits are likely to be gained from these methods, but unfortunately, if they are not successful in diminishing nightmares, another treatment pathway for the disturbing dreams should be considered.

Concluding Thoughts on Nightmare Treatment

One of the more fascinating discoveries we learned from the original landmark

IRT study in *JAMA* was finding out several years later that many nightmare patients were at the time actually suffering from undiagnosed sleep-disordered breathing. Even so, IRT produced stellar results. This information will prove useful in upgrading assessments and treatments to yield better results for our patients. Unfortunately, many experts from other fields of healthcare may be missing out on these connections by failing to explore these unexpected streams of knowledge.

In my opinion, these previously uncharted waters must now be more vigorously navigated, and we expect to learn about much larger adverse impacts generated by sleep and sleep disorders on conditions like PTSD and depression. For example, and of special interest to this chapter, you may recall we discussed RBD, or REM behavior disorder, in Chapter 9 on parasomnias, but we've not discussed RBD here. Perhaps you can guess why; IRT, as the best example, is not a treatment thought to work on the acting out behavior of RBD. More so, if someone used PAP therapy in an alleged RBD case and the bad dreams resolved, most likely the patient was incorrectly diagnosed with RBD. This refresher is mentioned here because RBD is a very different type of disorder and not really like nightmares. When RBD is in the picture, nightmare treatment should never be applied as a first-line therapy, and in most cases, it would probably not prove a treatment consideration.

Please keep two more related things in mind. First, if anything about your nightmares makes you suspicious of parasomnias beyond RBD, please go back to the review on parasomnias in the second half of Chapter 9. If pertinent, make an appointment to discuss your concerns with the appropriate doctor. Second, regarding psychotropic medications, drugs are often prescribed with the very best of intentions, but frequently make sleep worse. These drugs may interfere with more comprehensive treatment programs by misdirecting resources to the exclusion of sleep and sleep disorders. Finally, and on a good note, sometimes these drugs can provide unexpected benefits for your sleep. We'll explore a few of these points in the next chapter.

> ## Sleep Research Pearl #16

In the first decade of IRT research publications (1992–2001), considerable pushback on the validity and benefits of this self-empowering technique was pressed by two groups of experts. Because IRT worked on posttraumatic nightmares, numerous trauma and PTSD experts expressed concern that our approach was dismissive of the underlying trauma. They insisted IRT wasn't really what it claimed to be, that is, a mind's eye mental imagery therapeutic method, but rather, IRT was another form of desensitization or exposure therapy; they speculated the patients were spending a lot of time thinking about their nightmares, so over time the nightmares went away.

The second group comprised traditional psychoanalytic psychotherapists, for example, Jungian therapists who insisted elimination of the nightmares wasted valuable resources because the nightmare patients could no longer access the valuable dream content from their disturbing dreams since they no longer suffered from nightmares.

To all those who raised concerns or questions about IRT, we responded with one question of our own: "Do you think sleeping better after suffering from nightmares for years and often decades is a worthy therapeutic goal?" Why did we raise this question? Because "yes" was the deafening response we received from the vast majority of nightmare patients who decreased or eliminated their bad dreams. Now on the receiving end of sound sleep, they were ecstatic with this pronounced drop-off in disturbing dreams, not to mention their satisfaction with the ease of treatment. Moreover, making a large dent in their crippling fatigue, low energy, or sleepiness produced immediate gains in quality of life. Having failed so many prior therapies, including numerous drugs and psychotherapies, even PTSD therapies, their desperation brought them to our doorstep.

After treatment, we discussed with several of our patients the complaints lodged by these dream or trauma experts who disparaged IRT. The patients were not only stunned by such criticism, but also angry that healthcare professionals would not acknowledge their incredible gains from sleeping better by no longer being assaulted night after night in their dream worlds. Moreover, no patients developed "symptom substitution," the problem of new symptoms springing up or worsening after eliminating a different symptom. According to the dream and trauma experts who insisted IRT was not targeting the cause of nightmares, new symptoms were bound to emerge after the use of this "far-too-simple" therapy. In fact, the great news for nightmare patients was the decrease in nightmares led to improvement in several other symptoms.

To this day, many healthcare professionals know next to nothing about nightmare disorders, many have never heard of IRT or even the concept of treating nightmare disorders, and finally, many, many, many still scoff or otherwise dismiss this evidence-based non-exposure treatment because it doesn't fit their working niche as a psychoanalyst or trauma specialist.

IRT most likely works because of the way an individual "sees" a new set of images; these new images may trigger changes in the way the brain heals itself from bad dreams and nightmares. Ironic, then, that these experts cannot "see" the value of IRT.

CHAPTER 17

A Fresh Look at Psychotropic Drugs, Hypersomnias & Napping

What are the unrecognized relationships between psychotropic drugs and sleep disorders, and how does excessive sleepiness or napping behavior fit into my treatment plan?

Revisiting Medications

Psychotropic medications (drugs that target the brain, usually for mental health and sleep conditions)—including pills for depression, anxiety, PTSD, mood disorders, bipolar disorder, panic attacks, obsessive-compulsive disorder, sleep disorders, insomnia, and nonrestorative sleep—often stir up controversies about effectiveness and side effects. In my opinion, it's more important to ask, "Are psychotropic medications as potent as non-drug treatments?"

This question is not seeking to invalidate the necessity, potency, and utility of drugs to help certain patients in certain circumstances, whether in the short term or long term.

So, then, am I antidrug or biased against the use of psychotropic medications?

Not at all, if the prescribed drugs are used judiciously and yield clear-cut, very good to great results. In contrast, I want you to recognize when you engage a highly competent therapist (whether a mental health expert or a sleep specialist) head-to-head against a drug treatment, in the majority of instances (I acknowledge it might be a vast or slim majority), the nondrug treatment would prove superior to a medication(s).

Now here's the caveat you already know: finding an expert in mental health therapies or behavioral sleep medicine therapies is not easy. Sadly, many patients are faced with the tough choice to work with fair to good (instead of excellent to outstanding) mental health or sleep therapists versus sticking with a medication treatment yielding only average results. After all, if you only get average results from therapists and getting the same average results with a pill, why put in more effort with therapy?

A lot of patients, and especially professionals in these fields, would take issue with my viewpoint, and I am all for a debate. Regrettably, my sense is no debate is forthcoming from within large segments of mental health or sleep fields, because once professionals create a set of "authoritative standards of excellence," it takes years before they turn a critical eye back on these standards to earnestly examine how well their patients are served.

I can understand if the above sounds a bit too theoretical and certainly "political," but let me offer three practical corroborating points. First, when I spend time with expert mental health researchers and therapists, as well as similar sleep professionals, to discuss skills, competence, and results, which I have done on a regular basis for more than 30 years, I am regularly stunned (though now desensitized) by how many top-notch professionals of all stripes complain about mediocrity in their own fields.

Second, as a prime example that occurs over and over again, some therapists still employ the "talk therapy" discussed previously in the EFT chapters, which in its highly intellectualized form seems an outdated modality that rarely works except for extremely mild symptoms and routine circumstances. Talk therapy actually keeps more complex patients from recovery by maintaining their comfort level instead of challenging the individual to consider new ideas and insights.

And third, it is almost unbelievable how few behavioral sleep therapists actually exist in the field of sleep medicine, which means you could shop at 10 different sleep centers in one city and still not find a highly experienced sleep professional to work on the psychological aspects of insomnia. Moreover, *ad nauseum*, you can rarely find a highly experienced sleep professional that understands and treats UARS.

In contrast, I cannot say enough good things about highly competent therapists in sleep or mental health practices. If you are fortunate to find someone of this caliber, you will gain substantial progress in your efforts to manage and in some cases conquer your sleep disorders and psychiatric conditions, often through combination therapies that include medications. Lamentably, when you are assessing your own personal experiences or when you ask around, you will discover many professionals in these fields do not receive an A or even a B grade for their capacity to help the individual to solve or dramatically improve mental health or sleep health.

And to reiterate and assist you in your own exploration, too many mental health therapists often limit their practice to "talk therapy"—a method frequently viewed as professional malpractice by some psychology or psychiatry experts who now understand the need for more challenging approaches when interacting with their patients.

By *challenging*, I am not suggesting confrontation, although some therapies achieve success through such techniques. Challenging means patients are enlisted to do more exercises and homework outside of actual therapy sessions. In contrast, we now know various types of advanced therapies succeed in resolving mental problems in patients who failed other therapy programs where too much talking and thinking were emphasized in the therapy session itself. Instead, more advanced strategies teach precision techniques on how to feel and attend to emotions properly, or how to use the body during exercise and at work to relieve bodily tension, or how to use the imagination as the natural bridge between thoughts and feelings to gain more rapid insights into core emotional conflicts. These approaches—unlike talk therapy—lead to faster and more in-depth understanding of mental health difficulties, as well as providing lifelong tools a patient may apply in the future.

The same could be said about sleep therapists where so little is actually done to engage patients in how to use PAP therapy, or where the prescription pad pops up before the patients finish one short verbal paragraph about their insomnia.

I do not want to depress you by slamming some mental health and sleep specialists, suggesting you can only find mediocre care. My goal is to encourage caution and patience in selecting someone to work with in either field. A quick clue in searching would be to ask whether or not a certain practice for mental health and sleep problems gravitates toward medications. Specifically, when calling around or searching the Internet, start by asking this question sooner than later: "What therapies do you offer for my conditions besides medications?" The answers should prove revealing and expedite your search.

If you want to argue these medications must remain available as a reasonable Plan B, I'm fully supportive; however, why aren't there more efforts in disseminating the nondrug Plan A therapies instead? Plan A options in these situations are the advanced psychotherapies of which there are numerous, including *acceptance and commitment therapy* and *dialectical behavioral therapy*, two well-established, evidence-based methods. Many more are available, though not as well researched. And, EFT therapies are also highly effective.

In sum, mental health and sleep conditions may prove diabolically multifaceted, which paradoxically is why medications are so frequently not up to the task and yet so frequently prescribed. In so many cases, a medication is unlikely to address all the emotional or sleep difficulties that one individual experiences as he or she descends into a realm of darkness and despair. We as humans are just not smart enough to be able to scientifically produce a perfected chemical recipe to completely and irrevocably reverse all the misery from which mental health and sleep patients suffer.

What If My Only Option Is Medication?

Actually, medication is never your only option, but for sure, it could be the most expedient, reasonable, and appropriate option for an individual with acute suicidal feelings or depression so bad you are no longer able to function in your daily life. From our standpoint in the field of sleep medicine, we understand the need for acute psychiatric therapy, including the use of sleep aids for suicidal patients with unrelenting insomnia. Notwithstanding, we are concerned drug therapy is being pushed on patients willy-nilly before they have been evaluated for undiagnosed sleep disorders. To our eyes, it appears most physicians and therapists are unable to recognize these sleep comorbidities and the need for other treatment pathways.

As we near the end of the book, you may be wondering about or predicting how many depressed individuals or PTSD sufferers you know that are actually afflicted with a nonrestorative sleep problem caused by a sleep breathing disorder or a leg jerk disorder, not to mention their equally disabling insomnia or nightmares. To be sure, these people suffer from sleep disorders plus their mental health disorders, but if the sleep disorders were diagnosed and treated, concurrent benefits would be gained in the mental health realm. In some, mental health problems might all but disappear when it turns out the underlying source is sleep disruption, not simply the previously presumed psychologically or psychiatrically defined disorders.

If you offered a guess on the percentage of these individuals in which sleep disorders are "masquerading" as mental health disorders, I suspect your answer would be somewhere along the continuum of "a lot to a heckuva lot" suffer from disregarded, undiagnosed, and untreated sleep disorders. Which brings us to the questions you need to be raising and re-raising throughout your dealings with your providers: how and to what extent are these underlying sleep disorders worsening your mood, impairing your memory, and disabling your coping capacity? And do these impairments ultimately compromise your judgments and degrade your decision making, leading to overall corruption of your brain's efforts to function successfully day in and day out?

And never forget to ask about what's going on with your delta and REM sleep, or lack thereof, when trying to discern the mental health versus the sleep health contributions to your current psychiatric/psychological woes. There can be no question that fragmented REM or scarcity of delta sleep will make things worse, but you must press your various providers to pay attention to these critical stages of sleep.

As you begin or continue to monitor your experiences, behaviors, and attitudes to assess your mental state of affairs, now is the time to also ask yourself whether the medication is making a small, medium, or large difference in the quality of your life. If the answer is a small one, it would seem the right time for discussing new options with your prescribing physician or psychologist, as well as a skilled therapist, not to mention your sleep doctor, primary care physician, or other prescribing provider.

If you are gaining medium to large benefits from the medication, then the good news is you may have found the right combination of drugs or the single drug best for you. If so, there may be no bad news unless the results obtained from these drugs somehow steer you away from taking more than a fleeting glance at your sleep problems.

But These Drugs Help Me Sleep!

Do they? Are you sure? Just how certain are you pills help you fall asleep or help you stay asleep? Most importantly, how certain are you these pills improve the quality of your sleep? Are you getting more REM sleep or more delta deep sleep? Probably not. A considerable amount of research already shows many drugs prescribed to help sleep continuity are rated very poorly regarding sleep benefits, particularly when it comes to sleep depth.

The main reason for the low rating is drugs just do not work well when studied in large samples of patients over the long haul. Specifically, these drugs have not been perfected to work on the problem of insomnia or nonrestorative sleep in ways similar to the way an antibiotic cures bacterial infections or the way an antihypertensive pill consistently lowers blood pressure. To be absolutely sure, there are patients who swear by their use of Trazodone or Seroquel, and in some cases, we presume they are the fortunate cases actually getting deeper sleep, not just enhanced sleep continuity; nonetheless, not every user of these medications receives such pronounced benefits, yet providers continue to prescribe them without investigating the full scope of their impact on each individual's sleep.

Distinctions between drugs that really work well and those that sort of work is an essential point of understanding most mental health patients must chew on, swallow, and fully digest. In essence, as there are few perfected mental health medications, prescribing physicians cultivate the mindset of "well, at least it's something." But it may not be something for many people.

It may make things worse, especially if the drug interferes, as many do, with REM sleep and delta sleep.

When you understand this point of distinction, you will further appreciate (as if you hadn't already!) just how maddeningly complex mental health disorders can be and why reliance on medications exclusively for the vast majority of mental health patients, especially as it might relate to better sleep, often proves a false hope leading to more frustration and pain and, ultimately, desperation.

To be fair, I am not a big believer in looking at research studies from what's known as the public health perspective because it always misses out on the personally tailored effects a medication may provide to specific individuals. I completely, entirely, and honestly believe you if you declare Ambien works wonders. Not only do I believe you when you say it, I imagine in many instances the drug is truly yielding a very positive effect, including improvements in falling asleep and staying asleep, as well as in some cases improving quality of sleep.

In other words, some of these drugs produce near miraculous results in specific individuals, and for such patients I have no agenda to suggest they must find a way to sleep drug free. My point is you happen to be a fortunate soul when the drug is functioning as if it had been personally tailored to suit your biopsychosocial needs and that indeed is a wonderful outcome.

Such benefits are not the norm. If they occurred regularly, then there would not be so many mental health patients using not just one or two drugs, but often three to six drugs to allegedly combat or stabilize their mental health disorders or, in many cases, insomnia and nightmares. The multiple medication approach is often a sign of the weakness or nonspecificity of the medications. And when the multiple drug approach is seen among intractable insomnia patients, it is almost universally a sign of a patient too complex for the prescribing physician. Or the physician does not know how to identify other therapeutic modalities for the insomniac without relying solely on medications.

I must remind you as well that multiple drugs in an insomniac raises a huge red flag for an underlying physiological sleep disorder, most commonly

OSA/UARS or leg movement disorders, and in some cases, parasomnias.

Angles to Consider When Drugs Are Providing Relevant Benefits

Clearly, there's just no getting around the use of sedatives and hypnotics for some people for a multitude of reasons. What can we say about these standard approaches to guide your use?

Most importantly, do your best to find a physician, which could be primary care, internist, or family medicine, as well as a psychiatrist or prescribing psychologist who demonstrates a capacity for fine-tuning the use of medications. Often, they are the type who will zero in on key symptoms and then describe how certain receptor sites in the brain might respond well to a particular drug or how a specific symptom profile fits with a particular medication or combination of meds.

Though I will not provide specific drug recommendations here, I want to offer certain suggestions about their general use.

You have probably heard hypnotics or sedatives should not be used every night. That's correct in theory, but what if you are already using them every night? Either way, the big factors to analyze as soon as possible are the strengths and weaknesses of the medication and how long you see yourself sticking with this approach.

The most common benefit someone will notice from sleeping pills is decreasing the time it takes to fall asleep, whereas the biggest complaint is the persistence of awakenings at night. You know from learning about physiological disorders, the most likely reasons for awakenings are sleep breathing events or leg movements. So, this information could fortify your resolve to make more progress in treating your insomnia with a breathing device or a leg jerk medication because you are no longer confused about why you wake up. You have the reason(s) staring you in the face. What would you like to do about it?

I trust you see where this is headed. You are getting some benefit from the sleeping pill, but it may not be enough benefit. You appreciate the potential (even if just sporadic) psychological respite of greater sleep continuity, and that's great. Instead of getting frustrated by the lack of perfection from the pills, you could look in the physical direction and ask how to decrease the sleep breathing events or the leg jerks.

For sleep breathing problems, now when you are near bedtime, you don't just think about taking the pill. You also think about nasal hygiene, nasal strips, and delving deeper into enhancing or truly normalizing your nasal breathing. You might consider sleeping on your side or stomach, since breathing events are worse on your back. You could also lower the bedroom temperature since breathing is naturally better below 65 degrees Fahrenheit. If you strike gold or silver with a couple of steps that lead to improvement, you will be taking control over the problem instead of trying to overcome demoralizing feelings when the sleeping pills don't work as advertised.

Over time, most sleeping pills do not consistently get you where you want to be, let alone keep you there throughout the night. Therefore, why not work on your physical disorders all the while?

This model is very conservative. It's not asking you to rush out and get the sleep study and start PAP, although there are patients with severe, if not desperate, conditions that need to do so. This model is about helping you see how much more you can do for your sleep, not only to get better sleep, but also to realize you may not be as dependent on medication as you once thought.

This same perspective applies to leg movement disorders and in some ways more so, because as discussed in Chapter 9, prescribing of psychotropic medications for sleep disorders, specifically nightmares or insomnia, is often a case of mismanagement where the physician or other provider took no time to sort out the possibility of RLS/PLMD. Instead, the insomnia aspect was easily spotted on the radar, so the conventional wisdom was to start or add drugs.

Regrettably, in the area of antidepressants, which are often prescribed to either improve sleep quality, treat insomnia, or enhance sleep continuity, most practitioners do not realize how many of these drugs cause or worsen leg movement symptoms, both the restlessness of RLS and the twitchiness of PLMD.

In this scenario, the most important first step is to figure out your leg movement symptoms. Remember, someone with anxiety tends to think about anxiety "all over." As discussed regarding emotions, you can learn to pay closer attention to where *exactly* in your body you feel feelings. When you learn to pinpoint anxiety, for example in your throat, chest, stomach, or hands, it may open up the opportunity to sense "anxiety" in your legs or feet as well. If so, that's the beginning of knowledge and awareness of the possibility "anxiety" resides in your limbs, potentially a sign of RLS.

You can always look for physical signs too. Are your bed linens messy in the morning? Does a bed partner say you kick or otherwise move your legs a bunch during the night? Or do you seem to toss and turn quite a bit? All these factors suggest greater chances for RLS and PLMD.

With this knowledge, you would begin working with your doctors on vitamin or mineral deficiencies, the two most common being low iron levels, measured via the biomolecule serum ferritin, or low vitamin D. If you test deficient, then your next step is vitamin or mineral replacement, or both, as is often the case. In a matter of weeks or a few months, your sleep might improve just with these supplements. You might also try L-tyrosine as described in Chapter 9, though be sure to read the caveats as well regarding possible augmentation and impulse-control disorder in any dopaminergic agents. And you can now engage in a clear-headed discussion with your prescribing physicians on your desire to try one of the top medications for leg movements, again mentioned in Chapter 9.

All within a matter of days, weeks, or a few months, sleep quality might get better, awakenings might decrease, and sleep continuity may extend. Because you took control of the situation, you realized more was happening than could be fully treated with a sleeping pill. The sleeping pill helps, but it wasn't helping enough, so you used these strategies to push things forward.

In the case of leg jerks, it is not unheard of for the individual to gain such a good response to supplements or medications, they no longer need or want to use sleeping pills. And, in the circumstances of successful treatment of sleep breathing events, the same thing can occur, though it clearly takes longer as one has to factor in all the steps of testing and initiating a PAP machine or alternate therapy regardless of whether you are continuing or discontinuing a sleeping pill.

Summing up, where we wish things were right now is for all mental health clinics to be conducting research protocols like the one underway at the GGZ Drenthe Mental Health Institute in The Netherlands.[174] They are dividing up hundreds of patients into two separate groups, those who undergo standard mental health treatments including medications and psychotherapy, and those who receive mental health treatment plus thorough state-of-the-art sleep evaluations and treatment. The researchers clearly understand the serious lapse in the field of mental health, given their background statement, "Unfortunately, in mental health care sleep disorders are often poorly recognized and specific treatment frequently occurs late or not at all."

Such research will prove how invaluable sleep treatments are in the early going. No matter how late you are into the evaluation of your sleep disorders, now is the time to start treating them.

Another Role for Medications: Daytime Sleepiness as a Distinct Disorder

Among mental health patients, a substantial minority suffer from impairment due to daytime sleepiness from various and not always obvious causes. The underlying sleep disorder develops within the brain itself, through structural alterations (head injury) or functional changes (neurotransmitter deficiency), and this excessive sleepiness is termed *hypersomnia*.

Although hypersomnia conditions are uncommon, they are not rare, and since they mostly respond to stimulant medication therapy, we will identify the most relevant disorders if you happen to suffer from persistent sleepiness.

Most have heard of *narcolepsy*, which involves a strong physiological desire to sleep during wakefulness. In the worst case, a narcoleptic suffers sleep attacks and nods off in a matter of seconds, sometimes during odd circumstances like sitting at a table eating lunch or while making love. In some instances, "nodding off" is actually *cataplexy*, where the individual loses control of muscles and collapses. The collapse could be as simple as a droopy face or as dramatic as falling down. The narcoleptic is confused about cataplexy behavior because he or she is not actually falling asleep at the moment.

Of all the conditions described here, this classic form of narcolepsy is the most complicated and most difficult to treat. Not only might stimulants be prescribed to reduce (though often not cure) sleepiness, but antidepressants are often needed to stop cataplexy. One positive research trend is the narcolepsy diagnosis can be more rapidly obtained by examining the spinal fluid of the patients for a "hypocretin" deficiency, a very reliable indicator.

Posttraumatic narcolepsy involves symptoms similar to classic narcolepsy, though head trauma injuring the brain is the obvious cause. The good news is trauma-related narcolepsy is very likely to resolve over time, though it might take several months or a couple years compared to classic narcolepsy, which requires medication for one's lifetime.

Another disorder, *idiopathic hypersomnia* (IHS), indicates sleepiness due to an unknown cause, which generally means lots of different causes though they may not be easily identifiable. In our clinical experience, many IHS cases turned out to be UARS. Regardless, hypersomnia cases without an obvious cause occur, and many will benefit from stimulants or newer drugs that use a different pharmacologic mechanism to promote wakefulness. This area of research is very exciting because some new medications exhibit no abuse potential, compared to stimulants; and, therefore the drugs offer hope for much better and safer treatments. Wakix (pitolisant) is the new drug in this unique category.

All these hypersomnia conditions respond reasonably well to stimulant medications; rarely do they eliminate sleepiness. Nonetheless, stimulants radically improve the individual's lifestyle so they can often drive a car or hold down a job, two activities perhaps previously compromised. Indeed, classic narcolepsy is a debilitating condition if left untreated, and these individuals almost always suffer co-occurring psychiatric disorders, especially anxiety and depression.

A complete discussion of stimulant medications is beyond the scope of this book; nevertheless, if hypersomnia appears as a component of your sleep disorders and no one seems able to effectively treat it, then you will want to discuss hypersomnia with an experienced sleep doctor. Your search might take time because many sleep professionals do not receive much training or acquire much experience in managing hypersomnia disorders. As suggested above, pay attention to the new research on wakefulness-promoting pharmaceuticals now coming available as these options might eventually prove superior, and sleep doctors are beginning to prescribe these agents.

Mixed Depression and Sleepiness Conditions

A final hypersomnia condition, and perhaps the most frequent, involves the complex relationships and differences between low energy levels and depression. In this instance, the question arises as to whether a person can attack their mental health issues simply by adding more energy into the equation. We know depressed patients report low energy and fatigue, and some report excessive sleepiness (hypersomnia).[175] Clearly, these symptoms are hallmarks of untreated sleep disorders too. Yet, when no obvious sleep disorders like breathing or movement disorders are detected, then a possibility exists for co-occurring depression and hypersomnia. For the past hundred years, nearly everyone presumed the depression caused this hypersomnia.

Nonetheless, the depressed patient cannot easily sort out this puzzle when he or she has been treated with antidepressants for years and received mixed results. Furthermore, their sleep treatments do not play out in a simple or rapid way. In other words, fixing sleep disorders does not immediately filter out residual depression symptoms. Instead, over the long run, a trial-and-error approach extending months or years may be needed for these mixed cases to sort out the residual fatigue or sleepiness. We always encourage depressed and other mental health patients to work aggressively to solve sleep disorders, but it is usually only after the sleep treatment regimen is well established that a patient and a prescribing physician can successfully adjust medications—if adjustments are needed.

In the meantime, it sure would be satisfying to the depressed patient to gain more energy, which brings us to the question of what medications might help. In the forthcoming discussion, notice how we could be talking about narcolepsy, idiopathic hypersomnia, or the sleepiness of depression.

Compensatory Medications for Daytime Sleep Symptoms

Caffeine. Caffeine is probably the single most widely used stimulant in the world to treat depression given how many people don't have access to antidepressants versus how many people can drink a cup of coffee or consume other beverages or plants with caffeine or related agents. I wholeheartedly endorse caffeinated products as a means to improve energy, fight off sleepiness, and treat depression. While this approach may prove adequate in the long term for milder cases of depression, and in the short term for moderate depression, we wouldn't expect caffeine to be the optimal solution.

That said, we should also ask, optimal solution for what? If you are confused or unsure about how much of your low energy is depression and how much is untreated sleep disorders, experimentation with caffeinated products is in order and can range from hot cocoa and chocolate to green or white tea all the way up to black tea, coffee, espresso, and bolus caffeine drinks (think Red Bull) and other over-the-counter or herbal stimulants. I am not suggesting heavy dosages of caffeine as the best long-term solution, but keep in mind the more you benefit from caffeine, the more likely you are gaining valuable information about the likelihood of a strong physiological sleep component, most likely a sleep disorder, that underlies the sleepiness, fatigue, or low energy state.

Stimulants. Heavy-duty stimulants have been used in depressed patients as well as sleep disorder patients who suffer severe daytime sleepiness, the *sine qua non* of low energy in a sleep apnea patient. The use of stimulants, therefore, is another potent option to consider whether it's the depression or it's the sleep disorder or both causing the disabling low energy state.

Drugs such as Provigil, Nuvigil, Adderall, Strattera, and Ritalin, to name some of the most popular stimulants, have been increasingly prescribed over the past 10 to 20 years, which is a positive development because it means physicians and other prescribers are giving serious attention to the problems of daytime fatigue and sleepiness. We would like to see such doctors also recommend sleep studies for the vast majority of these patients, but it's obvious for now prescription pads receive more ink than referral pads. As relevant, some of these prescriptions could be written for Wakix (pitolisant) as noted above.

In a strange way, one of the most important considerations for stimulants and related agents is whether they actually help nighttime sleep continuity. As mentioned, sleep continuity is a very big deal because of its airtight relationship with the need for a psychological respite from the day's events. Individuals using stimulants may achieve greater productivity during the daytime and literally expend more energy through greater physical activity or exertion. Physical exercise or activity (think yardwork and laborious home repairs) often deepen sleep, and deeper sleep regularly yields greater continuity of sleep. All told, the stimulant user may notice greater productivity and satisfaction; he or she feels a greater sense of achievement at the end of the day and therefore a greater willingness to let go and relax when getting ready for bed. Obviously, the stimulant cannot be used too late in the day, which might result in sleeplessness.

Dr. Michael Perlis investigated the use of Provigil in insomniacs to see whether their increased productivity during the day would lead to greater improvement in sleep at night. Although the results were mixed, the thinking behind the research fits perfectly with the working theory that a sleep disorder patient would like to feel as if one has worked through the day and "earned" the right to a good night of slumber.

Those who struggle in their efforts during the daytime are a set up for a bad night of sleep. They don't deserve the bad night. Rather, the bad night is more predictable because of the inability to access a fully energized state during the daytime that leads to satisfaction in the waking hours.

The Universal Drugless Intervention: Napping

Napping behavior can prove highly beneficial or destructive, and in mental health patients there are many opportunities for both results to emerge. The biggest problem with daytime dozing is how naps worsen your ability to sleep well at night; moreover, napping may cause short- and long-term disruptions to your regular day–night schedule. Worst of all, if your nap is of the wrong type (to be explained below) you could wake up feeling very unrefreshed and sluggish and wondering why you even bothered.

Let's spell out the results of a good nap: you should feel refreshed, and whatever the dismal feelings you felt before the nap, now you should feel much more like getting up and accomplishing your next set of goals or tasks.

How do you achieve this good nap? Unfortunately, it is an incredibly precise intervention, so to speak, based on many individual characteristics. While it's true a good starting point for an insomniac is to take naps early and make them short, it's also true a lot of variation goes into these instructions, including some people needing longer naps and, conversely, others needing micronaps either early or late.

The crux of the matter turns out to be what the nap is doing to your brain during the period of sleep, and ultimately, we may discover a certain amount of "brain-washing" is going on even in naps as short as one minute. Whatever turns out to be the explanation, it is unequivocal some people can nap and wake up feeling gloriously refreshed, while others dread napping as they literally feel more depressed.

Taking into account all the above, the most important rule to remember about napping is whether or not you can use it as a potential life preserver. I am referring to that time of day when things are just so bleak or dark, or you are so tired and sleepy, or your motivation and energy are lagging so badly, you really don't care much about anything and desperately would like an escape.

In such situations, do not hesitate to use the nap, especially if you have learned to use napping in the past to get over the hump. When you nap, conduct relevant experiments to ensure the nap turns out to be a good one.

First and foremost, if you know or suspect you suffer from OSA/UARS, you must find the most appropriate position for napping. Consider all possibilities. Many individuals nap sitting upright with the chin to chest position. Others lean forward with the forehead on top of their folded arms. Some pick a side to sleep on, but one should do so with obvious elevation greater than 45 degrees from the plane of the bed or sofa. Before the nap, some apply nasal strips or use nasal sprays to insure nasal patency.

When you suffer from OSA/UARS but don't find the right position, your nap quality is much more likely to be poor, whereas if you find the best position coupled with the best timing, you greatly increase your chances for a refreshing nap. Personally, if I nap on my right side at 30 to 45 degrees, I usually awaken refreshed, with one major caveat. The longer the nap, the greater the need to use my OAT (the Metz appliance) or an AIRMAX nasal dilator during the nap; thus, I must control my nap duration before the start (that is, set an alarm).

What is the best duration? Generally, the closer you are to your bedtime, the shorter the nap must be. As a guide, after a rough night of sleep, I will occasionally take a 45-minute snooze before the noon hour, compared to a one- to five-minute micronap taken between 5 p.m. and 6 p.m., should a need arise in the late afternoon. For these shorter naps, I use head to chin sitting up position or leaning forward on a table with my forehead centered on my folded forearms.

These examples are a guide. I know of many troubled sleepers who daily must go back to bed to sleep in the morning for one to three hours, preferably using their PAP. Others take longer naps between 3 p.m. and 7 p.m., again with PAP, because of schedule issues that mandate this timing pattern.

Experimentation with position and timing is the only way to sort out your best napping experience.

Finally, beware of the longish nap later in the day that appears to serve no purpose. This form of napping heralds either a serious mental disorder such as depression or a serious hypersomnia condition, likely from an untreated physiological sleep disorder, most likely OSA/UARS or possibly IHS. Some people are cursed with suffering severe hypersomnia from both depression and sleep-disordered breathing. Bottom line, the napping in this instance is not serving much benefit but at least signals the presence of serious disorders needing more treatment, to be addressed sooner than later.

No doubt there are individuals who nap because of boredom, whereas others nap due to shift work. The circumstances may require professional consultation if the napping behavior eventually leads to disruptions in the quality of your life.

Integrating the Information

Summing up, for those who must use psychoactive medication or substances such as caffeine, activating antidepressants, or stimulants, judicious use may lead to a more satisfying lifestyle, culminating in a more satisfying sleep period. Use of medications and other agents directed at these goals may prove a veritable godsend for many individuals with mental health disorders. The question that emerges, and we trust this question comes up without delay, is whether the prescribing providers are paying close attention to the underlying sleep disorders so rampant in these patients.

Arguably, these insights are nothing to sleep on. Recognizing how medications may only serve as short-term solutions engages patients and their physicians and therapists toward a deeper exploration and more thorough analysis of sleep dysfunction. The sleep piece of the puzzle often turns out to be causing a much greater share of the distress than once imagined among those afflicted with mental illness.

Last, and of considerable importance to your well-being, all that's been discussed in this book and in this chapter seeks to connect the zzzots so you realize fixing your sleep could markedly improve your memory and concentration, as well as favorably influence your mood and coping skills. When these cognitive and emotional factors are functioning at an overall higher level, you typically gain greater skills in decision making and for judging what's best for your health.

In contrast, the combo of poor sleep and poor mental health compromises, contaminates, or corrupts these cognitive factors, causing worse memory and concentration and declines in mood and coping skills, thereby generating greater deficits in decision making and, ultimately, adversely affecting the judgments you make in your life.

Worst of all, mental health patients with sleep disorders greatly increase their risks for suicidal thinking and behaviors. And, it should be of great interest that nearly all sleep doctors who are working in the area of mental health know treating sleep disorders can improve a person's mood and thereby decrease suicidal thinking and behavior. While research is scant, a few studies have emerged in proving the value in treating sleep disorders in suicidal patients[176] along with the calls for more research.[177]

To reiterate, nothing to sleep on here. Go for it and evaluate and treat your sleep disorders as aggressively as you are able and as soon as you are able. These treatments have the potential to markedly enhance the quality of your life, or literally save your life.

Let me close by repeating some points about sleep physiology. All of the above may prove to be directly related to your capacity to achieve longer periods of REM or delta sleep or both, as well as higher quality of REM and delta. These deeper stages of sleep are likely to hold the keys to how higher quality sleep so positively affects the way you feel. And future research is also likely to prove that higher quality of sleep leads to greater efficiency and effectiveness in your overnight "brain-washing" operations mentioned early in the book. This cleansing function has been recently described as the "glymphatic system," which I will offer a final comment about in the Epilogue.

Sleep Research Pearl #17

When we researched so many connections between sleep and mental health, we were routinely engaged in discussions with hundreds of mental health professionals, some of whom were elite thought leaders at prestigious institutions. Several of these encounters involved top doctors at the highest ranked psychiatric hospitals in the United States, Canada, Europe and Israel.

Our vision was simple: if we really want to understand and follow what's going on in the sleep of mental health patients, what better place to do so than on-site in mental health clinics or hospitals? More than 20 years ago we talked initially with our local contacts throughout New Mexico, then in the ensuing years we spoke with hundreds of mental health professionals in numerous national and international venues, such as VA medical centers, private hospitals, university hospitals, private clinics, and specialized clinics for obesity, drug rehabilitation, or eating disorders.

Some of these conversations were brief, while others were extensive, including very preliminary development of a path forward. Yet, in all these conversations, despite acknowledgment and even some enthusiasm, each facility rejected any implementation due to the lack of financial reimbursement or the inability to integrate sleep health into their insurance-based system. Thus, the most prominent barriers were money and insurance-driven healthcare.

These primary issues explain why and how the mental health community continues to fall short in addressing sleep health in their patients. The connection between sleep and mental health is so intricate and of such magnitude, only by working together could we generate the kind of changes needed to help mental health patients receive top-notch sleep health care.

Out there, to be sure, there are many sleep doctors and technologists, as well as many mental health professionals and experts, who know this Truth with a capital T. Yet, because of the vast array of administrative hurdles in our current healthcare system, including the inability to get paid for any sleep services in a psychiatric or psychologic venue, we are currently at a dead end, figuratively and, sadly for some patients, literally as they are never going to be offered the sleep medicine care they so desperately need.

Over and over again, we discussed the idea of putting a sleep center or a sleep laboratory into these psychiatric or other specialty facilities. To this day, I receive outright rejections and unreturned phone calls. Forgive me for the drama, but this is madness, and somehow it has to stop before more lives are lost. Over the years, I have repeatedly heard the main excuse—"it's the system!" I'm old enough and experienced enough to know that professionals of all types run these systems, and the blame for this fiasco, in my opinion, rests squarely on the shoulders of those who should know better and who should want the best for their mental health patients. It is their task to fix the system; a system does not fix itself. Harsh, but true!

CHAPTER 18

AT THE END OF THE DAY, WHAT ATTITUDES ARE LIFESAVERS?

How can I use humor, work, and prayer to cope with my sleep disorders?

Changing Your Attitude Is Not So Easy

No matter how much we delve into the adverse impact of psychological and physiological sleep disorders on your functioning, thinking, and feeling, we must close out this book with very special resources beyond the clinical realm. We must turn our attention to universal assets all humans possess—precious gifts from our Creator that offer immense intrinsic value in warding off self-destructive thoughts and actions, and in the process, let us sleep.

Any resource that changes our attitudes and influences us to see things more positively is bound to move us away from self-defeating behavior and self-harm. And there are no greater human capabilities to employ than a sense of humor, a sense of productivity, and a sense of the ineffable, all of which have served mankind more than most other resources since humans first came into being.

Our capacity to laugh at things and to work at things, and our ability to appreciate a spiritual dimension in our personal reality, are time-tested variants of psychotherapy. For millennia, humans relied on humor, work, and prayer to see themselves through difficult spots. And, as luck would have it, any daily effort you enlist in bringing a smile to your face, taking pride in your achievements, or in pausing for prayerful reflection on your life generates tangible potential in aiding your quest for the healthy slumber you have been reading about in this book.

Prayer, work, and laughter are not substitutes for everything discussed so far, but they represent pathways sometimes ignored by mental health professionals and sleep specialists. In this closing chapter, we delve into these realms to demonstrate tried and true resources to calm your fears and move you toward positive steps in your daily life.

And, "closing" is the operative phrase here because these resources greatly increase your capacity to find closure at the end of day and bring peace of mind at bedtime. Emotional closure is a pivotal objective when seeking peace of mind at the start of your sleep period and while sleeping all through the night.

Can You Laugh About It?

A good sense of humor is worth its weight in therapeutic gold. For example, how many narcissists does it take to change a light bulb? Only one—as long as everyone is watching!

The awesomeness of jokes starts with the sudden change of consciousness you feel in the form of either the "tickle" somewhere on the inside or the smile changing the contours of your face. Did you feel either of these things when you read this joke? Perhaps you only felt the "tickle" in your mind or simply a little smirk across your lips.

Phase one of any joke is the split second where you do not think or feel the same way you were thinking or feeling just a second ago. Depending on how elaborate or potent the meaning or impact of the joke, personally or just generally, phase two lasts several seconds or minutes and sometimes much longer (especially if more follow-up jokes are triggered) because it redirects your energy away from negative influences.

Specifically, humor generates more impact if it strikes at the heart of a mental health issue in ways that relieve tension felt by the individual. Take the narcissist joke: it could be reasonably argued anyone undergoing a mental health crisis of whatever degree has adopted an acutely narcissistic view of his or her problems as they relate to current reality.

This statement might seem like overkill, but I am not suggesting every mental health patient is suffering a narcissistic personality disorder, where the individual has a tough time trying to think and feel about things from someone else's point of view. In the true narcissistic disorder, the individual's self-absorption is so intense that when asked, "Hey, do you know what time it is?" the narcissist looks at his watch and declares, "Why, yes, it's time for my lunch!"

Instead of a clinical disorder, an acute narcissistic perspective may take over any traumatized person's thinking, creating a self-absorbed state that seems quite normal due to the intense suffering already overwhelming his or her coping skills. However, if the self-absorption is not deflected or defused, there is a tendency for too much introspection to turn into a trance-like state where the traumatized individual spirals downward.

Self-absorption is a logical state of affairs when mental agitation or depression just cannot be relieved; in these circumstances circling the wagons seems sensible and appropriate. Yet, jokes and other forms of humor (*I Love Lucy* may be one of the most potent forms of psychotherapy ever devised) enter your consciousness through a figurative side door and release portions of the mental and physical tension you have been experiencing, which hopefully resets your attitude and possibly your mood in a surprisingly short span of time.

Which reminds me of my favorite *Lucy* scene, where she's trying to sell a vacuum cleaner she was tricked into buying. In falling prey to a clever salesman, she learns the sales pitch of throwing a dirt bomb onto a rug as she enters a new customer's apartment. The tenant is shocked, but Lucy hands her a ten-dollar bill and says, "If I can't sweep up all that dirt in two minutes, that's yours." A sly, knowing look spreads across the woman's face as she watches Lucy plug in the vacuum to sweep the carpet, but the vacuum's switch does not seem to work. Lucy says, "That's funny, I can't imagine why it doesn't work," to which the woman responds, "I can, the electricity was turned off—we didn't pay our bill."

Speaking of the Broom family, did you hear they had so much trouble sweeping at night, they were all on prescription sweeping pills and over-the-counter sweep aids. Eventually, they visited a sweep specialist at an accredited sweep center. After taking a careful sweep history, they were instructed to follow this age-old bedtime ritual: "Stop worrying and sweep everything under the rug."

Letting Humor Intrude into Your Everyday Life

Lots of experiences and feelings in our daily lives cannot be swept aside. "Reality" challenges us throughout the day. This reality, molded by our individual desires and perspectives, often collides with those who see things differently, then conflicts arise after which pain is not far behind. Pain may be physical, mental, emotional, or spiritual, and it is nearly impossible to go through a day without experiencing interpersonal conflicts intruding into your reality, and so much of mental illness shows up in our difficulties in dealing with other humans. Sometimes, it is straightforward abuse when another person directly inflicts a twisted reality on a victim, physically, mentally, emotionally, or even spiritually.

More commonly, pain arises from our inability to understand and cope with the differences between our own and other individuals' ways of thinking about things or doing things. In virtually every individual with a mental health issue, symptom, or disorder, a share of the problem arises through difficulties and conflicts with other people. This point does not indicate the other person caused the whole problem. More times than not, this other person is a *signal* or *marker* if the mental illness is especially prone to deterioration in the presence of the "other" person for reasons that may be obvious or not.

To be sure, genetics or biology also have great bearing on mental health, but despite what many mental health experts profess about the etiology and treatment of the common disorder depression, it is incontestable an enormous number of individuals who use antidepressant medication could discover alternate treatments or methods to improve their coping skill in day-to-day living.

A potent form of psychotherapy, believe it or not, teaches how humor is a very special antidote to pain. Whether it be learning to laugh at oneself or learning to laugh at certain experiences in life, a capacity to tap into the humorous side of reality correlates with your ability to strengthen mental health. Learning to look differently at your situation and recognizing there might actually be a way to laugh about it may go a long way in moving someone toward higher ground and a healthier mental perspective.

At minimum, the Internet is filled with humor sites, so if you want to give it a try, find one and read a lot of jokes before bedtime or in the middle of the night if awakened. If you like the results, also consider looking at humorous material at least twice a day and monitoring how it affects your mood, attitude, and perspective. It can't hurt unless you come across side splitters!

Still, there are many mental health situations, circumstances, and levels of distress that are so painful, humor seems out of reach. Where does someone turn in times so troubling?

Can You Work Around and Through It?

Work is its own psychotherapy, and arguably it ranks up there as one of the most potent, and some would say the single most potent, form of therapy for at least two reasons. First, by working, you are usually continuously interacting with other people, such as colleagues, coworkers, clients, consumers, and lots of other people, all of whom you variously like/dislike, love/hate, and find delightful/annoying to be around. In other words, work provides a rich environment for testing and refining your coping skills pretty much all day long. Enriching and strengthening your ability to adapt to and cope with life's daily stressors is a critical component of a healthy mind, and work often proves the optimal testing ground toward these ends.

The second and likely more important reason is how the nature of your work plays a huge role in creating or maintaining an identity for yourself in the world. This identity includes simple yet meaningful labels, like teacher, nurse, homemaker, mechanic, clerk, administrator, doctor, lawyer, engineer, janitor, baker, grocer, and the list goes on. Most relevant, building your identity is a complex process as you create a *persona* of how you act and appear as a teacher, nurse, lawyer, and so on.

For example, a teacher could be stern, passionate, funny, challenging, curious, unbiased, skilled, and a host of other traits, but there will usually be a few specific characteristics that stand out. A very passionate and funny teacher is going to be known by the students as funny and passionate, and therefore, the teacher will take pride in these traits.

Identity formation and maintenance—how you see yourself and how you want others to see you—provides one of the most centering or grounding experiences you will ever feel in your life for the simple reason that what you *do* on a day-to-day basis is in effect the daily story you are telling yourself about your place in the world.

As an aside, identity formation is a natural and healthy process and should not be confused with the recent term "identity politics," a contrived, unhealthy, and dangerous sociological development that has regrettably infected a number of institutions throughout our communities, states and nation, not to mention around the world.

Now back to our regularly scheduled program. Figuratively, work serves as a center of gravity for the overwhelming majority of adults. And the more things you become good at, or in some instances the few things you do very well, or in rarer cases the one or two things you do great, all lead a person to feel mentally fit and capable about himself or herself, at least in the work environment, which in many cases carries over beyond the job.

Of course, never underestimate the job of homemaker, which often proves more challenging and difficult than a host of so-called difficult and challenging occupations. Keeping a well-functioning home, raising children, and invigorating a healthy family life are right up there as the most important work in keeping neighborhoods, communities and societies operating successfully. These same points about developing your capabilities apply in the home, and a solid performance here unequivocally should lead to tangible gains in identity formation and character development, and sometimes more so than a paying job.

Mental health professionals may not emphasize how your work impacts your self-esteem. In real life, most of us gain self-esteem by demonstrating our capacity to do things, that is, manifesting our capability. When we do things, we are more likely to feel good about what we accomplished, and in many cases, we take pride in attempting to do things even if we did not accomplish all we set out to do. Doing things, to be clear, also includes good deeds that help others along the way.

While the concept of self-esteem is relevant as we must learn to love and respect ourselves, the notion you or others can simply feed your brain with positive thoughts and feelings only goes so far. In fact, your development over the course of your life typically hinges much more on either the effort or the accomplishments, or both, you attempt and achieve in work or in home life. Learning to be a capable person is what makes a person feel whole; and work and homemaking are two of the greatest arenas in which to expand your capabilities.

A great many individuals might develop the same process through other spheres like community involvement, religious commitments, or volunteer programs where strong dedication leads to pronounced capabilities. In all these situations, individuals almost invariably feel and believe they have served a purpose or contributed to a worthy endeavor.

What If You Cope Poorly and Lose Your Job?

If you do not cope well at work, then a worst-case scenario might be you quit or get fired from your position. Such circumstances, beyond the pain and anguish, may have negative consequences on your mental health, both in the short and long run. First, your center of gravity has been knocked off its axis, and second, you no longer are engaged in an environment to regularly use your coping skills. No doubt leaving a job might seem like the right decision at the time, and if another job is soon available, I am not suggesting you must always tough it out at the first one. But, categorically, be aware the longer you remain unemployed, the greater your chances for spiraling downward.

This decline in mental health is directly related to the loss of activity from no longer going to work regularly. If you are not *doing* regular activities such as work, in particular, your self-worth diminishes as you lose tangible ways to demonstrate your capability. These changes lead to a loss of self-respect, self-esteem, self-love, or whatever you choose to call it, because you no longer experience the daily injection of healthy pride you hopefully would be enjoying from a job done and sometimes done well.

Being out of work is a damaging and sometimes deadly affair above and beyond its disruption to your sleep patterns. It may lead to a degree of demoralization that causes or aggravates depression, triggers thoughts of suicide, and alienates the individual so much that reentering the workforce seems impractical if not impossible.

In no uncertain terms, it is imperative for such a person to return to any form of work imaginable as soon as feasible, notwithstanding mental or physical illness that might delay reentry. Even working a volunteer position without pay or other noticeable benefits will lead to intangible gains achieved by *doing* things on a daily or regular basis. In turn, this work may serve as the catalyst to finding a new job in your field or perhaps a new line of employment.

It's worth pointing out here a commonly overlooked fact about jobs and careers. Most working adults change careers as often as five to seven times throughout their lives. So, the above discussion, to reiterate, is not about having to stick with one job to prove something. The take-home message is that sticking with work wherever you find yourself working is an enormously powerful component in stabilizing mental health.

Unfortunately, many healthcare professionals do not seem to appreciate the unequivocal need for someone with mental health issues or disorders to find steady work. Whether it is working for yourself at home or working in a traditional business environment, a pathway for recovery almost always involves regular daily activities that lead you to put effort into things you *do*. While communities must always consider safety net issues affecting severely afflicted individuals, even in these circumstances the individual has more to gain by regular activities in some form of work, again whether for pay or through volunteering.

If you decide to arise each morning and walk around your own neighborhood, collecting trash and recyclable materials and transferring them to the proper bin, you will enhance your capability and likely gain dignity and self-respect, and take pride in your actions. Regardless of whether you receive any compensation or whether anyone else notices what you are doing, you will benefit by exerting yourself to do such things and feel the accomplishment of your work. I have witnessed just this type of behavior in my own neighborhood.

It is impossible to overestimate the value of work or working on something in your daily life. No matter how mundane or even boring you think work might be, it is in your best interest to look at all tasks—including, as noted above, housework, chores, so-called menial labor, running errands, changing diapers, cooking, cleaning, or mowing the lawn—with a fresh set of eyes.

For most, I encourage you to take note: your Creator gave you two arms and hands, two legs and feet and a heart and a brain, not to mention eyes to see, ears to hear, and a mouth to speak. Do you realize how incredibly fortunate you are to receive these blessed gifts? With these human resources you actually possess the capacity to work and to enjoy the fruits of your own labor. Wow, let's repeat that: with your very own mind and body, you have the ability to create things and do things in your environment to make your world a better place. Pretty amazing when you stop to think about the power of One.

Can You Pray About It?

We live in a different age regarding matters of religion and spirituality. We are both blessed and cursed by an abundance of information that leads many to assume we will eventually discover logical explanations for everything in the universe.

When I hear very smart people opine in this manner, including their commentaries on how old-fashioned and useless religion has become in their lives, my immediate reaction is to recall this quote attributed to Aristotle, "The more you know, the more you know you don't know," but honestly, I am surprised and disappointed that so many smart people forget this perspective. Said more harshly, they forget how much they don't really know at all. Even Aristotle, near the end of his life, according to several respected

Jewish historical records (although quite possibly apocryphal)[178] embraced not only the Creator but spent considerable time learning about Judaism.

My aim here is not to suggest adopting a religious program or even to believe in God (although I suggest if you are currently a nonbeliever, you might one day discover how such an approach to life may prove more rewarding than you previously imagined). My intention is to engage you to consider the probability of another dimension of reality that is broader, deeper, and more complex than our standard or logical or rational ways of thinking. As a starting point, you might consider what a pretty smart guy once said. Per Albert Einstein, "Imagination is the highest form of research."

Is this the imagination of the same imagery processes we have been discussing in this book? In part, yes, because the mind's eye possesses the remarkable capacity to build a bridge between thoughts and emotions. But these imagery skills are only a starting point, from which we may choose to embark on a journey to learn about deeper questions on the very nature of our existence and the meaning of our lives, doing so perhaps as Einstein implies by researching with our imagination.

Where to Begin?

The age in which we live is too noisy in just about every circumstance you can find yourself. And this "noise" interferes with our efforts to think and feel as well as to just *be*, which is why so many people struggle at first to find the wherewithal to gain a SOLO moment (see Chapter 13). Instead, we are caught up in too many tasks, chores, responsibilities, and distractions that frequently interfere with our most primary goals or objectives in living our lives. This can be the downside of work, if all you ever do is work!

Most people, nearly all, whether or not they know or acknowledge the point I am about to make, spend far too much time avoiding the universal truth, which is we are all striving to find meaning in our lives. This meaning is not as simple as, say finding a good job, although good work absolutely can help you find meaning in your life. Yet, here's a wild card to consider:

a bad job also helps you find meaning in your life. This process of finding meaning is even more important in today's world because so much of our time is eaten up by many other things that under the microscope frequently prove trivial or inconsequential, that is, literally and figuratively possess little to no meaning.

This subject is tricky, often goes undiscussed in the modern world of our "entertainment society," and, surprisingly, does not seem to be consistently addressed in mental health sessions. While there may be no hard data on this last point, I have encountered thousands of mental health patients in my sleep medicine practice of over 30 years and not often have I heard a patient describe how logotherapy was incorporated into his or her psychotherapy. *Logotherapy* refers to Viktor Frankl's theory,[179] first written about in his 1946 book *Man's Search for Meaning,* that we are driven to search for a life purpose or a meaning to one's life. Ironically, he developed portions of logotherapy through his survival in multiple Nazi concentration camps. In sum, religious and spiritual matters appear to be frequently overlooked by a large proportion of mental health therapists.

This concept regarding meaning or a spiritual dimension in your life may prove extremely important to you, whether you know it or not or whether you believe it or not. Put simply, if you know it and embrace it, and then make a strong effort to apply some aspects of this dimension in your daily life, chances are higher you will be better prepared to prevent serious and chronic mental health problems. Specifically, therapies oriented toward finding meaning and purpose in your life or helping you to consider your relationship with your Creator increase your chances for recovery and are usually more valuable than buying into the theory life is merely a random set of meaningless events, or worse, chemical reactions.

This information is the God's honest truth, even if you consider yourself an atheist. And, by the way, lots of atheists know and believe these same points because they too strive to find a purpose and meaning to their lives even though they do not embrace the concepts of a spiritual dimension.

The path forward may be uncertain. Do you start attending or increase your frequency of attendance at a church, a mosque, a synagogue? Or start volunteer work at a religiously oriented institution? Do you read special books to engage your mind more actively in spiritual discussions? Do you attend a 12-step program with its very strong emphasis on embracing a Higher Power?

Any step can serve as a beginning, and other possibilities exist beyond what's listed above. When I counsel someone in this realm, one of the first things I suggest is to consider the amazing attributes of what it means to be alive, and to reflect on what can only be understood, in my opinion, as the miracle of life. You are alive and filled with an abundance of resources. Doesn't it make sense to want to know something about why you are alive and what the meaning of your life is?

If you are willing to try just the smallest step, I would encourage you to find a favorite prayer or two and recite it at bedtime (over time with your eyes shut) just prior to your intention to fall asleep. All major religions offer prayers specific to bedtime and prior to falling asleep. Surely, these are worth sleeping on.

A Path Wisely Chosen

Undeniably, humor, work, and prayer are not the answers for certain individuals in whom a deeper wound inside prevents sustainable improvements in mental health and in sleep. Indeed, emotional closure seems unattainable; thus, no peace of mind is close at hand. These folks are almost never in a position to recover their healthy slumber.

This grave wound has scarred the individual and usually has been initially addressed by the therapist in relevant discussions about the trauma and how to treat PTSD. Even so, it's worth saying that despite the sincerity and efforts of so many therapists, it is well known far too many seemingly irreversible cases of PTSD simply do not respond well to most therapies, including advanced therapies like exposure or EMDR.

In some cases, these advanced therapies are not readily accessible to the patient. In others, the skills needed to effectively administer these highly efficacious advanced therapeutic approaches are lacking in some therapists either due to poor training, a lack of experience, or the outright inadequacies of the therapist, who may not possess a capacity to learn such sophisticated techniques. No doubt, many patients have walked away after reporting unsatisfactory experiences with various types of exposure therapies. As you might expect, such patients are also suffering horrible sleep disturbances that appear equally incurable.

What remains for this person? More drugs? More therapy? Humor? Work? Prayer?

While all these things should be considered again, what if the individual has tried them all with no results? Sure, it's reasonable to ask the individual exactly how the steps were applied, though it's usually a reasonable assumption some effort was attempted without success, so the patient lost motivation for any further attempts.

What next?

When encountering these circumstances, sometimes I will ask an individual, what if you found yourself stranded on a deserted island with all the survival resources you need, but you were alone, what would you do? Would you give up and starve to death or would you find a way to survive? What do you think would happen to your sleep problems? Do you really know what you would do or what would happen? If you would not try to survive, what does it tell you about yourself? If you know you would try to survive, what does it tell you about yourself?

This thought experiment may help some individuals gain a sense of perspective about the troubles they are struggling to overcome. Therapists employ such techniques when other standard therapies have not yielded benefits. And this technique is used with the hope it drives the patient into a brief introspection on what's at stake.

Where might this sort of nontraditional therapeutic encounter lead?

Two Paths Forward: Gratitude First

In my experience with trauma survivors in particular and various other patients with different types of intractable mental health symptoms or disorders, I have noticed two distinct pathways that sometimes create new momentum for patients in trying to recover from or at least alleviate to a degree their severe mental distress.

Each of these pathways, directly or indirectly, addresses the problems caused by the deep wound or scar. The first pathway involves the question of "Why did this happen to me?" Or, "Why is this still happening to me?" In other words, the person does not quite understand whether they "deserved" this set of problems or whether it's all just bad luck or bad genes.

Consider the epitome of this scenario in which Lou Gehrig, New York Yankees slugger, declared on July 4, 1939, a couple months after having to give up his beloved game of baseball, "Today, I consider myself the luckiest man on the face of the earth." He had been diagnosed with the disease amyotrophic lateral sclerosis and died just two years later. How could he possibly see himself as the luckiest man on the face of the earth?

How is such a mindset possible?

In part, when a person honestly appraises the course of his or her life, it is extremely rare to not find someone else whose life is considerably more problematic and miserable. While such comparisons never seem to serve as a long-term solution to any of life's hardships, their short-term benefits may prove stimulating, enlightening, and perspective-changing because the truth of such comparisons resonates with Lou Gehrig's statement.

Truly, I believe each one of us is incredibly lucky, fortunate, and blessed. The question is whether or not we are willing to look at our lives in this way to realize the curses, hardships, and suffering we experience really are a part, and yes, often a big part, of our particular life challenges. And no matter how painful the challenges, an individual may choose—eventually—to see such things as having made him or her into a better person.

As shocking as such ideas sound in the twenty-first century, where apparently all suffering is deemed nothing short of evil, the reality is the largest proportion of trauma survivors in particular (and of many other mental health patients in general) reap great benefits and rewards when they sincerely achieve this mindset—a mindset that sets them free from the past events that have plagued them for so long.

It does not mean the wound is healed or the scar is gone. It means the individual has grown to understand we all go through trauma, every one of us, big or small, young or old, strong or weak, and how we come out the other end is something we have some influence over, and we can choose to look at our hardships in new ways.

Choosing gratitude is a remarkably powerful antidote compared to feeling traumatized for the remainder of your life. Grateful people find it so much easier to close out the day, find peace at bedtime, and gain more restful sleep.

A Second Path: Forgiveness

The second pathway is more daunting because it not only might ask the two questions "Why did I deserve this?" or "Why is it still happening?" but also raises the stakes by placing a much greater burden of responsibility on the individual, who must now attempt to resolve any guilt or shame embedded in the deep wound by actively choosing to forgive.

The forgiveness here may be directed externally to others who harmed you, or it may be internally, where you forgive yourself for past deeds that have deepened the wound or kept it from closing.

Shame and guilt are the ugliest of emotions, and few people eagerly seek to spend time emotionally processing them, although some people, regrettably, learn to wallow in shame or guilt in highly destructive patterns difficult to overcome. While there are perhaps a minority who consciously enter this vicious cycle for unhealthy reasons, it's safe to say most people stuck in a shame or guilt cycle really don't believe they have any control over it or the means to extricate themselves from it.

To be clear, externally driven shame or guilt refers in part to the grudge you are holding against the person(s) or institutions that you believe wronged you and should be ashamed or feel guilty about what's been done to you. Your perception of such individuals or entities generate tremendous anger, if not rage, at those who harmed you, and sooner than later a very deep and demoralizing bitterness sets in and consumes you. Fueling all these negative feelings is the suspicion or belief the offender or assailant outwardly shows no remorse for the actions perpetrated against you.

Even if an apology were forthcoming, and even if the offender repeatedly apologized, it would prove insufficient to dislodge the grudge. The grudge usually comprises a mix of anger, fear, and sadness, as well as guilt and shame, which all now operate to fuel the mental health disorder to the extent no psychotherapy will resolve the matter.

Thus, the question emerges after so many unsuccessful attempts at therapy, medication, or other interventions whether the individual is willing to explore the possibility of forgiving this "enemy."

It's worth pointing out that religion, especially formal religion, plays a very useful role in this area of advanced emotional processing because religion almost always provides a pathway leading to acts of forgiveness or showing mercy on other people. Unfortunately, skeptics often mistakenly think religion is about instilling more guilt and shame in the individual, and while that is distinctly possible in certain settings, most religions strongly preach the value of forgiveness because they recognize the self-destructive powers of a grudge.

Diving Inside

Internal shame and guilt are more difficult to assuage for the obvious reasons. You were the one who performed the troubling or destructive behavior, and thus you are the guilty party. As such, your guilt is very likely to bring on more than a small dose of shame to double-team you with that worst of combinations: guilt-shame.

Sometimes, there would seem to be no way out of this problem because if, in the worst case, you destroyed someone's life either through death or through a crippling effect on their physical or mental abilities, you are directly reminded none of this damage can be reversed, or if partially reversible, it's usually limited.

The universal question then becomes how much punishment must you inflict on yourself in order to believe sufficient justice has been meted out? And the corollary, of course, is how long do you need to be punished?

Again, most people shy away from guilt and shame even though directly confronting these ugly emotions is better for your health, often removes a great burden, and relieves a great deal of emotional tension. Nonetheless, when the avoidance of or aversion to shame and guilt stands in the way, it signals the unbearableness of dealing with these two highly charged emotions.

In the simplest example, for purposes of clarification, you commit a minor misdeed and naturally feel bad about it; you bumped into someone who then dropped her groceries. You confess or apologize, and you proceed to assist in the cleanup. Yes, you immediately felt guilt, shame, or embarrassment, but these same feelings caused you to act and repent, so to speak, and then you redeemed yourself. In totality, you actually feel better than if you had run out of the supermarket to hide. Instead, you openly admitted you had done something wrong or hurtful and then responded in the healthiest of ways.

With deeper wounds involving deeper shame and guilt, it is never this simple. Indeed, as the best possible guide, just review some of the most popular and intense movies that reveal in the final third of the picture how the protagonist finally comes to grip with the terrible guilt and shame that's been squeezing his or her brain and body. Only near the end of *Good Will Hunting* do we see Matt Damon's character finally breaking down and crying about his relationship with his dad, after which Robin Williams' character finally helps him to confront what's basically been destroying his soul and offers the truth of the matter, several times, "It's not your fault."

This is a great example of the deep wound buried alive, as it were, inside the mind and body, but the phrasing "It's not your fault" clearly does not work for lots of people because in fact it was their fault, or at least strongly appears to be.

Which brings us back to a far greater challenge of forgiving yourself for something bad, hurtful, or harmful you did to someone else or perhaps yourself. How do you ever forgive yourself?

The Most Difficult Journey

Everyone knows something about the idea "love conquers all," but does anyone think the negation of the phrase ever brings fulfillment? Do you ever think or feel hate or spite or envy or jealousy conquers all? Surely not. Yet, these are just a few of the bitter emotions that fuel an external grudge or internal grudge and prevent someone from choosing the path of forgiveness.

Oddly, when a person struggles to forgive himself or herself, the biggest block may be the emotion of self-hatred, fueled by guilt and shame so intense and so out of control.

Obviously, working through this story is going to be a long one, equivalent by analogy to writing your own book, perhaps your autobiography. Worse, there are no shortcuts I am aware of because even if you hope for a special moment of epiphany, spiritual grace, or just something knocking you over the head and waking you to a new reality, the truth of such a change almost always requires painstaking detail and a journey of considerable length. Even then, you still might need a special wake-up call.

Perhaps you have already trekked a long way down this road. Given how many people put sleep issues at the bottom of their to-do list, maybe you already had a reasonable head start by the time you picked up this book. Perhaps you have put forward some efforts to confront the guilt or shame for past deeds. No matter where you find yourself on this journey, self-forgiveness frequently feels like a distant land on another planet in some other galaxy, if not some other universe.

In my experience, for this story to gain a happy ending, I believe the one solution that might be attempted revolves around the ability to find something more important in life than your own life. Sounds odd, I know, but for at least some period of time, which might be a month or many months or might stretch into years or longer, placing your emphasis on a life outside your own may provide the time for a natural healing that may occur for reasons beyond which can logically be explained.

Devoting yourself to God or a child or grandchild or other loved one or to your community or to the planet or world peace, or anything else that brings passion along with loving compassion, will serve to bring you outside of yourself. As indirect as this method seems, it has served millions of individuals down through the ages once they realized they could no longer change the past or could no longer struggle with the attempts to self-heal.

Forgiveness is not easy, but it is usually easier when you realize how badly the grudge (or self-grudge) is holding you back in your life. To forgive someone else or forgive yourself for past misdeeds is hopefully not something you need to wait to express on your deathbed. Better to forgive now so you can live the life you were always meant to live.

Closing Remarks

It is said we live in difficult times. After all, when can you remember so much divisiveness and polarization on just about every issue of the day? When can you remember a time when relationships were severed with your friends or family over different points of view? When was there a time when virtually the whole world was told to stay inside or wear a mask outside?

Nevertheless, you still possess the senses and mental faculties to decide how you want to see the world, and you possess the skills to learn how to cope in the healthiest of ways as you live your life in this increasingly upside-down world. Increasing your capacity to create a balanced life will improve your mental and physical health, enhance your daytime work and other activities, and hopefully lead to a more satisfying sleep experience. Gaining and holding on to the most positive attitude is one way to withstand the "slings and arrows of outrageous fortune" seemingly so common in this crazy world.

A final way to help, though some may think too simplistic, are the words in Irving Berlin's masterpiece sung by Bing Crosby in *White Christmas*:

> *"When I'm worried and I can't sleep*
> *I count my blessings instead of sheep*
> *And I fall asleep counting my blessings.*

When my bankroll is getting small
I think of when I had none at all
And I fall asleep counting my blessings."

In the Bible, in what we call the Torah or the Five Books of Moses, near the end of a 40-year journey in the Wilderness, just outside the Promised Land, Moses exhorts the Israelites to "choose life."[180]

I encourage you to count your blessings and choose life.

Sleep Research Pearl #18

A special Sleep Research Pearl to end the book awaits you in the Epilogue, and you don't want to miss out on this brief discussion on how our current understanding of practical sleep issues like napping, hours of sleep, and regulated sleep schedules might lead to a newer understanding of the biological activity in sleep, yielding an even better understanding of and capacity for a sleep quality the existence of which, perhaps, all of us have never imagined possible.

EPILOGUE

DREAMING OF SUPER SLEEP

You know I favor a *sleep quality* model as the be-all, end-all to piece together your sleep puzzle much more than the *hours of sleep* model. I have reiterated almost exclusively a strong proposition to assess the quality of your sleep to discover how sleep disorders wreak havoc with your slumber.

Our model of care seldom aligns with conventional wisdom practiced in the field of sleep medicine. For example, I emphatically believe mental health patients should be offered the opportunity as early as possible to evaluate and treat their physiological sleep disorders like sleep breathing and sleep movement conditions instead of being incessantly told, if not compelled, to address psychological aspects first. And, your sleep problems need to be addressed as independent disorders, not as secondary symptoms of mental illness. If serious, evidence-based assessment and treatment can only be provided by sleep medicine specialists, then the mental health community owes it to its patients to refer as promptly as possible. Likewise, sleep medicine specialists not only must increase their receptivity to help these afflicted individuals but also must recognize their need for more services and hands-on care than a typical sleep apnea patient.

We discussed at length the problem of UARS and the difficulty obtaining a proper assessment and treatment for this subtle form of sleep-disordered breathing—a diagnosis routinely ignored, neglected, or rejected by a large contingency of blinkered sleep professionals. Making matters more complicated, we delved into the necessity of using advanced PAP machines like ABPAP and ASV to eradicate pressure intolerance while treating UARS, and posited some patients may improve delta and REM sleep with advanced PAP. Again, all these points are at odds with sleep professionals who mistakenly insist CPAP is the silver bullet.

I also downplayed the importance of normalizing day/night schedules for bedtime and wake-up time because in my clinical experience a naturally occurring schedule to suit your lifestyle often emerges after addressing your sleep disorders. Optimizing the quality of your sleep leads to a new, spontaneous, and healthier schedule that may exhibit more range than the fixed regimens endorsed by behavioral sleep specialists.

Last, we placed major emphasis on psychological treatments involving key components such as mind's eye imagery, emotional processing skills, and fine-tuned modifications to current CBT-I practices. Most of these therapeutic interventions are not offered in sleep centers, including CBT-I, where scant resources are available for this highly effective therapy. Even in mental health circles, many of these therapies are not provided.

In sum, our approach to sleep disorders has taken us down several pathways, any and all of which are not widely disseminated within professional circles of sleep medicine, psychiatry, or psychology, and yet these pathways can and do lead to dramatic improvements in sleep, and hopefully, large benefits to your mental health. Specifically, everything summarized above unequivocally should yield a positive impact on your sleep quality. Big gains are more obvious with the treatment of OSA/UARS and leg jerks, but large gains from learning to process emotions more effectively can also be realized. In fact, long-term gains from becoming a skilled emotional processor often prove a lifesaver for more than just sleep issues.

Notwithstanding this salient and health-giving paradigm, and analogous to our discussions about delving deeply into our emotions to discover new insights, here is the time we must raise one last set of questions, both from the standpoint of future sleep research as well as for advances in sleep therapies.

Where does this search begin? First, I always start by asking, are we looking deep enough into the sleep problems we are treating? Personally, I am always curious and always experimenting with my own sleep, which on occasion has guided or inspired some ideas we've researched. Thus, the most obvious question I ask myself is whether something deeper than sleep quality is to be found.

When heading down this pathway multiple times through the years in my efforts to learn more, I often found myself returning to the very intriguing sleep behavior we discussed briefly in Chapter 17, namely, napping. Napping is very near and dear to me as it got me through 35 years of life, from age 13 to 48, when I suffered moderately severe undiagnosed and untreated UARS and mild OSA. Not only did I try to learn everything I could about napping, I also experimented with various approaches to napping.

Yet, to this day, napping behavior leaves me puzzled. Why are some naps better than others? How is it possible you could feel great after a one-minute or five-minute nap but feel worse after a 30- to 60-minute nap, or *vice versa*? Since a huge proportion of the population reports highly variable napping experiences, doesn't it seem odd how these responses to naps go against the traditional view "more sleep is better?" Bluntly, why would shorter naps create a better response than longer naps? On the face of things, it makes no sense. If sleep duration is the be-all, end-all of sleep health, as is obsessively pronounced by so many sleep professionals as well as popular media, then wouldn't longer naps make you feel better than shorter ones? And, how do we possibly explain why some naps provide relief immediately upon awakening, others bring relief more gradually and of course some provide no relief or make things worse?

So, napping catches my eye because this idiosyncratic behavior perhaps will lead to a new clue about another core element in our understanding of sleep. Could this missing link, so to speak, explain how or why shorter versus longer hours of sleep at night do not consistently predict how well you will feel the next day, beyond what we know about our sleep quality explanation? Could a new core element explain why a person naturally might need to go through periods of sleeping longer or shorter hours over a stretch of time because his or her mind-body is operating differently at different times? Could this missing link reveal once and for all the most accurate and beneficial way to adopt a sleep schedule personally tailored to you? And, finally, what about catching up on sleep to rectify past sleep debt? I trust you gather from all the treatment discussions, we absolutely can erase some of our sleep debt in the aftermath of months and years of bad nights of slumber due to previously untreated sleep disorders, but is there a deeper factor in catching up that might define "good" catching up versus something else?

In medicine we love the word *parsimony*, or *parsimonious*, to express the idea of finding a good hypothesis or theory with the simplest or most unifying explanation. Can one thing, just one thing, explain most or all of a research hypothesis? Or, in the case of an individual patient, does one disease explain all that's going on? Does a patient suffer a chronic cough because he smokes, suffered a viral illness, has risks for lung cancer, and works outdoors in a polluted city?

We assume all four factors are in play, but as we learn more about a patient and see him or her regularly in clinic, we eventually hope to find the most important and parsimonious cause if one is to be found. What if years after the onset of the chronic cough, a savvy lung doctor recommends a blood test and discovers alpha-1 antitrypsin deficiency. At this point, we probably now have the very best and most parsimonious explanation for the chronic cough, as this rare disease affects the lungs, liver, and other organs as well as causing a chronic cough.

Thus, parsimony can be extremely important if we were missing something for years that would more accurately draw the whole or nearly the whole picture. With new and more precise knowledge, we can direct more precise care.

In our sleep world, is there an underlying, parsimonious factor we might be missing about sleep quality?"

I still believe sleep quality is the essential clinical piece to solving one's sleep puzzle. However, in recent years, I cannot help but wonder whether there's something still deeper and likely related to the glymphatic system (the healthy brain-washing system applied most actively during deep sleep and mentioned just a few times in the book). It has occurred to me as well as others that the biological waste accumulating in our brains could be the very reason we go to sleep. The waste builds while awake, and only through sleep can it be properly "rinsed" away.

Along these lines, we know the glymphatic system is much more active during sleep, and apparently more efficient during deeper or perhaps consolidated sleep. Thus, what I would like to leave you with is the idea it may not be enough to simply obtain the highest quality of slumber. It may be your sleep quality gains are also activating the glymphatic system in the most efficient ways.

So, if you treat all your sleep disorders, gain markedly enhanced sleep quality, and feel great throughout the day, then this point is largely irrelevant. But what if you achieve high sleep quality and don't feel as great as you expected? What would explain this lack of benefit?

To my way of thinking, it seems very likely we will one day learn how to measure the impact of the glymphatic system and hopefully recognize how well sleep quality is facilitating its waste-removal activities; and, perhaps we will discover a better functioning glymphatic system provides a clearer explanation for why we feel better after sleep as well as throughout the day. Moreover, current research already speculates a poorly functioning glymphatic system as a key link to dementia, which generates interest for nearly everyone.

I believe sorting out these connections between sleep quality and glymphatics will get us much closer to answering the questions posed about napping as well as other sleep issues. For example, do short naps produce great results not because of the brief sleep duration, but rather because brief functioning of the glymphatic system removed just enough waste products from the brain that were driving the immediate problem of sleepiness or other cognitive declines in the middle of the afternoon? Would longer naps not be as effective if the individual suffers from an untreated sleep disorder, which has more time to flare up during the longer sleep episode and thereby interfere with or compromise the functioning of the glymphatic system?

All these points suggest even greater complexity and less parsimony, because a brief nap would seem to permit only sufficient time to enter superficial sleep and not delta or REM. Moreover, it appears delta is the place where glymphatics work best, although I would speculate we will discover a pivotal role for REM sleep as well. Then again, what if a theory about sleep consolidation and not just sleep depth explains the power of a brief nap, assuming it fits into the category of excellent albeit brief consolidation.

Finally, we also want answers to the question: do we go through periods of longer sleep or shorter sleep because of a "sleep need?" Or is the change in duration directly tied to how much time the glymphatic system needs to power wash the brain? And will research on the glymphatic system reveal to us once and for all whether the notion of a normalized day/night schedule needs rigid enforcement—as so frequently advertised by experts, professional and amateur alike—or will we realize a fair degree of variation works just fine when sleep quality or sleep consolidation is so high the glymphatic system operates at high efficiency?

I am most eager to sleep on these questions and perhaps research them in the coming years. Looking for answers in this realm just might bring us to the place many have dreamed about, including myself, where we attain something we shall name "Super Sleep."

Until then, sleep well and prosper!

APPENDIX A

TROUBLESHOOTING GUIDE: ADVANCED PAP PEARLS

Introduction

This supplement is your go-to, how-to PAP guidebook. Reference this information often to identify and solve problems. Look for online resources as well, but please note very few sleep professionals possess expertise, training, or knowledge in dealing with advanced PAP devices. They might have great tips for solving a mask or leak issue, but their commentary on PAP is usually directed at CPAP or APAP (auto-CPAP).

To be certain, auto-CPAP is still CPAP; whenever you breathe in or out you still receive the same pressure. APAP ranges between two pressures, for example 5 of CPAP up to 10 of CPAP. Depending on your position or stage of sleep, the device may detect the need for higher or lower pressure, but unlike bilevel devices, the only benefit is the raising or lowering of "fixed" pressure. No matter the specific CPAP pressure along this range, it's always the same problem of breathing out against the same pressure you breathed in. Bilevel eliminates this problem by automatically lowering pressure when you breathe out. If you breathe in 10, you could breathe out against 6.

Also, a special reminder, refer to the beginning of Chapter 7 for the Pearl of Pearls (page 80) on imagery distraction to overcome adaptation issues with the mask or pressure sensations. Imagery distraction used early and often during adaptation proves highly advantageous for most mental health patients attempting PAP therapy.

The Work in Progress

Imagine starting a new medication your doctor declares will make you feel better, but then before gaining benefits you feel like you are experiencing something just shy of the trials of Job. Whether the medication treats cancer or depression or arthritis or restless legs or leg jerks, the drug's side effects overwhelm you to the point of wanting to give up. While all evidence points to the medicine's potential to cure or improve your condition, the adaptation period feels exasperating and demoralizing, if not painful, due to new symptoms feeling like "the cure is worse than the disease."

This analogy encapsulates the early, mixed experiences of many PAP therapy patients. PAP sounds like a great idea up until the point you stick an unwieldy, odd, and uncomfortable (sometimes painful) mask on your face and then air is forced into your nose and throat.

To help navigate through this initial process including barriers, missteps, and difficult adjustments let's troubleshoot now, because virtually every sleep apnea patient reports glitches with the mask or the air pressure, and these in turn lead to other glitches, nuisances, and annoyances.

Let me remind you about dealing with DME/HME companies, insurance carriers, and government regulators. Do not be surprised to find yourself gnashing your teeth as these entities prove more of a hindrance than a help in your efforts. Remember the adage the squeaky wheel gets the oil.

If you are the kind of person who pays strict attention to details, your adaptation may proceed rapidly and smoothly. If you are the type of person who might need a lot of coaching and support for your Big PAP Adventure, you may need patience, because one to six months is how long it might take to get everything running optimally.

A key point about this supplement is the overlap with many concepts in the earlier chapters, but now we will drill down much deeper into precise coaching steps of a type you would receive any day of the week if you were visiting our sleep center. Unfortunately, a lot of information you are about to learn is not standard fare at the majority of sleep centers, perhaps because most centers do not conduct research on PAP therapy patients or because they don't use advanced PAP equipment.

Our combination of research into the fine points of advanced PAP and our hands-on experience with thousands of mental health patients using PAP has created a system in which greater than 90% of sleep apnea patients who fill a prescription for the device eventually go on to use PAP.[181] My own use of PAP therapy since 2002, including trials with just about every device and mask on the market, has greatly expanded my appreciation for the struggle as well as my capacity to successfully coach PAP patients.

Mask Type, Style, Fit, and Comfort

It cannot be repeated enough: the mask must be comfortable! Without a comfortable mask, you will never wear PAP regularly. For a more sensitive person, consider using the nasal pillows mask; several types apply minimal to no actual contact to the remainder of the face, that is, the nasal pillows sit only in the nose, and the headgear works to minimize anything else touching your skin, or the headgear straps are so thin their presence fades rapidly.

The greatest mask of this type, the Breeze, is no longer readily available, but for someone who wants absolutely nothing touching any part of the face, this mask might be worth searching for online. It operates as a semicircle on top of your head, held in place by the leverage between the nasal pillows in the nostrils and the back of your head. If no other mask works for you, try to track down the Breeze.

Another option new to the market is the Bleep, patterned after the Breeze, but even more noninvasive as it creates ports outside instead of inside the nostrils. It looks to be a game changer for many patients because it works without any headgear. For more details, check their website, www. bleepsleep.com. It still shows some kinks in the system, but they appear to be working diligently to perfect the mask.

The major drawback to nasal pillows is the emergence of mouth breathing, a complication arising in many OSA/UARS patients, either as part of their sleep breathing symptoms or as a side effect once exposed to pressurized air. You would think mouth breathing requires a full face mask (FFM) to encircle both the nasal (nose) and oral (mouth) airways. For many people, the FFM proves the best solution, but for those with claustrophobia or other anxieties or sensitivities about an awkward covering on their face while sleeping, the

FFM is a nonstarter, turning off many otherwise willing patients. We'll return to mouth breathing shortly.

Starting in a place (sleep lab, sleep clinic, DME setting) that permits you to try all types and styles of masks until you find one or two comfortable models is the ideal. The mask technology industry is expanding exponentially to meet this problem, and most sleep lab technologists possess considerable experience and familiarity with all the nuances of this vast assortment. You just need a sleep tech willing to work with you to pin down the most comfortable choices.

Unfortunately, this preliminary encounter may lead to a conflict between the sleep staff at the sleep center or sleep lab and the staff at the DME/HME. What if the mask recommendation is not identical at both locales? Such disagreements occur often. If you spent a whole night in the sleep lab, though, using PAP therapy and trying on different masks to test comfort and fit, does it make sense you would find a better mask spending 15 to 30 minutes with a DME specialist who does not even hook you up to a PAP machine or even let you lie down in a sleeping position? The short and long answer is "no." Occasionally, DME will employ superior staff compared to sleep lab techs, but 80% to 90% of the time, you will gather the most reliable information from your interactions with sleep techs.

Notwithstanding, if you suffered a bad night in the sleep lab, perhaps you were not fitted with the right mask.

Watch Out for Myths About PAP Adaptation

It also cannot go without saying: your very first attempt at PAP therapy will prove next to impossible at finding the perfect long-term pressure settings or the perfect mask. Can you see the potential for how frustrating this experience would be? You've just spent an entire night in the lab (trying to sleep in an odd environment with uncomfortable sensors attached all over your body), you fill your script from the DME company for the machine and the mask (often taking weeks for insurance approval), and then when the equipment finally arrives at your home, you cannot tolerate the mask or the pressures. Worse, the mask or pressures seem uncomfortable to the point of degrading your sleep. Figuratively, this is the scenario of starting a new medication with great upside potential, but your battle with the side effects feels like a crushing blow to your hopes for improved health.

What would you do next? You are supposed to ring up the DME and ask for immediate assistance. Why? Because your insurance dollars are not simply paying for the PAP equipment. Built into the coverage, allegedly, is an allotment of time paid to the DME to provide support for your efforts to use the device. While the DME could prove helpful once you learn to identify more of your own personal idiosyncrasies in using PAP, unfortunately in the early going DME staff will not prove adequate in getting you over the hump unless you work with a special type of DME company, often locally owned or committed to going the extra mile.

We'll return to these connections regarding the DME and the sleep center to gain insights and information you need to successfully manipulate your mask fittings and pressure settings. For now, let's get back to masks, and close with this essential reminder: if your mask isn't comfortable, you have the wrong mask! And no amount of mythology based on conventional ~~wisdom~~ nonsense should dictate that you "just have to get used to it."

Mask Leak and Seal

As much as comfort is crucial, if you gain comfort but the mask leaks from a poor seal, your efforts may be hampered depending on the severity of the leak. Mask leak is a surprisingly complex issue to which many sleep centers and labs, as well as DMEs, do not seem to give a great deal of attention; many sleep professionals hold to the perspectives of the mask manufacturers, who often describe leak in terms of "a reasonable amount but no more." This phrasing is extremely misleading because with our patients we routinely find the optimal approach is zero leaks.

Nevertheless, zero leak is a confusing point because there are three types of leaks:

- normal leak to ventilate carbon dioxide
- nuisance leak that disrupts sleep
- objective measurable leak, compromising your best response to PAP

Carbon dioxide ventilation is the normal "leak" the PAP device measures and removes from the leak calculation; this real-time leak is usually not viewable on your device. When you are looking at the leak number on your PAP screen, it does *not* include this normal blowing off of carbon dioxide (CO_2), which is released through port(s) you see and hear on the front or sides of the mask.

Exhaling (breathing out) is how you expel CO_2 from the body, so if a mask port were blocked or your mask had a defect, CO_2 would build up. Such a defect makes it impossible to use the mask because your natural response triggers rapid hyperventilation similar to running a race where you can never catch your breath. As the CO_2 is stuck inside the mask, the brain keeps you breathing faster and faster to expel it.

For most, the mask gets ripped off within a few minutes (or seconds) of trying to use it, whether you are asleep or awake at the time. This situation is only dangerous if you suffer from other lung conditions where you already experience difficulty exhaling CO_2. Don't worry, though, as many patients with COPD, asthma, and restrictive lung diseases use PAP all night without developing problems with the mask. Besides, all masks now have the appropriate port systems to release the necessary amount of exhaled breath. Only if the mask is tampered with in some way could this serious malfunction arise.

Again, this type of leak is normal and has no bearing on the types of leaks that cause problems adapting to the mask; the two other leak issues are both abnormal, need to be monitored regularly, and must be resolved in timely fashion, but they have nothing to do with CO_2, so while not dangerous, they will seriously hinder your efforts to use PAP.

Nuisance Versus Objective Leak

The distinction between these two leaks (nuisance and objective) are blurred as they may overlap for any given patient; both nuisance leak and objective leak are measurable, more or less, and nuisance leak is more of a qualitative problem, whereas objective leak is more quantitative.

Nuisance leak is the more important when you first attempt PAP because it will annoy you so much, you will cease use. The best example of nuisance leak is a well-fitting mask that nonetheless leaks from a tiny area on the sides of the bridge of the nose. If pressurized air is ejected on one or both sides of the nasal bridge, it will shoot straight into your eyes. An enormous number of people stop using PAP therapy because of nuisance leak to the eyes, despite it causing a very small objective leak, so small, in fact, it might not register as a leak on the device screen. Tell that to your eyes!

A quick way to solve leaks targeting the eyes is to find a soft, stretchy sock with a comfortable surface and apply it as a second "mask" to cover your eyes without putting any pressure on your eyelids. Obviously, an eye mask might work as well as long as you integrate it with the PAP mask and headgear straps. This jerry-rigged system might sound cumbersome but actually fits rather comfortably if you finesse it. I like the sock approach because I can weave the ends into the headgear straps on the sides or back of my head to provide additional comfort when I need to tighten the headgear.

Another common leak occurs on the cheeks when using the FFM style. This problem feels unresolvable and is especially annoying because the leak easily turns into the disturbing sound of a "mask fart," fortunately without odor. The noise almost always awakens the PAP user, but if it doesn't, it will awaken your bedpartner, who will then elbow you to fix it.

To solve cheek leak be sure you correctly fit the mask. Going back to the original dilemma of sleep center versus DME, you may discover one place recommends a large FFM, and the other insists you need a medium; eventually you may discover, only one of these sizes solves the mask leak at your cheeks, but it sure would have been nice to know the correct size the first time around.

Making matters more finicky, the real problem may be the headgear. You might have needed large headgear with the medium mask or medium-sized headgear with the large mask. Working hands-on with an experienced sleep tech is the best place for a finessed evaluation.

This scenario also proves expensive because most insurance carriers only cover mask replacements every three months. If you select the mask from the first titration test and then discover two weeks later the cheek leak does not abate, you would either need to pay out of pocket (often a few hundred dollars) to obtain a new size mask or wait it out for the next 10 weeks before insurance covers the new one.

At our center and at some DME companies, loaner programs address this snafu with the goal of finding the right mask so at the three-month mark the next prescribed mask will be the right one to solve leak. On the other hand, just imagine how many people give up on PAP because of the wrong mask at the outset (which they did not realize was "wrong") coupled with their lack of resources to get the "right" mask as soon as a problem is identified. Tons of OSA/UARS patients simply put their devices in the closet, never to be used again, or only revisit the issue when the insurance coverage becomes available again. Quite the medical system flaw!

Again, you might discover you want to start with nasal pillows or nasal (covers the nose) mask type at the outset because the leak problems are more readily eliminated. Yet, even these masks cause difficulties due to irregularities of anatomy, such as the degree of indentation on the bridge of the nose, the puffiness or hollowness of the cheeks, facial hair above the lip, and the vertical or horizontal dimensions of the face.

Mask Liners

One of the best solutions for nuisance leak is the RemZzzs mask liner system. There are other mask liners systems as well; the Pad A Cheek system offers a well-known product in the field. We use both systems, but we had the most success with the RemZzzs because you can work with them more fastidiously to produce more precision in addressing how the liner is layered onto the mask to resolve the leak problem.

Mask liners are an interesting invention; they can eliminate the nuisance leak yet also cause either slight worsening or improvement in the objective leak. In the early going, this paradox proves irrelevant because stopping nuisance leak allows you to use PAP therapy, whereas objective leak shows less influence on your ability to use the device. Rather, objective leak prevents you from achieving optimal PAP results because you are losing pressurized air needed to treat sleep breathing events. In other words, short-term you must solve the nuisance leak, and then long-term address objective leak. We'll discuss objective leak next because it also relates to mouth breathing.

Mouth Breathing

Did you know a natural reflex exists to open your mouth to breath when you suffer air blockage through your nose? In other words, mouth breathing while asleep is its own confirmation you suffer from a sleep breathing disorder. Even if you only mouth breathe when you suffer a cold, then on that particular night you are also experiencing a sleep breathing disorder. The ironic thing about mouth breathing is it does not resolve the problem it's attempting to solve. It provides air since none was inhaled through the nose, but the oral airway proves inadequate in pulling enough volume to normalize breathing. Again, the oddity of mouth breathing, despite being a natural reflex to help you breathe, indicates pathology best understood as a component of sleep-disordered breathing.

When pressurized air is channeled into the nose, sufficient air volume overcomes the blockage in the nasal airway. PAP therapy resolves OSA or UARS and may resolve mouth breathing. But if pressurized air causes its own discomfort, a new reflex emerges in the mouth, which opens and releases the extra air. *Irony Alert: you are treating a disorder that triggers mouth breathing, yet the treatment of the disorder may trigger mouth breathing.* As you would expect, this latter type of mouth breathing commonly occurs while breathing out (exhalation).

Regardless of the old or new causes of mouth breathing, it must be dealt with effectively, or both nuisance and objective leak will continue as major barriers. Most PAP users gain rapid awareness of mouth breathing because of the annoying sensation of dryness in the mouth, either prior to PAP or soon after starting. Dry mouth is your most reliable signal of mouth breathing, but for those without this symptom, mouth breathing can be detected in the sleep lab by a trained sleep tech.

The two most common treatments for mouth breathing are the FFM or a chinstrap. The latter device is a circular strap running from the top of the head to the chin; it is tightened to nudge the mouth closed, but not so tight as to cause tension and soreness in the teeth or jaw muscles. Successfully applying a chinstrap means you will breathe through your nose with PAP, which then creates options for over-the-nose and nasal pillow masks. Most sleep apnea patients find nasal masks most comfortable at the outset. However, take notice of timing here; surprisingly or not, a majority of patients eventually find the FFM more comfortable, and some use a chinstrap with the FFM; you will learn why momentarily. In other patients, dry mouth is caused by oral hygiene issues, including dehydration. Don't hesitate to use OTC products like Biotene or Xylimelts, and drink more water.

Advantages of Full Face Masks (FFM)

Use of the FFM is certainly more difficult for the obvious reason too many points contact the skin, creating more leak opportunities, which makes it seem silly to start this way. Moreover, use of FFM proves paradoxical because it was originally advertised as an over-the-nose-and-mouth device sufficient to deal with mouth breathing. Yet, this logic does not hold up because, as above, mouth breathing produces a lesser volume of air flow, and thus breathing events persist. As we now understand, the real goal of the FFM is to discourage mouth breathing by giving the patient the security to open the mouth (the reflex) only when necessary. However, over the course of the night, the goal is for mouth breathing to be minimized while nasal breathing is maximized.

Got it? Yeah, I didn't think so. Don't worry, it gets worse!

A more subtle and potentially more relevant problem is how mouth breathing almost always changes the angle of the jaw. Experience for a moment your lips closed, but then feel the sensation of dropping your jaw (but keep your lips touching). If you are unclear on this exercise, look in the mirror. As an aside, for fun, start noticing some features in your face that perhaps indicate your age; then several weeks or months after getting solid results with PAP, look again to notice how you look younger, a very common cosmetic benefit and something nice to look forward to!

Back to your jaw. What happens the moment you open your mouth and drop your jaw? Usually, it looks like a pronounced double chin or a facial expression of dullness, or both. With the jaw dropped, place your two index fingers on the point just in front of your ears (the temporomandibular joint, or TMJ). Now repeat the motion of the jaw dropping and lifting back to normal and go back and forth. Notice the increased degree of difficulty breathing through your nose in the dropped position compared to normal position. At the same time, notice with your lips still sealed you are not mouth breathing when jaw dropping.

From all the above, it should be clear mouth breathing itself is not the only part of this problem; rather, it is a sign of a much more pronounced problem in which the angle of the jaw opens, the tongue falls toward the back of the throat, and then breathing is further obstructed. If you put it all together, then you will not be surprised to find out many sleep apnea patients using the FFM also need the chinstrap to prevent jaw dropping, even if no mouth breathing was evident.

At our center it is extremely common for patients using the FFM to also use the chinstrap. I have used the combo many times. The urgent question before you is whether you really need to go through all the trouble of using the FFM? Why not select a nasal pillow or a nasal mask plus the chinstrap and forgo the FFM? The answer requires time to sort out. Many patients do use a chinstrap with every sort of mask and still achieve good to optimal results, but regrettably, this level of success may never be achieved among those who insist on only trying the nasal masks without a chinstrap.

Subtle Mouth Leak

The obvious reason for failure with the nasal masks is that air still can leak through the mouth without gross mouth breathing. This final phase of assessment is usually called mouth leak, or sometimes mouth sputtering, in which the amount of air leaking is much smaller, yet still problematic, compared to true mouth breathing. In the olden days, patients were instructed to place a small, narrow piece of tape covering only the middle third of the lips, top and bottom, in an attempt to train the individual to keep the lips closed. Now we realize a more involved process is effective, and it goes by the scary name of "mouth taping."

Air Blasts Triggered by Mask Leak

Before moving to mouth taping, we need to discuss one final problem caused by air leak. Recall if the leak is large enough, then the amount of actual pressurized air getting past your upper airway has been reduced. This decrease means you are getting insufficient air to treat sleep breathing events. Nowadays, many PAP devices have auto-adjusting algorithms that detect this loss of air and send a new blast into your nose and throat. The result is the patient awakens and notices a smothering sensation as if drowning in air.

Unfortunately, many patients never receive this education. Instead, they are led to believe or talk themselves into believing their pressures are too high. But the real problem is not high pressure; it's large leak that triggers higher pressure via the blast of air, which was merely attempting to compensate for the technological perception of diminished airflow.

A ton of PAP users quit PAP after just one of these air blasts without ever finding out the simple leak explanation. If a patient does talk with sleep support staff, the individual will insist on lowering the pressures, which theoretically could help as the next air blast after the next leak would be a smaller volume of air. Nonetheless, the patient should be directed to address the mask leak issue that caused the problem. This effort might require a quick trip to the

DME or sleep center or sleep lab to find a solution to the mask leak issue.

Bottom line, try not to overreact to an air blast scenario. Yes, it can be exceedingly uncomfortable, if not scary. But the problem is not the air pressure; it's the mask leak. By all means, if you become very nervous about the air blasts, you definitely want pressures to be lowered as much as possible until the mask leak can be fixed. And make sure you also give equal if not more attention to solving the mask leak issue.

Mouth Taping

No, not duct tape! Although—you might be surprised how many people try it.

What you need is a drugstore brand of "gentle paper tape." Initially, you might be comfortable only covering small sections of your mouth instead of the whole opening. Undoubtedly, you must feel secure in attempting this step, and you need to feel comfortable with your exit strategy. The best approach is cutting a strip long enough to extend beyond the boundaries of your mouth and then twirl the ends of the tape into "quick-release" safety tags, which obviously are not sticking to your facial skin.

If you suffer a sudden bout of panic, anxiety, or claustrophobia, or some physiological issue such as stomach indigestion that increases the chance for reflux or vomiting, the quick-release twirls are grabbed in an instant and the tape removed a second later. Even more expedient, gentle paper tape is so thin you can poke your finger right through it if an urgent situation arises. On the other hand, if the paper is so thin you feel air coming in and out, cut a small piece of linen material and attach it to the sticky side of the tape, so your lips are now pressing up against the cloth material instead of the adhesive. Clearly, you must be comfortable with such steps and confirm you are using these materials safely as you don't want to swallow or inhale the added material. For these reasons, working with sleep professionals, especially experienced sleep technologists, will prove invaluable.

Finally, among sleep apnea patients who use both a full face mask and chinstrap, some also tape their mouths to prevent mouth breathing or mouth leak. Though we would wish this complex array of steps proved unnecessary, the truth is some patients never attain an optimal response to PAP until they conquer mouth breathing, mouth leak, or mouth sputtering. Though mouth taping is a last resort and somewhat scary, in select patients it really seals the deal (pun intended) for those who could never find any other way to prevent air leaking through their lips.

PAP Mode

This is the biggest of the biggies, so I will repeat: most patients will be encouraged by their sleep doctors to start using a device known as CPAP, where the C stands for *continuous* and delivers the same pressure all night long, whether you breathe in or out, lie on your side or back, or enter a deeper or a lighter stage of sleep. I very rarely recommend starting with CPAP unless you are forced to by your insurance. APAP was mentioned, but now I want to note it can be used with an expiratory pressure relief setting, or EPR. With this setting, you get slightly lower pressure on expiration, so technically it's like bilevel. The catch is the pressure drop only reaches 3 units; if you breathe in 10 units, it only drops to 7 units breathing out. While potentially beneficial, most auto-bilevel and ASV devices provide greater swings in pressure and are more comfortable as well as more effective. In particular, for someone with anxiety, an EPR drop to 7 down from 10 on APAP may feel inconsequential, whereas drops of 4 units or greater might be needed for maximum relief, comfort, and enhanced results.

Despite the pervasive and arguably ill-informed conventional wisdom to prescribe CPAP devices, in 2005 we stopped virtually all these prescriptions in favor of dual pressure modes. Then, in 2008/2009 we prescribed still more advanced devices—particularly those manufactured by the ResMed corporation, which were designed with greater technological sophistication to improve the comfort level and the objective response to PAP therapy by more aggressively eradicating flow limitation.

These devices possess auto-adjusting features, and the two most common ones are ABPAP, for *auto-adjusting bilevel*, and ASV, for *adaptive servo-ventilation*. You would like to get started with one of these two key PAP modes instead of wasting time, effort, and resources on CPAP or APAP. We'll focus on both advanced models so you get the gist of why they are better as well as how to persuade your sleep center staff to prescribe advanced PAP in place of standard CPAP or APAP.

Auto-Adjusting PAP Pressure Devices, Part I

Just like a diabetic who attempts to monitor levels of glucose and then changes the dosage of insulin as frequently as every day, the human airway does not function in a static manner to receive only one fixed dose of pressurized air. In fact, no medical technological treatment has yet been created to respond perfectly to this problem, and, regrettably many sleep professionals do not even recognize it as a problem as they believe in a one-size-fits-all model and prescribe fixed CPAP to most of their patients.

You would think it rather obvious daily or nightly factors could easily alter the needs of the human airway in attempting to remain wide open: nasal congestion, different sleep positions, and changes in temperature or humidity are just a few, but the biggest ones are based on the fact that you simply do not breathe the same when your sleep is lighter or deeper or when you are sleeping in REM stage instead of NREM stages.

These ideas prompted manufacturers of PAP equipment to produce auto-adjusting devices that might detect a physiological need to lower or raise pressure settings. By analogy, when you talk with your doctors about virtually any medication, the same type of discussion unfolds: "Under these circumstances you might want to raise the dosage of your diabetes drugs," or, "under these circumstances you might want to lower the dosage of your antidepressant," and so on. Yet, this kind of discussion emerges haphazardly in our field of sleep medicine and sometimes only when the squeaky wheel begs for oil.

Remarkably, the device manufacturers are leading the way in achieving symptomatic relief previously unobtainable with CPAP or APAP devices. Let me say that again: private and independent businesses have everything to gain or lose, and they are the ones making the technological advances to give you better sleep. Yet, the vast majority of sleep professionals ignore these advances. Free market capitalism is a great thing, but apparently the sleep medical profession needs to be pulled kicking and screaming into the twenty-first century.

With auto-adjusting features and the sophisticated algorithms in ABPAP and ASV, you will almost immediately notice greater comfort, but more importantly, after just one night of sleep, you will often notice higher quality slumber. If you recall our earlier discussions, you must find a way to convince your sleep center to bring you back to the sleep lab to manually titrate these advanced devices even though the device is set to the auto mode.

This step is essential because the algorithms inside the devices are good to very good, but they are not consistently excellent to outstanding. They cannot respond flawlessly to every change in your breathing, so it is imperative for the device settings to be precisely set by a sleep technologist watching your sleep and breathing in the lab. When these settings are more precisely calculated, the algorithm works more effectively because its window of pressure ranges matches your specific needs.

Compare riding a bicycle with three speeds to one with 10 to 15 gears; you know how much smoother the pedaling feels with the latter. Most of the time, you are not going to use all 15 gears; yet there will be a range that works best for you and feels most comfortable depending on the circumstances.

A *manual* titration of an *auto*-adjusting device will find the most effective range in the sleep lab. Unlike a bicycle where you could in fact experiment with different ranges yourself, the precision settings of these devices are much more reliably determined under the watchful eye of an experienced sleep technologist, as often as every year or two to maintain high quality, finely tuned solutions.

Auto-Adjusting PAP Pressure Devices, Part II

If you like technology, this section will help you appreciate how these devices work to better your sleep; this information may arm you in your efforts to persuade your sleep physicians to let you try one at home or in the lab or hopefully both sites.

ABPAP and ASV use systems to literally track your breathing, breath by breath, and thereby create rolling averages of what can be understood as your breathing metric or measure. These metrics are not all the same in each device. With one type, the metric measures the shape of your airflow curve, whereas another device measures the volume of each breath. Still another device may possess a capacity to analyze the collapsibility of the airway. It may surprise you to learn we don't know for sure how each device performs with precision because algorithms are proprietary intellectual property; therefore, to protect their interests, manufacturers reveal only generalized information on algorithms.

Nonetheless, your breathing is sensed, and the algorithm gauges a range between normal and abnormal breathing. It is easy to sense when someone stops breathing, but it is much more difficult to sense when breathing degrades into a subtle flow limitation event. Please review Figure 5.4 here to make sure these points are clear.

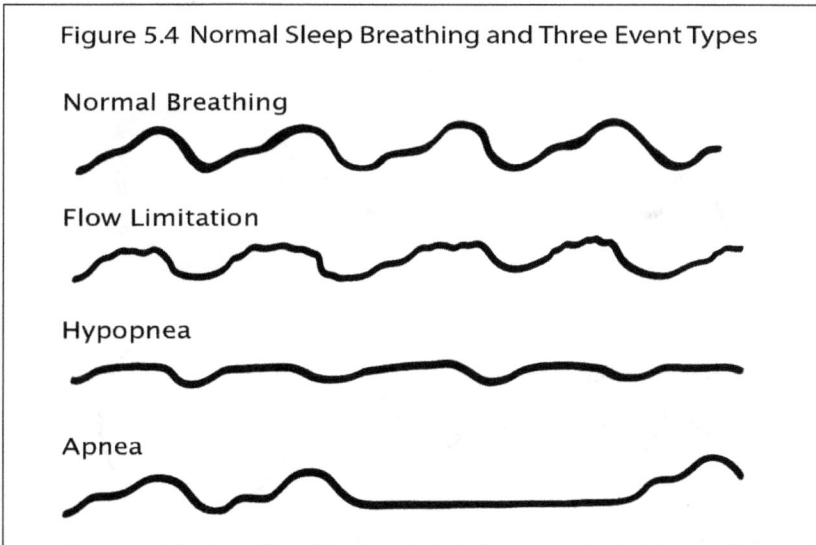

Figure 5.4 Normal Sleep Breathing and Three Event Types

Normal Breathing

Flow Limitation

Hypopnea

Apnea

Figure 5.4 The four shapes range from well-rounded (normal breathing) to extremely flattened. Three sleep breathing events show increasingly severe flattening, indicating increasingly smaller air volume.

If you consider the differences between the three main breathing events—apneas, hypopneas, and flow limitations—it would be interesting for you to guess which type of event is the most difficult to treat because this knowledge helps you understand the critical value of the auto-adjusting technology, as well as the need for more time spent in the sleep lab. You may recall we first posed this exercise in Chapter 6. It's useful to review Figure 6.1 again because you might be in the midst of working with your sleep center.

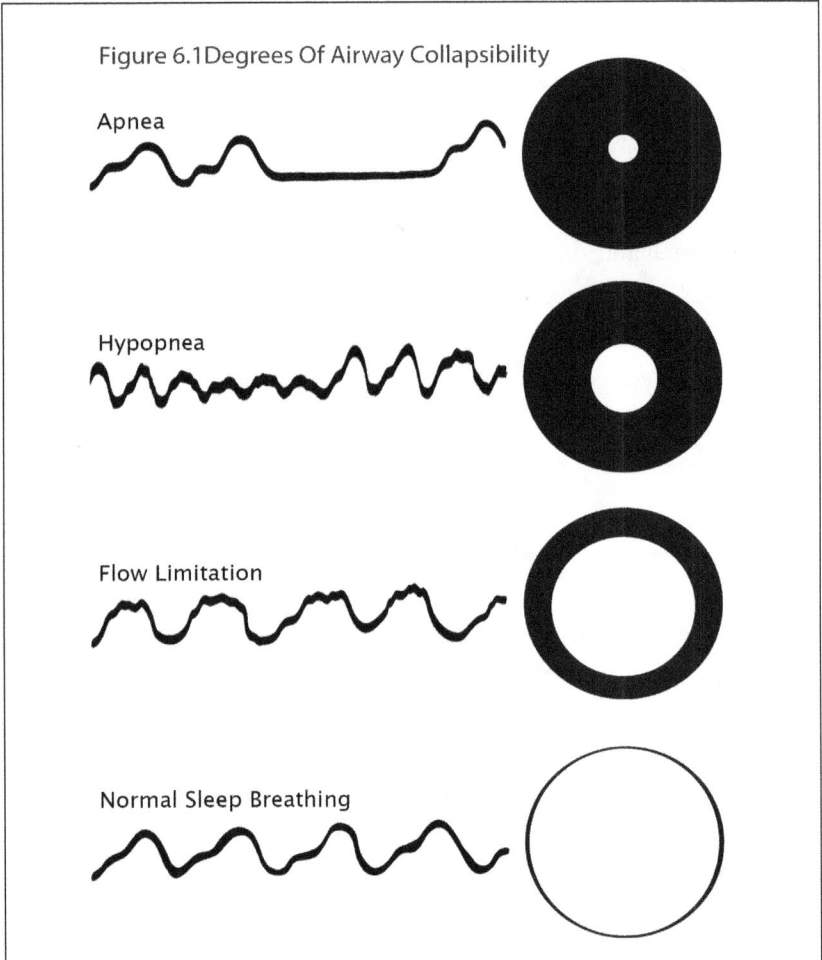

Figure 6.1 Degrees Of Airway Collapsibility

Apnea

Hypopnea

Flow Limitation

Normal Sleep Breathing

Figure 6.1 The lines on the left side depict tracings of three types of sleep breathing events along with normal airflow at the bottom. On the right side, looking from top to bottom, the cross-section views show increasing air space volume as the collapsibility steadily decreases.

Ironically or not, the apnea is the easiest to treat because you only need a little pressurized air to overcome it; usually, at low pressure the apnea turns into a hypopnea, where you lose 50% of air flow instead of 100%. In other words, a breathing event is still occurring, but now the pressurized air has decreased its severity.

Think of the apnea as a closed airway; when you give it just a bit of pressurized air, you are opening the airway some, but not all the way. The residual breathing pattern appears as a hypopnea, which can then be treated by delivering a higher level of pressurized air. This increase in air opens the airway further but does not yet make it normal.

If you guessed the hypopnea is now converted into a flow limitation, then you understand the dynamics of treating sleep breathing disorders. In other words, if you next want to treat the flow limitation, then still higher pressurized air is needed to fully open the airway. Clearly, flow limitation needs the highest of all pressures.

As the pressures increase to the highest levels, it becomes more difficult to stabilize the airway to fully normal patency because this higher pressure is more difficult for the human body to tolerate, at least upon initial use of PAP.

Now, after reviewing the schematics in Figure 6.1, you see how the airway space gets larger with each successive increase in pressurized air, starting from apnea until airflow is fully normalized. Only when you arrive at normal airflow do you see the largest open space compared to apnea where the spaced is the most closed down.

So far, so good. However, what happens when you cannot tolerate the higher pressure to eliminate flow limitation? As you recall from the earlier discussion, again in Chapters 5 and 6, instead of normal airflow looking well-rounded for all parts of breathing in and out, as shown in Figures 5.4 and 6.1, only the top half looks rounded, while the bottom half of the airway shows a wobbly appearance, meaning it is responding inconsistently to the higher pressures while you breathe out. This problem was defined earlier as *expiratory pressure intolerance*, or EPI, although some in the field of sleep medicine call it *pressure intolerance*. Please review Figure 6.2 to observe the fluctuations we're discussing here.

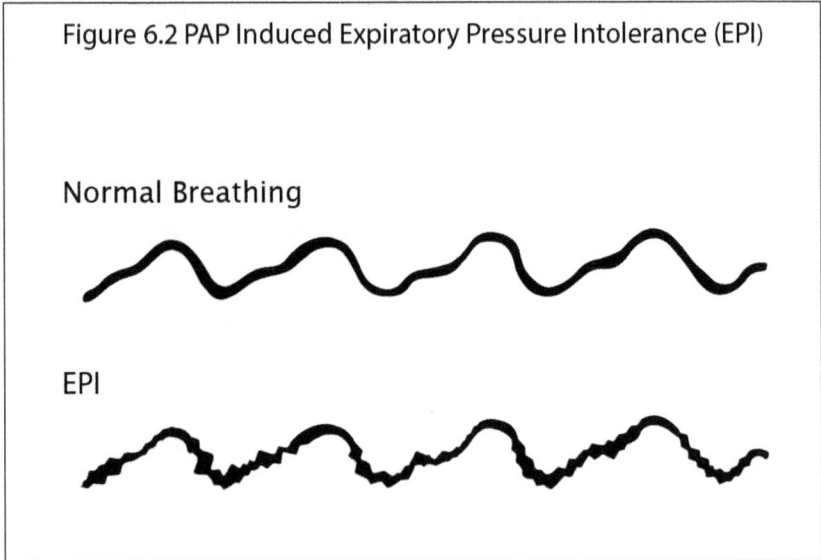

Figure 6.2 Expiratory pressure intolerance (EPI) is a subtle change on the airflow tracing, and the sleep technologist must be trained to accurately identify EPI and to adjust pressurized air accordingly.

EPI typically occurs while you are trying to breathe out against the pressurized air coming in. We will return to this topic shortly because the presence or absence of EPI often determines whether you gain an optimal response to PAP. In some patients, the degree of EPI severity determines whether you are capable of adapting to PAP. This knowledge also assists your efforts to receive a prescription for an advanced PAP mode, which, by the way, is the most effective solution for eradicating or preventing EPI.

Auto-adjusting technology scrutinizes these four patterns of breathing and continuously sorts out the degree of pressure needed to resolve as much abnormal breathing as possible and turn it into normal breathing. As you would expect from the above, auto-adjusting technology eliminates virtually all apneas and hypopneas with relative ease; in fact, it works so well some sleep professionals are persuaded to prescribe the device without ever testing the patient in the sleep lab. Indeed, there are patients who have reported very good to dramatic improvements just by starting out with an auto-adjusting device without ever having been tested in a sleep lab.

Sounds pretty awesome, doesn't it? Well, yes, it is awesome, especially if you are a fairly classic sleep apnea patient where the overwhelming number of breathing events comprises apneas or hypopneas. When more UARS flow limitations enter the picture, more scrutiny is needed. And mental health patients in particular, for reasons that are not clearly understood, appear to manifest a greater proportion of UARS flow limitation events than classic OSA patients.

To reiterate (see Figure 6.2), when the pressures increase to higher levels, the airway overreacts, fighting back, if you will; and instead of a fully open passageway, the airway remains in a constant state of flux between EPI and a semblance of normal breathing. The net result is usually pronounced disruption to sleep.

In a nutshell, this specific description explains why CPAP fails so many mental health patients: because this wobbliness is invariably occurring only during one phase of breathing—exhalation. To reiterate, CPAP is just one fixed pressure delivered at the same level, whether you breathe in or breathe out, but your body only needs the higher pressure when it breathes in, whereas the same pressure delivered when you breathe out causes this intolerance, or EPI. EPI goes to the heart of the problem of how CPAP fails so many patients and how auto-adjusting bilevel technology can rescue so many patients.

Auto-Adjusting PAP Pressure Devices, Part III

Many sleep professionals are wary of aggressively treating UARS flow limitations for two separate reasons. First and foremost, many sleep doctors and techs simply do not understand or appreciate the importance of these subtle breathing events; therefore, they give sparse attention to this component during a diagnostic or titration PSG. The second reason is all the negativity unleashed by insurance carriers, especially from Medicare, who seem to reject the very idea of UARS despite tons of research validating how it affects your sleep.[182] Put these two forces (ignorance and rejection) together with the practical matter of attempting to titrate out flow limitations (potentially triggering EPI with CPAP), and you can see why it makes more sense to let sleeping RERAs (respiratory effort-related arousals, another "sciency" term for flow limitation) lie. Sleep technologists complicate matters more because they may have their own biases either in favor of addressing flow limitation or ignoring it.

All these problems could be resolved in a matter of seconds by learning how to titrate out the RERAs while at the same time preventing the onset of EPI. Such results are conveniently achieved by learning to titrate auto-adjusting algorithms in the sleep lab; and to be clear, it is the manual titration of the auto-adjusting algorithm that achieves these results in far superior fashion compared to sending someone home with an auto-adjusting device with which the patient was never evaluated in the lab.

In sum, what you have learned in these three short sections on auto-adjusting devices is potentially a game changer when attempting to start and use PAP. Things really are this straightforward, but it requires the cooperation and implementation from the sleep professionals with whom you are working. Even if you print out and show them these three sections, they may choose to reject these ideas, at which point I can only suggest looking for another willing sleep professional in your area.

Truly, your effort is worth its weight in golden slumbers. Pushing ahead to receive a manual titration of an auto-adjusting device in the sleep lab may prove one of the more powerful steps, if not *the most* powerful step, you will ever take to solve your sleep breathing disorder. So, do not sit back and simply accept an opinion based on outdated evidence that restricts you to the use of outdated CPAP devices. Use this knowledge to gain an advanced PAP device, one that is more likely to provide you with the *rest* of your life.

Tips for a Successful Sleep Lab Titration Study

When you reach this step, you don't necessarily gain more control over your care plan, so it's useful to prepare by clarifying any specific goals you want to accomplish. Even then, the best laid plans may go awry. Nonetheless, if you are suffering from one big issue, you want to clarify in your own mind how best to communicate this problem.

For example, suppose your biggest issue is chronic mask leak. You might experience all types of leaks involving the way you fit the mask to your face, the impact of your body position on mask stability, and the real possibility you've already tried more than a handful of masks. How would the sleep lab help you find a solution to this nagging problem?

The good news is most sleep techs show a lot of motivation and skill in solving leak problems, and the very best sleep techs may surprise you by taking one really intrusive step to solve the problem on the night of your sleep test. Can you guess the step?

The secret is a great sleep tech will "step" right into your sleep lab bedroom while you are sleeping to very quietly lean over you and actually listen or feel for the air leaking out; and the tech must also observe where the leak springs from by close inspection of all contact points between mask and skin.

These same great sleep techs will inform you of their intent to enter your bedroom during the night, and you can also take the initiative, letting your sleep tech know your comfort level in following this procedure. Moreover, to be blunt, if you are suffering an intractable mask leak issue, conceivably the only way to accurately identify the source is through the eyes, ears, and hands of a very capable sleep tech who knows the most professional and skilled ways to conduct a sleep study titration.

Arguably, solving intractable mask leak issues is one of the most important reasons for returning to the sleep lab. Additional issues must also be dealt with through this hands-on approach or through technological manipulations. The following bullet list of items will help you prepare better.

- *Sleep lab bedroom environment.* Bring special pillows you use at home. If temperature sensitive, clarify what you can add or subtract in the way of blankets, comforters, and so on, to adjust accordingly.
- *Struggles with masks.* The sleep tech is typically working with one or two other patients, so your access to changing out masks may not go

as smoothly as you would like. Therefore, the best time to sort through masks is before lights out. Or, you might fare better by requesting a special daytime mask-fitting appointment a few days prior to the sleep study, or else clarify how much mask-fitting time you will receive before lights out on the night of the study.

- *Confusion about mask types.* In your search, you may discover an interest in many different types, such as nasal pillow, over-the-nose, and full face. Given the amount of time of the study, ranging from seven to 10 hours, try to find three masks to attempt and arrange them with the sleep tech in a ranked order, starting the night with the one you predict will work best. Don't hesitate to stick with the best one all night if you are doing great, but if you are not clear on the results, instruct the tech to give you trials on the other two for a couple hours each.

- *Mouth breathing, taping, and chinstraps.* If at all possible, you want to try some or all these steps before a repeat sleep lab study because there are fine points to each application and fine points to solving problems. Again, a great tech will find the best chinstrap and show you the best ways for mouth taping, but this issue and these procedures could increase anxiety, so try to learn more about your own reactivity prior to the next study.

- *Pressure changes.* As described earlier, minor adjustments to pressure could yield marked improvements in the response to PAP, both objectively and subjectively. While some pressure changes feel too strong, others feel too weak. The more you use PAP at home, including experimenting with small pressure adjustments, the easier you will discern how pressure feels in the sleep lab. And don't hesitate to ask or clarify with the sleep tech whether the inspiratory pressures are rounding the airflow curve to eliminate flow limitation events.

- *PAP-NAP.* As discussed in *Sleep Research Pearl #7*, this procedure is another lifesaver for those who simply cannot resolve one or more of these adaptation issues described in this section. Most sleep centers are familiar with the PAP-NAP concept, but may not conduct it in part because so much confusion remains about billing and reimbursement for the procedure, despite the fact that Medicare typically pays for it. When your issues seem intractable, don't hesitate to request a PAP-NAP at your sleep center.

• *Leg jerks.* More discussion is presented below on leg jerks. The one point to mention here is whether the sleep tech will need to visually confirm any changes in this condition by observing you on the video at your sleep study. Leg jerks are supposed to register on limb sensors, but some patients manifest subtle movements that must be confirmed by close visual observation. If you suffer more subtle movements and are trying to clarify the diagnosis or determine whether medications or supplements are working, you should invite the sleep tech to step in a few times during the night to check on leg movements.

• *REM and delta sleep.* Last and not least, although many sleep centers have policies about standards for sleep tech communications with patients, you should unequivocally let your sleep doctor and your sleep tech know how curious you are to learn how PAP affects your REM and delta. Some centers are beginning to loosen up their rules and engage patients to review aspects of the computer tracings. If so, that's a fine time to ask about how well REM was consolidated and how much delta was generated. If the tech is not permitted to discuss these elements, request the info verbally or in writing from the sleep center; you really would appreciate knowing how these critical stages of sleep responded to the new pressure settings attempted in the sleep lab.

Tracking Progress Through Changes in Sleep Quality and Insomnia

More factors are coming up, but now is the right time to emphasize the best ways to track your progress. It's one thing—one very *big* thing—to get the equipment properly functioning as early in the process as possible. Finding the best mask, best PAP mode, and best pressure settings makes things so much easier.

That said, many will struggle with even the best equipment, and then there will always be those forced to go through the standard process of initiating care with CPAP, failing it, and then arguing and appealing for advanced PAP. These appeals are very mixed. Some people have the door slammed in their face. Others require protracted appeals lasting three to six months. The fortunate ones find sleep professionals who, after listening to your complaints, pause, reflect, and then realize you really need a better treatment option.

As you proceed, for your benefit and for your communication with sleep professionals, it is imperative to use the right terms to explain your progress the right way.

First, unfortunately, most sleep professionals are obsessed with how many hours you use the device. If you are using PAP six to eight hours per night, you will find some sleep doctors telling you how great you're doing and care not a whit about your actual response. Because you never know how the sleep professional might respond, try to take control of the conversation from the get-go by focusing on any changes in your sleep quality and in your insomnia.

In starting this conversation with the sleep doc or sleep tech, you could note you are not seeing much change in either your quality of sleep or the disruptions in your sleep (insomnia). If the doc turns the conversation to how many hours of use, hypothetically you might say "I'm getting about three hours per night, so shouldn't I notice any improvements during those three hours?" This type of exchange may put sleep professionals back on their heels if they are too obsessed with the number of hours you sleep.

More to the point, you can also declare (when regrettably true), "I only get three hours because I feel like I'm sleeping worse with the device, so I take it off and then sleep better for the next three hours without it."

These examples are not in anticipation of you suffering a poor response. Rather, these pointers, when relevant, will guide your communication with sleep staff who may not practice sleep medicine at the highest levels.

To be sure, you want and expect (and we hope) you can report soon after initiating PAP you are sleeping deeper, feeling more refreshed when you wake up in the morning, and clearly noticing fewer awakenings (insomnia) during the night. One of the huge changes common to successful PAP users is the report of "falling back asleep faster" after awakenings, which is an incredibly satisfying milestone to achieve in the early going.

The good news is improvement in middle-of-the-night insomnia is exceptionally common in PAP users because PAP is restoring your unconscious confidence to no longer worry about sleep breathing as pressurized air is now protecting you. In short, you go back to sleep both because you are confident it is safe to do so and because your breathing feels more stable with PAP.

One caveat arises if you develop a bit of anxiety after an awakening. This anxiety may amplify the pressurized air sensation in some individuals, making it more difficult to return to sleep. If so, consider using the "ramp" button on your device to temporarily lower pressures for five to 30 minutes (you decide). As pressures start lower and gradually ramp back up to your normal settings, you might find it easier to fall back asleep. Some need to use the ramp function at bedtime as well.

Sleep quality, insomnia, and improvement in daytime energy are the most powerful variables you want to track and also communicate to your sleep staff, letting them know one way or another the extent of your progress.

Other variables can also be tracked, including trips to the bathroom (nocturia), morning headaches, dry mouth, attention, concentration, and memory. Speaking of which, if you believe you will have difficulty tracking or remembering how you are progressing week to week, then please start a daily diary in your phone, computer, tablet, or on a piece of paper to identify the targets you want to track. Then use this tracking system every single day, regardless of whether it was a good or bad night of sleep. If you use specialized software to assist in tracking sleep, like OSCAR and SleepMapper designed for PAP users, these usually provide a note-taking portal or tab where you can collect your insights after each sleep period.

Last, when insomnia persists, don't hesitate to return to Chapters 10 through 15 for more psychological strategies, including CBT-I, to solve unwanted sleeplessness. You also will find more insomnia tips in Appendix B, which follows this one.

Tube Placement

Turning back to more mundane matters, tube placement should not be a big deal to many patients, but it becomes a big deal if the setup in your bedroom prevents you from organizing equipment easily. The single best system, and one that most patients find difficult to arrange, is a "headboard" approach, but it's worth looking into because it essentially solves all issues regarding tube placement and access to the device.

The "headboard" style means finding or building a bookshelf-like structure, perhaps a bookshelf itself, placed at the head of the bed. With the types of PAP devices now manufactured, this shelving's depth can be as narrow as six to 10 inches. It can be whatever design, size, or height you choose, but the goal is to make one shelf on a plane close to level with the height of your bed; a few inches higher or lower than the bed is fine. The place to set the device on the shelf should be at least one to two feet wide for easier maneuvering. The system allows you to reach above your head to touch the control panel of the PAP device, and you can also lay tube slack on the shelf as well.

Most people for convenience choose a system on one side of the bed, as you would use when travelling and sleeping in a hotel or someone else's home. The side system can work, but if you are getting entangled with your tube or it otherwise seems to disrupt your sleep, then the headboard approach is worth the trouble to install.

Tubing is designed to be very flexible and, to my knowledge, it is virtually impossible for it to wrap around your neck in a dangerous way. Still, some who are more restless sleepers than others may complain of tube entanglement. To repeat, it is very difficult for tubing to become unsafely tangled because of the special way it is constructed.

If any sort of tangling experience occurs, it would immediately raise questions about other factors in play, such as persistent breathing events or leg jerks, which are causing the restlessness and then, in turn, tube tangling. Both these conditions cause people to move a lot in bed; the breathing compromise causes you to reposition your upper body constantly to find a better way to breathe, and the leg issue through its own actions causes lower body movement that may eventually trigger tossing and turning. Return to Chapter 9 for more on leg movements, check the additional notes below on the connection between leg jerks and air swallowing (see Aerophagia), and take note of more summarizing info in Appendix B.

Humidifier

Heated humidification is the best approach for most, and research has clearly shown a heated humidifier single-handedly could make the difference between using and not using your device. Strangely, heat humidification was not the norm with PAP therapy as recently as 10 to 15 years ago (that is, 25 to 30 years after PAP was introduced), but technological advances have unequivocally demonstrated a humidifier as an essential asset.

Most do well breathing humidified air from the PAP device. Some complain heated water makes the air too warm, and others occasionally suffer the accidental condensation of water inside the tube, which then flushes all the way through into the mask. This latter event is very upsetting because for a moment you might actually experience the horrible sensation of breathing in water, namely, drowning.

Once we go through the basics of humidifying the air, you should be able to avoid such occurrences and gain great benefit from humidification. Without humidity, the air will dry out the mucus membranes in your nose, mouth, and throat, but if the heated air proves problematic, you can simply fill your humidifier tank with water but never turn on the actual heating element. This *pass-over humidification* approach runs the air over cold water and still yields a moisturizing effect.

Most PAP devices come with a humidifier directly attached or built into the machine, and in most instances, this proves sufficient for your needs. In the past, there were stand-alone humidifiers clearly superior to the humidifiers directly attached to the device, and occasionally, there is still a need to use a stand-alone device for individuals whose water supply depletes too quickly.

The stand-alone humidifiers often have larger canisters to accommodate the need for more water for the whole night.

Most humidifiers offer multiple settings for how high to warm the water (a temperature setting) and how high to set the moisturizing effect (humidification). You must play with these settings over a period of days or weeks to figure out what works, and it is very much to your advantage to spend the time doing so. Then again, most if not all machines have an "auto" setting for humidification, and surprisingly or not, this approach often provides excellent results without needing any tinkering whatsoever.

One extra consideration is the impact on your own body temperature. If you set the temperature higher, you may discover the need for fewer bed linens and covers. For some, this warming benefit is quite nice if they previously were too cold during the sleep period. Many insomniacs complain of cold hands or feet, and this change in temperature may improve or solve this problem. Of course, if you like sleeping in a cooler environment, this benefit might turn into a side effect as you need to find a way to stay cool when using heated humidification.

The greatest benefit is no longer awakening with dryness in your airway. Humidification may also exert a beneficial influence on your nasal passages, reducing congestion, although as discussed in the section on chronic nasal congestion, individuals with untreated nonallergic rhinitis (NAR) may experience worse symptoms when first exposed to pressurized air. Therefore this issue must be monitored closely for those with NAR.

With humidification, there is a greater chance you will keep the mask on longer. Patients who suffer dry mouths or noses or throats are likely to rip off the mask in the middle of the night without realizing why, or awaken with an awful drying sensation and then remove PAP for the remainder of the night.

Overall, when adjusting your humidifier settings, do not necessarily start with the default values unless it is set to automatic, in which case it's reasonable to try auto before tinkering. Keep in mind research has shown cooler temperatures promote better breathing; therefore, if you can keep humidifier water temperature under 70 degrees, it may yield better results.

However, resolving the drying effect is the more important objective, so configuring the temperature and humidification to meld perfectly is where to focus your attention.

In my practice, some patients keep increasing humidification settings when they believe their persistent dryness is from poor humidification, whereas the real problem is unrecognized mouth breathing. If your settings are in the midrange of humidification intensity, and your temperature settings are in the 65- to 75-degree range, yet you feel dryness, you must determine whether mouth breathing is the real culprit.

Please note different settings are needed for different seasons. One of the most common times for a "drowning" episode occurs in the summer in a well air-conditioned room. A lower room temperature causes the tubing from the PAP device to chill to a lower level, which then condenses the water vapor on the inside, resulting in rushing water through the tube. The same might occur in wintertime if you keep your house heater off and the room temperature below 65. The simple solution is to wrap up the tube or buy a tube sleeve to sustain the moisturized air. Some tubes may come with their own insulation or other stabilizing material to prevent this problem.

Humidifiers require tinkering, like so many other aspects of PAP, but the effort usually makes a difference in your results and in your capacity to consistently apply the device all night long.

Aerophagia, aka Air Swallowing

Air swallowing, or *aerophagia*, is an occasional to common side effect when using PAP therapy, which usually manifests as bloating in the stomach. It can be a deal breaker for those afflicted severely. Less common but unsettling symptoms include post-PAP belching or gas.

In the worst-case scenario, abnormal anatomy regarding the esophagus (the upper tube leading to the gut) and the trachea (windpipe) may predispose an individual to swallowing air or feeling the specific sensation of pressurized air forced into the stomach. Those who report this sensation are almost always aware of swallowing air while awake; that is, when in bed and not yet asleep they feel air entering the stomach. This situation is the worst case because there is no obvious cure for the problem, and there may be limited, risky, or complicated surgeries proposed to alter the anatomy in an attempt to prevent the condition.

In my career, I have seen at least one of these very unfortunate cases in which an individual reported severe and painful bloating, which in turn prevented adaptation to the device and therefore no benefits from using PAP therapy. His ENT physician indicated an abnormal anatomical alignment of the trachea for which he could not offer surgical recommendations. At the time, he went on disability for untreated OSA.

Fortunately, this severity is extremely rare because most causes of aerophagia can be identified and treated with solutions ranging from simple mask adjustments to the use of medications for specific conditions that appear to trigger air swallowing while asleep.

Periodic limb movements (PLMD) or leg jerks, as discussed at greater length in Chapter 9, appear the single most common cause of aerophagia. Yet, we find nothing in the published literature about this phenomenon or the pathophysiological mechanism of how it unfolds. Nonetheless, the simplest, albeit speculative, mechanism is leg jerks produce an arousal that triggers the reflex to swallow.

I believe strongly some connection of this sort must be occurring because in greater than 90% of aerophagia patients who were treated for leg jerks, air swallowing resolved completely. In subsequent titration sleep studies, patients' leg jerks had diminished, and they reported immense relief from the resolution of aerophagia symptoms.

The second most common cause of aerophagia involves mask issues. For example, if a person uses a full face mask yet still mouth breaths during the night, air swallowing may ensue. In a related matter, if the individual suffers moderate leak, the PAP device will produce compensating and very annoying bursts of extra air pressure. If so, the burst might trigger a swallowing reflex even when you don't awaken from these events.

Solving both mask leak issues and mouth breathing simultaneously could be the essential steps to prevent aerophagia. We often use chinstraps with patients on full face masks to prevent "jaw drop." And although this combination feels quite bulky at first, we have been surprised at how many people immediately reported improved sleep, less leak, and some reduction in aerophagia.

We worked with a patient recently who had severe esophageal disease, including dilatation of the esophagus, and in our discussions with her gastroenterologists we were very pessimistic about how to reduce her aerophagia. The doctor was equally pessimistic about attempting any surgery. While ruminating about how to tell this poor old lady the bad news, I learned one of our very proactive sleep technologists had just met with her a week earlier and recommended the use of a chinstrap. A few days later, I happened to answer the phone in the sleep tech control room, and it was the same patient, who eagerly told me how the chinstrap had eliminated all the air swallowing, and now she was gaining real benefits from PAP therapy.

Other mask issues may come up, triggering aerophagia. For example, someone using nasal pillows or a nasal mask can still swallow air. We have seen some reduce aerophagia with chinstraps or a mouth taping procedure. Most conservatively, if you do not show leg jerks objectively on the sleep study, then your standard should be to investigate and resolve any issue with mask fit, mask comfort, mask leak, and mouth breathing as the most likely means to diminish or eradicate aerophagia.

The third most common causes are the separate or combined effects of reflux or rhinitis (nasal congestion). Patients with esophageal reflux clearly suffer greater sensitivity and altered functioning in this anatomical space that lies so closely to the windpipe. Whether it's a specific reflux episode or something else related to reflux pathophysiology, many patients report a decrease in air swallowing shortly after treating their reflux with appropriate medications.

A fascinating and little-known fact about reflux is it triggers the "nonallergic rhinitis response," the NAR condition we discussed at length in Chapter 8 where a buildup of mucus and other congestion unrelated to allergies arises throughout the nasal and oral cavity. Although I am no expert on this pathophysiology and do not know whether it has been studied from a sleep-oriented perspective, it is reasonable to presume someone with congestion in the back of the throat (for example, post-nasal drip) will engage in more swallowing than normal. In this instance, reflux triggers the rhinitis, which increases mucus production, which increases swallowing. If this mechanism emerges when someone is attempting to use PAP therapy, we believe reflux-induced NAR is triggering swallowing episodes leading to aerophagia.

Any form of rhinitis may be a factor in aerophagia, whether allergic or nonallergic, and therefore we recommend aggressive treatment of these conditions not only to prevent potential air swallowing, but also to facilitate an airflow stream with less turbulence due to a clearer oral-nasal passageway.

As detailed in Chapter 8, we had particularly good luck in using the antihistamine nasal spray azelastine for nonallergic rhinitis, as well as the older spray known as ipratropium (Atrovent). The former comes in several brand names such as Astelin or Astepro, but there are other antihistamine nasal sprays under other brand names that also work. Atrovent would be the most common name for the ipratropium nasal spray. We use nasal steroid or cromolyn sodium sprays and various nasal rinses for allergic rhinitis. As described in Chapter 8, we've recently learned of patients using OTC xylitol-based nasal sprays gaining excellent results in treating NAR.

In sum, aerophagia may not only diminish the benefits a patient receives from PAP, but as the severity of bloating and gas worsens, it eventually causes patients to cease use. Although the overall proportion of cases of aerophagia in the PAP population is unknown and likely small, it is a very big deal to those who suffer the problem. The good news is the largest proportion of aerophagia sufferers find clear-cut solutions.

Weak DME Program

As discussed in Chapter 7, the greatest wild card, which also usually serves as the weakest link in your efforts to progress, is the quality of care received from the durable medical equipment (DME) or home medical equipment (HME) company that manages the sale of your equipment and its resupply of your headgear, masks, tubing, filters, and other parts like humidifier chambers.

These DMEs (or HMEs) are notorious for poor to mediocre service. One of the biggest drawbacks is few companies specialize in sleep apnea equipment. Instead, the sleep "division" may be operated by one or two people, whereas the remainder of the staff might be working on all other home medical equipment needs for other patients (wheelchairs, crutches, oxygen concentrators, and so on).

Even though a DME sells medical equipment, they all suffer at least two strikes against them from the get-go. First, due to burdensome overregulation from the government, particularly Medicare, these typically small business enterprises (either home grown or franchises) must waste excessive time completing a maze of paperwork to fend off audit problems from insurance carriers. This regulatory disease infects the sleep center as well because they must communicate with the DME to supply pertinent medical records to justify the patient gaining coverage for the PAP device. Then, the DME must navigate through the insurance company's bureaucracy to gain approval for the coverage.

Strike two is a DME is not really a company designed to deliver medical care. Think about crutches for moment and how little time is spent teaching someone to use them, not to mention how briefly the patient uses them. In contrast to the minutes needed to learn to use crutches, PAP takes an individual 10 or 100 or 1000 times that amount. Worse, no patient actually learns to use a PAP device at a DME company; in fact, many DME facilities still do not hook up the device and turn on the power when instructing a patient on how to use it.

Many DMEs do not create office space to let the patient lie down on a bed or cot or sofa to replicate the proper positioning of the mask or headgear as would be used at home in bed. In reality, patients learn to use PAP in the home environment through trial and error and through the professional environment of the sleep center and laboratory, where your home experimentation could be supplemented by experts solving specific fitting and pressure setting issues.

It is obvious to all sleep doctors that DME participation in PAP distribution was a bad idea from the outset. Instead, the process should have been designed to better coordinate with sleep centers where staffs possess much greater expertise. Indeed, the DME should have been designed to operate within the sleep center. But because Medicare insists too many physicians must be greedy or corrupt, these government agents could not fathom the idea of physicians selling PAP devices to their patients on the specious grounds devices would be sold to patients who do not need them. To be sure, there are bad actors who serve up rotten apples that spoil the barrel. But this government designed solution has caused untold misery in the field of sleep medicine and caused harm to hundreds of thousands, if not millions, of patients by creating a serpentine network that in and of itself thwarts patients' efforts to use PAP therapy. Of course (no surprise) this widespread PAP failure costs the government more money due to the devastating effects of untreated OSA/UARS in amounts far greater than any known evidence of greediness or corruption in the field of sleep medicine.

A third strike may enter the equation if you are unlucky enough to work with a DME company who has employed a respiratory therapist—the usual agent to set up the PAP device—with limited background in sleep medicine. What do I mean by limited? As described earlier, consider a sleep technologist who spends 2000 hours per year directly working in the hands-on environment of the sleep lab to help sleep apnea patients adapt to their devices. Two thousand hours! A respiratory therapist may have never spent more than a couple nights in a sleep lab, and that night was only for observation and training purposes and nothing more. Thus, the respiratory therapist's job is more about knowing the mechanics of the device, how to set the pressures, and over time, perhaps learning how to properly fit different types of masks, but none of this expertise derives from a scenario in which the patient is actually sleeping with the device.

Tell me, who would you trust more to provide care and knowledge in learning to adapt to PAP therapy?

Finally, to reiterate, DME/HMEs are greatly burdened by government regulators, who have also placed heavy restrictions on insurance carriers. The net result is DMEs must deal with a bucketful of minutiae, usually trivial, to satisfy rules intentionally designed to make it more difficult for you to get your device and supplies.

Am I really suggesting this triad of administrative wizards (DME, insurance, government) want to thwart your capacity to obtain a device? Perhaps directly, no; but indirectly, yes! Here's the reason why: in recent years there has been an emerging negative consensus (originating from insurers and the government) that too many people are prescribed PAP devices, which is costing too much money. In fact, some institutions would like you to believe the epidemic of sleep disorders in general and sleep apnea in particular has been blown way out of proportion.

This point of view emanates from the deeper problem of how much society disrespects sleep and therefore discounts the value of sleep treatments. Medicare, as one prime example, looked at this issue a few years ago and claimed the rapid expansion of PAP prescriptions had to be investigated. In addition to looking at all device prescriptions in Medicare patients, they also looked at all the sleep lab tests conducted related to the prescriptions being written. They even went so far as to publish and distribute the number of sleep tests each sleep doctor was conducting in order to embarrass those individuals who were conducting the most procedures.

Since 2015, the tack taken by government regulators, largely through Obamacare, or what we affectionately call the "Unaffordable Care Act," the latest approach is to bog down the insurance carriers and DMEs with so much extraneous paperwork that PAP device approvals will be rejected at record rates. The government will declare these efforts are necessary to avoid waste, fraud, and abuse, but without sounding conspiratorial, the government must know their efforts will deprive tens of thousands of individuals from ever receiving a PAP device, which then makes Medicare's bottom line look better—or actually much worse when you factor in all the patients who end up hospitalized for the cardiovascular diseases that follow when OSA/UARS is untreated.

As cynical as these points sound, be prepared when dealing with your DME/HME company to encounter innumerable delays in obtaining your device, or subsequently, your supplies. Be especially prepared for not being able to receive an advanced PAP device such as ABPAP or ASV. And finally, be prepared for incessant efforts to take away your device when you do not use it on a regular basis (defined by the government as four hours per night on five nights of the week).

The DME puzzle is a major barrier to the care of sleep apnea patients and appears to be getting worse as we move toward increasingly socialized medicine, which invariably means greater bureaucracy, leading to lower efficiency or productivity, which then almost always leads to lower quality of care. To top it off, you also experience more aggravation, as well as wasting more time and effort in working with DME institutions as part of your treatment package.

While virtually all sleep apnea patients must deal with this nonsense, the process takes its toll on more vulnerable patients, those with disabilities or with mental health problems, so I want to alert you to be vigilant as the process unfolds, because the bumps in the road will affect nearly all patients at some level.

Finally, if you are fortunate enough to have choices, either in your own location or through access to online PAP suppliers, keep these options in mind at the first hint you are not receiving quality care from your initial experience with a DME. It is a verifiable fact that patients are constantly begging or attempting to change to a different DME company within the first several months or first year of the contractual relationship.

If you are lucky to find a single person at your particular DME who appears helpful, and this person stays working at this DME, chances are high you will get reasonably good to outstanding service. But if you discover your DME suffers from high turnover rates among its staff, this instability is a telltale sign you should be thinking about looking elsewhere.

Sleep Professionals with Limited Experience

In another matter directly bearing on your DME relationship, a major obstacle to care is working with sleep professionals at a sleep center who simply do not have the time, energy, or motivation to learn and practice at the highest possible levels of sleep medical care. For numerous reasons, quality of care among doctors varies greatly, and sleep medicine specialists are no exception to this rule. Because sleep medicine is perceived so simplistically by so many inside and outside the field, chances of encountering individuals who do not go the extra mile are lamentably quite high.

To be fair, this problem in sleep medicine is largely a function of ignorance because sleep medicine is such a relatively new field. As such, in attempts to gain respect from other medical fields, the sleep field powers-that-be often embrace more conventional wisdom than you might see in other specialties. As the best example, a whole lot of sleep medicine specialists, due to their initial training in pulmonary or internal medicine, do not have a natural or comfortable feeling about working with mental health patients with sleep disorders. They are conflicted because they want to provide sleep medicine services but then start off on the wrong path by incorrectly presuming psychiatrists and psychologists should be able to solve your sleep problems by restoring your mental health.

In other words, they do not see the pivotal role to be played in solving problems like insomnia and even nightmares by treating your sleep breathing and sleep movement disorders.

As a corollary to this problem, most sleep centers do not provide insomnia treatment services by someone trained in the evidence-based, psychological principles used for chronic insomnia, such as CBT-I (Chapter 15). Fewer still know anything about imagery distraction methods (Chapter 11) or emotion-focused therapies (Chapters 12–14). Instead, most sleep medicine specialists gravitate toward sleep aids, prescription or over-the-counter, and when these drugs fail, as they so often do, they are at a loss on how to proceed.

This narrow drug focus is in fact just a drop in the bucket. A similar constrained philosophy carries over into the "average" sleep doctor's efforts to treat depressed patients suffering co-occurring sleep apnea. Patients with depression are one of the more difficult—some would say the single *most* difficult—groups of sleep patients to manage, because their foresight and planning skills have been weakened by the depression such that they cannot consistently engage in all the steps needed to use PAP, including something as simple as cleaning their mask and tubes every morning.

Cleaning steps might seem inconsequential, but they are not. If the tubes and mask build up grease and grime, then sooner than later the equipment will not function at the highest level. If the mask starts leaking, the depressed patient may not have strong enough cognitive skills to recognize the problem was caused from a lack of regular cleaning. Soon thereafter, the depressed patient actually quits using the device, claiming intolerance to a leak. When this individual returns to a sleep center (assuming there is a return) often a year or more later and after it has finally been discerned by the patient or a family member that sleep is deteriorating, only then at the follow-up appointment would the doctor or sleep tech help the patient sort out the causative factor, namely, a lack of mask cleaning triggering the leak.

You certainly understood from the pages before this appendix that consistent efforts are essential to help psychiatric patients with sleep disorders. Regrettably, the most common sleep center you encounter may not demonstrate a strong appreciation for attacking this special set of issues in these patients. And it's not just a one-size-fits-all problem; rather, never having understood the inextricable links between sleep and mental health issues, this long-standing ignorance prevents sleep professionals from recognizing the necessity for greater attention to detail. Many sleep docs would candidly admit they do not wish to work with mental health patients and that they did not sign up for this level of complexity. Such attitudes carry over to many sleep centers, and there is no easy way around this unfriendly perspective, despite the very friendly nature of the vast majority of sleep doctors I encounter at professional meetings.

My strong words here are intended to prepare you for these encounters, mostly so you might spot the problem as quickly as possible and then begin looking for a new sleep specialist. When a new specialist is not available, it would behoove you to find ways to communicate with your sleep staff to see if they appreciate the additional services you may require to successfully treat your sleep disorders. In the worst-case scenario, what often happens is the sleep center and the DME take turns bouncing you back and forth, hoping the other institution is somehow going to solve your problems.

In the best-case scenario, it may prove invaluable to work only with sleep doctors or sleep techs who themselves are currently using PAP. When a sleep professional has the background and experience of using PAP personally, there's considerably greater potential for him or her to know more about the various quirks interfering with adaptation and progress. They may know many tricks and tips to help you because they have so much direct problem-solving experience through personal troubleshooting.

Last, you can always consider Internet resources because nowadays there are an enormous number of sites directly dealing with problem-solving for sleep issues related to PAP therapy, or there are individual videos put together by people who have lived and breathed through the experience. One of the best sites is www.cpaptalk.com. You may also find the information you are looking for at our website www.barrykrakowmd.com, where I provide educational support on an individual or group basis, or through my Substack newsletter at www.fastasleep.substack.com.

A Final Reminder on Pressure Setting Changes

Over the course of the first year, or much sooner, once you've gotten a good feeling about how all your equipment works, you may be ready to attempt your own pressure setting changes, as mentioned earlier.

This action may seem odd, depending on your relationships with healthcare providers, so to give a quick example, imagine a diabetic needing to change the dosage of his insulin that he takes at bedtime. Would the individual know enough to make the change, or would he need to visit with the doctor? The short answer is either way could work depending on the individual's ability to make prudent decisions. With insulin, a bad decision, as in far too much insulin, could prove life-threatening. In this case, the individual must be clearly trained and very comfortable taking the reins.

The insulin example contrasts sharply with your ability to make changes in your PAP pressures because you could almost never cause a life-threatening change in your settings. The one obvious exception would be to set the pressures way off-mark and no longer be able to tolerate using your device. If in this instance you were a heart patient and could not use your PAP, you might suffer serious problems. For example, a PAP machine can reverse some cardiac arrhythmias. Without the device the arrhythmias could return.

As described earlier, the kind of pressure changes you might make would be perceived as miniscule. Remember, we use the term "units of pressure," and the degree of change would often be as small as 0.2 units to 0.4 units.

Before you make such changes, you must first receive instructions either through your DME or through your sleep staff. Once they show you how to change the settings, your goal is to monitor your progress on a weekly, monthly, or semiannual basis to determine whether your sleep is as good as it gets.

The main point is little changes of pressure settings can make a surprisingly large difference. I described earlier how I have personally altered my settings with changes as small as 0.2 to 0.4 units and received substantial benefits.

The key is to closely monitor changes in sleepiness, trips to the bathroom, mental sharpness, and overall energy. When you experience a worsening of sleep quality, that's the time to consider small changes in your pressure settings, whether you do it yourself or seek assistance from your sleep center support staff.

Last and not least, technology continues to offer new innovations in managing your sleep breathing disorder. You could download the OSCAR software at https://www.sleepfiles.com/OSCAR/ to view flow limitation. My personal experience with OSCAR is that it may underestimate flow limitation events. Nonetheless, using something to view and track these events can guide you to recognize whether you are moving in the right direction. Moreover, with OSCAR you can actually look at breath-by-breath analysis, which means over time, you could probably sort out whether your pressures are rounding the inspiratory airflow curve. With obvious EPI, I believe OSCAR does show some of these fluctuations on the expiratory limb of the airflow curve.

Another technology is the use of various headbands to attempt to track sleep. I'm not referring to wristband technology here, although that too might prove accurate in the future. The headband technology attempts to determine deep versus light sleep or REM versus NREM sleep. Again, accuracy here is inconsistent, but if you get a feel for using this information, you might notice trends that indicate you are moving in the right direction.

Going forward, we anticipate tons of home monitoring systems becoming available for individuals so they can actively manage their own sleep breathing disorders with very high proficiency.

Pillow Talk

In closing, I want to encourage you to literally and figuratively reflect and clarify how you wish to position yourself going forward with PAP therapy. Literally, how would you position yourself in the bed? Figuratively, how well positioned are you to move forward with and stay the course with this invaluable but not so easy to implement physiological therapy?

How to lie in bed is frequently overlooked. If you were a politician, you could just as easily lie in bed or standing up, but seriously, how you situate yourself in the bed could seal the deal or prove a deal breaker. Misconceptions about your positioning also aggravate a problem here, as in an inexperienced DME staff advising you only to use PAP on your back (supine). This view is nonsense. You can sleep with PAP in any position you choose: on your side, back, stomach, or a combination, as well as changing your position all night long.

A difficulty arises in figuring out the bedding support system to make your position work, including the relevant factors of mattress, mattress topper, sheets, blankets, comforters, and pillows. The last category often proves most pivotal in your efforts. Here's a personal example. When I first used an FFM, I wanted to continue my decades-old pattern of sleeping on my stomach—the prone position. For my first six years using either nasal pillows or nasal masks, I only needed to rotate my head to one side.

With the FFM, lying on my side caused huge leaks. So, I applied a multiple pillow system to create a special "pocket" to place my head face down without the mask smushed against the sheets. The first pillow rested under my chest and abdomen, providing an elevated position. Then two more pillows formed the sides of a triangle with the top of my first pillow as the base. Inside the empty space of the triangle, my head and mask would fit. However, the space needed for this pocket cannot let the head and mask drop too far. The key was to create enough elevation so the mask could fit downwards, but the pocket had to be a tight enough fit to prevent the mask mashing up against the bed sheets. It might touch the mattress without pressing into it. I slept this way for more than a year until my ease of use and comfort with the FFM was so natural, I gradually removed many of the pillows and discovered I could simply rotate my head to one side or the other, using no pillows at all, or very thin pillows.

Bottom line, whichever position you use, think first about how you like to sleep and then try to come up with a system to aid your placement. Manufacturers of bedding and related materials are now inventing their own "CPAP pillows" with various contours to create ease in adopting certain positions, notably for side-sleepers, but there are products in the marketplace for just about any sleep position.

Last, I want to mention a recent discovery—the value of a featherbed. If you haven't seen one recently, it's a cross between a sleeping bag and a comforter and also slightly resembles a duvet. The beauty of the featherbed is it's not just a mattress topper. Rather, you can rearrange the featherbed into virtually any position to create unique spaces for your head, neck, and PAP mask. If you struggle with all other regular bedding or specialized CPAP pillows, check out the featherbed option because you can form it into virtually any shape you need to match your best sleep position for PAP use.

Taking the big PAP step truly is a big step. I don't say it to scare you off. I say it to realize that while going slow in the beginning is optimal for most, over the long run PAP is a large commitment that definitely "repositions" your sleep lifestyle. Nearly everyone who receives a good to great to outstanding response to PAP ends up embracing the system, but this psychological turning point is often predicated on receiving obvious benefits from the better night of sleep. If your symptomatic relief is minimal, it is very difficult to maintain a long-term relationship with PAP. I've seen less than a handful of patients in more than 30 years of clinical experience who stuck with PAP simply because they were convinced it was great preventive medicine for their heart. No other benefits were ever appreciated, but they stuck with it nonetheless. This perspective is so rare, it's hard to believe it occurs.

Therefore, finding a way to get benefit is crucial because then you will commit to changing your sleep lifestyle in a more dedicated fashion. That said, your "position" in life going into this great adventure will influence your commitment. If you are single and worried about the unromantic side of PAP, it's bound to influence your motivation. If you're married and PAP interferes with your spouse's sleep, it can turn into another deal breaker. Then there are those with shift work or other irregular schedules where it's too complicated to get everything set up night after night when you are *not* sleeping night after night. And, finally, for those using psychotropic medications on a regular basis, it would be great if the drugs help you adapt to PAP, but adaptation only gets you halfway home. What if you adapt well but you cannot appreciate any improvement in symptoms, in full or in part, because of the effects of the psychotropic meds on your sleep?

All these scenarios are common and greatly impact how the individual moves forward with PAP therapy. I left these particular items for last because I strongly encourage you to reflect on these aspects so they do not interfere with your efforts going forward.

PAP is truly a modern medical miracle. I hope it will prove so for you and your sleep.

Finally, don't hesitate to contact us at www.BarryKrakowMD.com to set up a sleep coaching appointment.

APPENDIX B

Quick Start: Sleep Dynamic Therapy Pearls

Introduction

Nowadays, we know many skip around in a book. This section has been written for those who need a short overview or "quick start" on how *Life Saving Sleep* (an expanded version of our original *Sleep Dynamic Therapy*) is organized to treat both mental and physical sleep disorders.

For those who have read the whole book through, you are already primed to never underestimate the role of physical sleep disorders as the most likely underlying factor in your sleep complaints, and how bad and broken physical sleep exacerbates your psychological sleep disorders as well. We explained sleep breathing and sleep movement problems to encourage you to seek help at a local sleep center for appropriate testing.

With few exceptions, treating your physiological sleep disorders may prove the single most important intervention you need to reverse the downward spiral of deteriorating mental health problems or suicidal ideation. Waiting or delaying assessment and treatment of physical sleep disorders frequently stalls out your progress toward gaining better sleep. Moreover, it may take extra time to convince your doctors and therapists to refer you to a sleep medical center. Don't wait!

In the chapters on psychological sleep disorders, a new mental framework, the *TFI system*, was introduced. And more details on the *TFI system* are found in my *Sound Sleep, Sound Mind* book. In *Life Saving Sleep*, we explored how the mind's eye naturally engages in imagery prior to falling asleep, so you can use mental imagery at bedtime or in the middle of the night to rapidly fall asleep or return to sleep. Then, we worked on emotional processing techniques because you learned how emotional residue from the daytime often leads to racing thoughts at night. Last, we finished up with the "thinking" approach to insomnia where you learned about cognitive-behavioral therapy and specific steps to shift your sleep patterns and rapidly break vexing cycles of poor sleep schedules, difficulties falling or staying asleep, and overcoming fragmented sleep.

This content reflects an enormous amount of information to bite into, chew on, swallow, digest, and absorb; so, let's use this special appendix to gain a good overview of *Sleep Dynamic Therapy* and provide specific steps right now to address both your physiological and psychological sleep disorders in whatever sequence you choose to apply them.

First Rule: Sleep Quality Rules

Above all else, it is essential to pay attention to your sleep quality. Embracing the quality model rapidly ramps up your understanding of physical and mental sleep disorders. This approach is the fastest highway to success because targeting any aspect of sleep quality immediately achieves improvements in sleep and daytime functioning. Accepting the truth about sleep quality may be the most important first step any individual can take simply because it removes so much past confusion in thinking about your sleep problems. When you feel clear about a sleep quality paradigm, you are ready to move forward in any way you choose.

For those struggling with the sleep quality idea, you might ask what holds you back from seeing or appreciating this perspective. The most common barrier is the use of psychotropic medications for sleep problems, which block bad sleepers from even understanding the nature of good versus poor sleep quality.

These individuals use medications for a sustained period of time, months or years or longer. Initially, they started on drugs to help initiate sleep or prevent awakenings at night, although these specific insomnia complaints do not explain the nature of their sleep problems; that is, insomnia complaints do not logically connect the zzzots to the quality of slumber. Instead, the problem was superficially "diagnosed" as not being able to fall or stay asleep. In fact, a huge proportion of patients define their problems as sleep initiation and sleep continuity problems, not sleep quality problems. Such terms are accurate descriptors of how you experience your sleep, but these very terms are so incomplete they lead to more confusion instead of enlightenment.

Snooze Flash: These sleep complaints, otherwise known as *sleep onset insomnia* or *sleep maintenance insomnia*, are absolutely tied to sleep quality issues in no less than 99% of cases. But if you were steered toward the sleep continuity theory, you will end up on medications; then, if the drugs prove effective to some extent, you will continue down these pathways, zeroing in on sleep continuity only. Eventually, you would develop or fortify your sleep quantity obsessions.

There is no easy suggestion to break through this confusion. You cannot just stop the medications, and you may not be in a position to taper off of them gradually, because these drugs may be helping in other ways. However, you can plant a seed in your brain to question the benefits of these medications as they relate to your sleep quality. Talking with your healthcare providers is essential to insure safety.

Most importantly, you could start by asking yourself how you feel when you wake up in the morning and how you feel during the first half of the day? If the drugs really are working well, enhancing sleep continuity and also adding depth to your slumber, you should wake up refreshed and notice less daytime fatigue and sleepiness for the first half of the day at minimum.

Do you notice these improvements or not?

Most patients taking multiple psychotropic medications for sleep purposes cannot confirm these drugs enhanced their sleep quality. This lack of clarity should be the first clue to help recognize a sleep quality problem remains unresolved. If this picture reflects your circumstances, then take the next step and question whether sleeping pills are doing anything beyond attempting to address sleep initiation and sleep continuity. Usually, you see some gains getting to sleep and perhaps staying asleep with drugs, but are you gaining any restorative, high quality slumber? That's a good start for people confused about what pills are supposed to do.

Once you are satisfied you suffer from a sleep quality problem, the next big decision is whether you want to attack one or more of your sleep quality issues on the psychological front or the physiological one. For anyone struggling to get started, it proves easier to begin in the one place that makes the most sense to you, which usually means with a mental treatment or a physical treatment, but not both simultaneously.

While you could choose both paths simultaneously, this approach appears more difficult for someone confused about sleep quality. So, let's tackle some specific steps to guide you down one path or another.

Starting with Sleep-Disordered Breathing Is Usually the Best First Option

Nasal Hygiene and Sleep Positions. As you might expect, consider an SDB treatment first if you seek rapid gains. You may feel better within days, and a window will be opened into a new way of understanding your sleep problems. Then again, most people imagine this step means starting with PAP therapy or the oral appliances discussed earlier. That's not the case, please read on.

If you have the means and resources to start at a sleep center, that's great, but if not, consider a conservative approach, one that invariably yields rapid benefits. Previously, we talked about nasal hygiene in Chapter 8, and it turns out these steps pack an enormous bang for the buck; they cost little compared to advanced treatments, and most people report improvement with something as simple as nasal saline rinses.

You would be well-suited to start a nasal hygiene program if you already suffer from obvious, chronic nasal congestion or sinusitis. Use all strategies described in Chapter 8 combined with a review of my free video series on nasal breathing called *The Nose Knows* at https://barrykrakowmd.com/top-videos. Pay particular attention to distinguishing between allergic and nonallergic rhinitis, because the former permits as many treatments as necessary, whereas the latter means you must restrict therapy to usually just one or two options, otherwise you will overstimulate the nose and aggravate congestion.

Many individuals suffer both allergic and nonallergic rhinitis, which necessitates finding a delicate balance when combining drugs. The marketplace offers newer dual-purpose nasal sprays with steroids and antihistamines.

Although more expensive, this drug combo may prove ideal for both allergic and nonallergic rhinitis. Or, you could purchase each medication separately for a cheaper price. Also, neti pot rinses and xylitol-based sprays can prove helpful.

When using nasal strips and/or nasal dilators, stick with them for several months to clarify benefit. In a study we conducted a decade ago, some needed to use strips for three months before confirming the value. A few patients had to cease use of nasal strips to finally realize the impact on their sleep, that is, once they stopped the strips, they noticed the immediate worsening of sleep quality and greater daytime fatigue or sleepiness. In contrast, many report next day improvement after the first night with a nasal dilator.

Last, it is worth evaluating your sleep position. If you tend to sleep on your back, which makes sleep breathing worse, experiment with sleeping on your side or stomach. These latter positions reduce SDB severity, but it takes time to train yourself to avoid sleeping on your back. Several devices to train you are on the market at various price points. If you discover avoiding supine sleep (on your back) makes a large difference, it would be worth your time and money to pursue this path. Chapter 8 lists a few of the new devices that show good results; expect more to come to market soon.

As a final tip, the Internet is constantly advertising new ways to deal with nasal breathing. While some items are purely gimmicks, there might be something new just right for you.

Weight Loss. Weight loss is rarely a valid first treatment option for the simple reason it is so difficult to lose weight. Moreover, even if you lose weight, par for the course is you regain it in a matter of weeks or months. It is regrettable how so few weight loss strategies work, usually resulting in lost time, lost effort, lost money, but not lost weight.

That said, a point of fact worth remembering is a 10% weight loss (from current weight), irrespective of whether your current obesity problem is mild, moderate, or severe, will actually decrease your sleep breathing disorder and most likely increase the quality of your sleep.

This point ought to motivate newly diagnosed sleep-disordered breathing cases. Who wouldn't love to forgo using a PAP device at the outset when all they would like to achieve, right now, is a 10% loss of weight? Sadly, it does not work out this way. Most people who are overweight cannot easily lose 10% of their weight or keep the 10% off once lost. Moreover, while 10% weight loss decreases SDB severity, it does not cure the problem.

If you could achieve such results, then by all means starting with weight loss would be reasonable. Even if you are successful (and you should take immense pride in your actions if you succeed), you will still need more treatment for your SDB going forward.

Starting with RLS and PLMD Treatments: A Reasonable Option

We have worked with a great many patients who cannot bring themselves to start with sleep breathing treatments, mostly because they can't "see" the condition. Even when someone else hears them snore or stop breathing, it remains an invisible condition as they never experience it in real time.

Restless legs and leg jerks may occur more visibly than sleep-disordered breathing. For one thing, if you suffer from these jumpy feelings in your legs, you notice the sensation while awake. And, when you are kicking your legs—dancing in the sheets—sooner or later you may wonder why your bed linens are in complete disarray in the morning. These visible signs of leg movements may motivate you to treat these disorders first.

In patients with mental health conditions, targeting RLS or PLMD early could prove beneficial, notwithstanding mental health professionals who provide services and prescriptions yet rarely spot RLS or PLMD. Instead, this unusual disorder looks nearly identical to an anxiety problem, in part, because patients with RLS manifest more anxiety symptoms as well as depression symptoms.

No surprise, when an RLS patient presents for help at a clinic or hospital, untrained eyes do not realize the anxiety is coming from the uncomfortable sensations in the individual's legs. Likewise, a fair proportion of RLS patients are only capable of sensing their anxiety as a whole-body experience instead of just in the legs. Indeed, in some cases of anxiety, the detection problem is so compromised the individual only reports "feeling" the anxiety in the mind (similar to the description of weak or poor emotional processing in Chapters 12–14). As you can imagine, many patients end up on medication for a generalized anxiety disorder (GAD) instead of a drug to treat RLS, the potential cause of the anxiety.

The drugs for RLS/PLMD are listed in Chapter 9, but keep in mind most mental health providers do not routinely think to prescribe them and instead recommend drugs for anxiety. It is not uncommon for an RLS/PLMD patient to be placed on anxiety drugs, like benzodiazepines (Valium, Librium, and so on) for more than a decade before another medical professional with a background in sleep sorts out the leg movements as the real source of the anxiety. Worse, some antidepressants used to treat anxiety or depression or both frequently worsen leg jerks.

The key point is to recognize RLS/PLMD could literally walk/run/ drive you nuts, and you might be currently using medications aggravating the leg movement symptoms. With all this potential for exacerbating your sleep problems, it would be invaluable to start your treatment by looking at leg movement symptoms before you proceed with sleep breathing treatment. But you must remember the important caveat that treating sleep-disordered breathing first in many patients eliminates leg movements, both RLS and PLMD, though more so the leg jerks while asleep and less so the restless feelings while awake.

For any leg movement symptoms, start with a serum ferritin test; if it is below the 50 ng/ml to 75 ng/ml range you might only need iron supplements to treat the condition. Also test for vitamin D and magnesium levels. While the latter is rarely abnormal, the former is often low or borderline in many RLS/PLMD patients, and vitamin D supplements may improve leg movement symptoms. Otherwise refer to the medications and supplements in Chapter 9 and discuss your choices with your primary care physician, psychiatrist, or prescribing psychologist. While all these RLS/PLMD drugs cause side effects, the great news is these meds most commonly work at low dosages, so side effects occur less frequently. Nonetheless, be sure to check out the information in Chapter 9 about the growing concerns on the augmentation side effect that may occur particularly with the dopaminergic drugs as well as the additional concerns about the onset of impulse-control disorders with these same medications.

Starting with Imagery for Insomnia: A Great First Choice

Insomnia could easily be your first choice for treatment. So many sleep patients recognize insomnia symptoms for the obvious reason they occur while you are awake and trying to fall asleep or trying to return to sleep. Whether the trouble is at bedtime or after an awakening, the problem is the same—difficulty in falling asleep when you wish to sleep.

Imagery is the absolute best choice for first efforts to combat unwanted periods of sleeplessness because imagery aligns directly with the way your mind tends to fall sleep, as described in Chapter 11. Imagery techniques can be learned and applied rapidly—literally the first time you are trained to use your mind's eye; tonight, you can apply imagery steps to fall asleep, and, more often than not, you will fall asleep, oftentimes faster than using a sleeping pill unless you are currently heavily dependent on sleeping pills.

An important point about imagery skill is you do not need to create photographic memories in your mind's eye. Imagery for insomnia is about using a guided daydreaming landscape, and the content of the images may comprise virtually anything: prior or upcoming vacation; walk in the park or in the hills; memorable scenes of your children or grandchildren playing; driving on a scenic highway; or simply visualizing the furniture in your house or, believe it or not, in your own bedroom. And don't forget any potential fantasy trips to Venus, Mars, or Jupiter.

In all these instances, just a few images are all you need, not perfect replicas of these things as in a photograph.

Imagery is extraordinarily powerful, and to maximize this potency you must access your natural tendency toward daydreaming or using your mind's eye on a daily basis. Repetition will help you achieve the exceptional benefits of imagery distraction night after night.

I have instructed many patients on imagery skills, from very young to very old, and most people understand imagery immediately. The largest proportion of insomniacs can and will apply imagery as soon as they learn it. Some profit by spending a few minutes in daytime practice for a week or so before tapping into the mind's eye at night.

If, however, you suffer from the blank or black screen effect when trying to visualize things in your mind's eye, best to skip this step now (you can always return to it later) and move on to CBT-I. In the meantime, you could spend some training time by looking at picture books, doing puzzles or playing Colorku as these activities move you in the right direction to use imagery for sleep.

Last, recall the discussion in *Newer Advanced Strategy* at the end of Chapter 15 on the combination of imagery and nonlinear thoughts as another variation to consider.

Starting with CBT-I for Insomnia: A Reasonable Option

CBT-I is a great system, especially for someone who likes a more intellectual or rational approach to insomnia. CBT-I points out insomniacs think of sleep as a task to perform and try too hard to achieve it. CBT-I helps you appreciate the value of starting out with a "less is more" attitude, which can yield rapid and huge benefits. The cardinal principle then is as follows: **do not spend time in bed not sleeping because doing so teaches you to not sleep in bed.** Instead, retrain your brain to link the bed with the feeling of sleepiness, which then leads to sleep. Thus, the real trick is not about *trying* to go to sleep; the real mission is to recapture the feeling of sleepiness that *lets* you fall asleep when your head hits the pillow.

When you embrace CBT-I, you commit to spending less time in bed initially so as to restrict your sleep, which in turn generates greater intensity in your feelings of sleepiness. As an example, if you nap every day, even for just 10 or 15 minutes, you are using up some sleepiness that could have been generated at bedtime. CBT-I would ask an insomniac to quit napping for a week or two to see whether this specific change yields more sleepiness at bedtime and thus a faster onset of sleep.

The most difficult step in CBT-I is what to do in the middle of the night when you awaken and cannot easily return to sleep? In contrast to difficulty with sleep onset, where you could indefinitely postpone your bedtime until you feel sleepy, it is more emotionally vexing to agree to arise from your bed at night, leave the bedroom area, and wait for sleepiness to return. This stumbling block is large because it is counterintuitive to the commonly held belief more time in bed somehow yields more time asleep. It does not! In fact, more time in bed awake leads to more time awake in bed, and ultimately less sleep.

Insomniacs believe vacating the bed is sure to subtract from sleep hours. This conundrum, in fact, explains why so many people reject CBT-I or, if tried, give up when this middle-of-the night situation emerges. There is no easy way around this situation if you want to follow a hard-core CBT-I program.

As described in Chapter 15, CBT-I can be softened, making it more palatable in the early going, so please refer to the specific steps to decrease the intensity of your efforts and experience. CBT-I has worked for millions of insomniacs, but it does not work for everyone, usually because they cannot emotionally embrace the concepts. If so, it might prove more feasible to reconsider the EFT approach to insomnia.

Starting with Emotion-Focused Therapy for Insomnia: A Challenging Option

Starting with emotion-focused therapy for insomnia is not for the fainthearted! It truly is an excellent and often essential path, sooner or later, especially among those who appreciate getting to the heart of the matter. Emotional work is of course intense, yet the yield is remarkably satisfying. For many, emotional work is also spiritual work, which means you would be confronting deeper personal issues about the state of your life and your relationships, including your relationship with your Creator.

Emotional therapy could begin with a simple step like checking in with how you feel every few hours in a day until you begin to embrace the natural emotional experience of sensing and acknowledging your emotions nearly all day long without feeling overwhelmed by them. Said another way, a key point in emotional development is to recognize you can indeed learn to tap into your feelings all day long without being run over by them.

Arguably, a simplistic yet accurate definition of mental illness is the inability to process your emotions day in/day out as a healthy experience or in a way that does not cause you to crumble or disintegrate. This latter term (dis-integrate) is a good one to ponder, because a person tends to feel very integrated and whole upon achieving the skill to consistently work through emotions as a learning and productive exercise. Thus, dis-integrated feelings are the opposite of effective emotional coping and lead a person to feel like his or her life is a jumbled mess.

Learning to spend time with emotions is the secret to learning how to feel and otherwise experience emotions, which by the end of the day leads to some emotional closure, the absence of racing thoughts, and pleasurable sleepiness at bedtime, all of which dissolves insomnia into nothingness.

Beyond this simple perspective, there are many advanced emotion-focused therapy techniques to be considered, but the most important thing to reckon with in your search is to avoid "talk therapy." Sadly, this form of therapy is a common technique provided nowadays among mental health professionals.

It is an unfortunate state of health culture that talk therapy remains such a common approach to mental health care because "talking" is a much lower level of therapy. It tends to work only for very mild mental health symptoms, those not having taken on a chronic character. For example, you are in conflict with your boss for the past three months only, and you need to chat with an independent person to discuss and clarify the steps you need to improve the relationship. Such a conflict might respond well to talk therapy, but if the conflict has been recurring for years and with different bosses, then it is a chronic condition that will require a much more intensive therapy, such as EFT or other relatively newer emotion-informed approaches.

Generally, when therapy sessions recur as two talking heads, there is a high probability for emotions to be left out of the dialogue unless the therapist specifically asks the individual to pause from speaking and instead pay attention to what is being felt, somewhere in the body, not just the head. Emotion-centric therapists routinely ask the patient to describe their emotional experiences to guide the dialogue. Such therapies as Greenberg's *emotion-focused therapy* or Peter A. Levine's *somatic reexperiencing* are two well-known therapies that go far beyond the talk therapy model of care.

Finding a professional with this type of training and approach to mental health care holds the potential for dramatic changes in emotional reactivity and subsequent improvements in emotional processing. The patient typically notices immediate reductions or cures in chronic insomnia. Learning to sleep like a baby again is consistent with learning how to process emotions so well during the day that emotional closure occurs night after night.

Starting with Insomnia: Last Choice: Alternative Medicine (External Solutions)

Some patients cannot get past the idea sleep problems must be addressed with medication. My point is not to judge; rather, I want to be clear that if you must start with a medication, it is far better to consider a supplement or over-the-counter medication because the chances of you becoming dependent on or, even worse, addicted to the drug are much less than if starting with prescription sedatives or other sedating agents such as antidepressants.

Remember, seeking to improve sleep continuity is the most common reason patients use a medication, accompanied by the mistaken belief more sleep hours guarantees improved sleep quality. Thus, a drug that works great on sleep continuity, which many prescription sedatives can achieve for a while, will make it more likely the patient keeps using the drug night after night even if sleep quality does not improve.

Nonprescription pills, supplements, or herbal remedies may yield enough relief to move in the right direction while you work on other sleep disorders—the real source of your sleep problems. For example, many patients use low-dose melatonin for years and receive some benefits. When these patients visit a sleep center, they discover it is much easier to taper off the melatonin when other sleep disorders are treated. Or they may discover continuing the melatonin works well for them while using PAP therapy or treating leg jerks. In contrast, with a similar scenario involving drugs like Ambien or Lunesta, the individual may face a serious struggle attempting to taper off these prescription sleeping pills.

Why is this issue such a big deal? Simply, prescription sleeping pills are much more likely to interfere with the depth of your sleep and therefore prevent you from ever attaining an optimal response from your sleep disorders' treatment regimen. Chances are high you have already tried prescription sedatives or other sedating psychotropic medications, and some patients will already be hooked on them despite years of mediocre results while using them.

For all these reasons, starting with a less intense drug therapy such as herbal remedies, over-the-counter sleep aids, or supplements like melatonin or magnesium is a better way to start a medication approach if you must start with an external treatment.

Starting with Nightmare Therapy

Last, let's introduce a unique circumstance for the individual suffering from chronic nightmares. It is remarkable how many individuals with the combination of mental health and sleep complaints also suffer chronic disturbing dreams and nightmares. For the most part, the typical patient will not report nightmares as the major sleep disorder. Yet a sizeable number do in fact describe nightmares as the worst thing during the night, because vexing dreams trigger daytime fears about going to sleep at bedtime or about returning to sleep after a nightmare awakening in the middle of the night.

Nightmares really are a primary sleep disorder, and among mental health patients in general or those with concurrent suicidal ideation, nightmare problems are quite prevalent and distressing enough for the individual to tackle this problem first. In just the past few years, more research is clearly associating nightmare problems with suicidal thinking; and, as a result, more research studies are underway with the specific intent to determine whether treatment of nightmares will reduce suicidal behaviors or thoughts. In fact, some of this research explores nightmare treatment as first-line therapy.

If you now return to Chapter 16, you will learn about the surprising advances in the field showing six different pathways to treat chronic nightmares, compared to about 50 years ago when the total number of treatments basically added up to zero.

In my own clinical experience, I have seen fantastic results in those individuals who chose to start by addressing chronic nightmares. Overcoming this condition appeared to open a doorway to a global realization for the necessity to treat all sleep disorders. In these patients, nightmare treatment proved the perfect quick start.

Since entering the field of sleep medicine in 1988, working with psychiatrists on nightmare treatment research, I gained more years observing patients undergo nightmare therapy compared to any other sleep disorder treatment. Seeing astonishing therapeutic results time and again, I can give a ringing endorsement for the first-step use of Imagery Rehearsal Therapy.

APPENDIX C

LIST OF REFERENCES

1. Reynolds CF, III, O'Hara R. DSM-5 sleep-wake disorders classification: overview for use in clinical practice. *Am J Psychiatry* 2013;170:1099-1101.
2. Jessen NA, Munk AS, Lundgaard I, Nedergaard M. The Glymphatic System: A Beginner's Guide. *Neurochem Res* 2015;40:2583-2599.
3. Underwood E. Sleep: The Ultimate Brainwasher? Science . 2013. 10-17-2013. Online Source https://www.science.org/content/article/sleep-ultimate-brainwasher.
4. Walker MP, van der Helm E. Overnight therapy? The role of sleep in emotional brain processing. *Psychol Bull* 2009;135:731-748.
5. Ju YS, Zangrilli MA, Finn MB, Fagan AM, Holtzman DM. Obstructive sleep apnea treatment, slow wave activity, and amyloid-beta. *Ann Neurol* 2019;85:291-295.
6. Ju YS, Ooms SJ, Sutphen C et al. Slow wave sleep disruption increases cerebrospinal fluid amyloid-beta levels. *Brain* 2017;140:2104-2111.
7. Krakow B, Ulibarri VA, Romero EA. Patients with treatment-resistant insomnia taking nightly prescription medications for sleep: a retrospective assessment of diagnostic and treatment variables. *Prim Care Companion J Clin Psychiatry* 2010;12(4):e1-e10.
8. Krakow B, Ulibarri VA, Romero E. Persistent insomnia in chronic hypnotic users presenting to a sleep medical center: a retrospective chart review of 137 consecutive patients. *J Nerv Ment Dis* 2010;198:734-741.
9. Krakow B, Ulibarri VA, McIver ND. Pharmacotherapeuti failure in a large cohort of patients with insomnia presenting to a sleep medicine center and laboratory: subjective pretest predictions and objective diagnoses. *Mayo Clin Proc* 2014;89:1608-1620.
10. Wu D, Tong M, Ji Y et al. REM Sleep Fragmentation in Patients With Short-Term Insomnia Is Associated With Higher BDI Scores. *Front Psychiatry* 2021;12:733998.

11. Scullin MK, Gao C. Dynamic Contributions of Slow Wave Sleep and REM Sleep to Cognitive Longevity. *Curr Sleep Med Rep* 2018;4:284-293.

12. Pesonen AK, Gradisar M, Kuula L et al. REM sleep fragmentation associated with depressive symptoms and genetic risk for depression in a community-based sample of adolescents. *J Affect Disord* 2019;245:757-763.

13. Krakow B, Germain A, Tandberg D et al. Sleep breathing and sleep movement disorders masquerading as insomnia in sexual-assault survivors. *Compr Psychiatry* 2000;41:49-56.

14. Krakow B, Melendrez D, Warner TD, Dorin R, Harper R, Hollifield M. To breathe, perchance to sleep: sleep-disordered breathing and chronic insomnia among trauma survivors. *Sleep Breath* 2002;6:189-202.

15. Krakow B. *Sound Sleep, Sound Mind: 7 Keys to Sleeping through the Night.* New York: John Wiley & Sons, 2007.

16. Sarah Kershaw. Following a Script to Escape a Nightmare. *New York Times* 2010. https://www.nytimes.com/2010/07/27/health/27night.html.

17. Daniel Goleman. Tormented by Nightmares? Rehearse a Different Ending. *New York Times* 1992. https://www.nytimes.com/1992/06/24/news/tormented-by-nightmares-rehearse-a-different-ending.html?smid=url-share.

18. Margaret Talbot. Nightmare Scenario. *New Yorker.* 2009. 11-8-2009. Magazine Article https://www.newyorker.com/magazine/2009/11/16/nightmare-scenario.

19. John Cloud. Nightmare Scenario: Bad dreams can do more than ruin a good night's sleep. Scientists are finding new ways to control them--and improve the health of mind and body. *Time.* 2012. 7-9-2012. Magazine Article http://content.time.com/time/subscriber/article/0,33009,2118290-3,00.html.

20. Krakow B, Hollifield M, Johnston L et al. Imagery rehearsal therapy for chronic nightmares in sexual assault survivors with posttraumatic stress disorder: a randomized controlled trial. *JAMA* 2001;286:537-545.

21. Krakow B, Johnston L, Melendrez D et al. An open-label trial of evidence-based cognitive behavior therapy for nightmares and insomnia in crime victims with PTSD. *Am J Psychiatry* 2001;158:2043-2047.

22. Kellner R, Neidhardt J, Krakow B, Pathak D. Changes in chronic nightmares after one session of desensitization or rehearsal instructions. *Am J Psychiatry* 1992;149:659-663.

23. Krakow BJ, Melendrez DC, Johnston LG et al. Sleep Dynamic Therapy for Cerro Grande Fire evacuees with posttraumatic stress symptoms: a preliminary report. *J Clin Psychiatry* 2002;63:673-684.

24. Krakow B, Hollifield M, Schrader R et al. A controlled study of imagery rehearsal for chronic nightmares in sexual assault survivors with PTSD: a preliminary report. *J Trauma Stress* 2000;13:589-609.

25. Krakow B, Tandberg D, Scriggins L, Barey M. A controlled comparison of self-rated sleep complaints in acute and chronic nightmare sufferers. *J Nerv Ment Dis* 1995;183:623-627.

26. Krakow B, Melendrez D, Ferreira E et al. Prevalence of insomnia symptoms in patients with sleep-disordered breathing. *Chest* 2001;120:1923-1929.

27. Neidhardt EJ, Krakow B, Kellner R, Pathak D. The beneficial effects of one treatment session and recording of nightmares on chronic nightmare sufferers. *Sleep* 1992;15:470-473.

28. Krakow B. Nightmare complaints in treatment-seeking patients in clinical sleep medicine settings: diagnostic and treatment implications. *Sleep* 2006;29:1313-1319.

29. Krakow B, Romero E, Ulibarri VA, Kikta S. Prospective assessment of nocturnal awakenings in a case series of treatment-seeking chronic insomnia patients: a pilot study of subjective and objective causes. *Sleep* 2012;35:1685-1692.

30. Krakow B, Melendrez D, Lee SA, Warner TD, Clark JO, Sklar D. Refractory insomnia and sleep-disordered breathing: a pilot study. *Sleep Breath* 2004;8:15-29.

31. Krakow B, Ulibarri VA. Prevalence of sleep breathing complaints reported by treatment-seeking chronic insomnia disorder patients on presentation to a sleep medical center: a preliminary report. *Sleep Breath* 2013;17:317-322.

32. Gieselmann A, Ait AM, Carr M et al. Aetiology and treatment of

nightmare disorder: State of the art and future perspectives. *J Sleep Res* 2019;28:e12820.

33.   Morin CM, Benca R. Chronic insomnia. *Lancet* 2012;379:1129-1141.

34.   Schutte-Rodin S, Broch L, Buysse D, Dorsey C, Sateia M. Clinical guideline for the evaluation and management of chronic insomnia in adults. *J Clin Sleep Med* 2008;4:487-504.

35.   Wu JQ, Appleman ER, Salazar RD, Ong JC. Cognitive behavioral therapy for insomnia comorbid with psychiatric and medical conditions: a meta-analysis. *JAMA Intern Med* 2015;175:1461-1472.

36.   Youakim JM, Doghramji K, Schutte SL. Posttraumatic stress disorder and obstructive sleep apnea syndrome. *Psychosomatics* 1998;39:168-171.

37.   Krakow B, Lowry C, Germain A et al. A retrospective study on improvements in nightmares and post-traumatic stress disorder following treatment for co-morbid sleep-disordered breathing. *J Psychosom Res* 2000;49:291-298.

38.   Krakow B, Ulibarri VA, Romero EA, McIver ND. A two-year prospective study on the frequency and co-occurrence of insomnia and sleep-disordered breathing symptoms in a primary care population. *Sleep Med* 2013;14:814-823.

39.   Krakow B, Ulibarri VA, Romero EA, Thomas RJ, McIver ND. Adaptive servo-ventilation therapy in a case series of patients with co-morbid insomnia and sleep apnea. *Journal of Sleep Disorders: Treatment and Care* 2013;2:1-10.

40.   Krakow B. An emerging interdisciplinary sleep medicine perspective on the high prevalence of co-morbid sleep-disordered breathing and insomnia. *Sleep Med* 2004;5:431-433.

41.   Krakow BJ, McIver ND, Obando JJ, Ulibarri VA. Changes in insomnia severity with advanced PAP therapy in patients with posttraumatic stress symptoms and comorbid sleep apnea: a retrospective, nonrandomized controlled study. *Mil Med Res* 2019;6:15.

42.   Krakow B, Melendrez D, Pedersen B et al. Complex insomnia: insomnia and sleep-disordered breathing in a consecutive series of crime victims with nightmares and PTSD. *Biol Psychiatry* 2001;49:948-953.

43.   Krakow B, Melendrez D, Sisley B et al. Nasal dilator strip therapy for chronic sleep-maintenance insomnia and symptoms of sleep-disordered breathing: a randomized controlled trial. *Sleep Breath* 2006;10:16-28.

44.   Krakow B, Melendrez D, Sisley B, Warner TD, Krakow J. Nasal dilator strip therapy for chronic sleep maintenance insomnia: a case series. *Sleep Breath* 2004;8:133-140.

45.   Krakow B, Haynes PL, Warner TD et al. Nightmares, insomnia, and sleep-disordered breathing in fire evacuees seeking treatment for posttraumatic sleep disturbance. *J Trauma Stress* 2004;17:257-268.

46.   Krakow BJ. Physiologic sleep disorders among treatment-responsive depressed patients with residual cognitive and physical symptoms. *J Clin Psychiatry* 2007;68:1444-1445.

47.   Krakow B, Krakow J, Eberle F. Polysomnography in sleep maintenance insomnia patients. *Ann Clin Psychiatry* 2007;19:53-54.

48.   Krakow BJ, Obando JJ, Ulibarri VA, McIver ND. Positive airway pressure adherence and subthreshold adherence in posttraumatic stress disorder patients with comorbid sleep apnea. *Patient Prefer Adherence* 2017;11:1923-1932.

49.   Krakow BJ, Ulibarri VA, Moore BA, McIver ND. Posttraumatic stress disorder and sleep-disordered breathing: a review of comorbidity research. *Sleep Med Rev* 2015;24:37-45.

50.   Reist C, Gory A, Hollifield M, Krakow B. Potential benefit of sleep assessment prior to PTSD treatment. *Psychiatry Res* 2018;262:354-355.

51.   Krakow B, McIver ND, Ulibarri VA. Respiratory arousal control needed for insomnia OSA patients-authors' reply. *EClinicalMedicine* 2019;17:100207.

52.   Krakow B, McIver ND, Ulibarri VA, Nadorff MR. Retrospective, nonrandomized controlled study on autoadjusting, dual-pressure positive airway pressure therapy for a consecutive series of complex insomnia disorder patients. *Nat Sci Sleep* 2017;9:81-95.

53.   Krakow B, Ulibarri VA, McIver ND et al. Reversal of PAP Failure With the REPAP Protocol. *Respir Care* 2017;62:396-408.

54.   Krakow B, Melendrez D, Warner TD et al. Signs and symptoms of

sleep-disordered breathing in trauma survivors: a matched comparison with classic sleep apnea patients. *J Nerv Ment Dis* 2006;194:433-439.

55.   Krakow B, Melendrez D, Johnston L et al. Sleep-disordered breathing, psychiatric distress, and quality of life impairment in sexual assault survivors. *J Nerv Ment Dis* 2002;190:442-452.

56.   McIver ND, Krakow B, Krakow J, Nadorff MR, Ulibarri VA, Baade R. Sleep disorder prevalence in at-risk adolescents and potential effects of nightmare triad syndrome. *Int J Adolesc Med Health* 2018;32(1).

57.   Krakow B, Artar A, Warner TD et al. Sleep disorder, depression, and suicidality in female sexual assault survivors. *Crisis* 2000;21:163-170.

58.   Mysliwiec V, Gill J, Lee H et al. Sleep disorders in US military personnel: a high rate of comorbid insomnia and obstructive sleep apnea. *Chest* 2013;144:549-557.

59.   Krakow B, Germain A, Warner TD et al. The relationship of sleep quality and posttraumatic stress to potential sleep disorders in sexual assault survivors with nightmares, insomnia, and PTSD. *J Trauma Stress* 2001;14:647-665.

60.   Krakow B, McIver ND, Ulibarri VA, Krakow J, Schrader RM. Prospective Randomized Controlled Trial on the Efficacy of Continuous Positive Airway Pressure and Adaptive Servo-Ventilation in the Treatment of Chronic Complex Insomnia. *EClinicalMedicine* 2019;13:57-73.

61.   McCall CA, Watson NF. A Narrative Review of the Association between Post-Traumatic Stress Disorder and Obstructive Sleep Apnea. *J Clin Med* 2022;11.

62.   Colvonen PJ, Rivera GL, Straus LD et al. Diagnosing obstructive sleep apnea in a residential treatment program for veterans with substance use disorder and PTSD. *Psychol Trauma* 2022;14:178-185.

63.   Lyons R, Barbir LA, Owens R, Colvonen PJ. STOP-BANG screener vs objective obstructive sleep apnea testing among younger veterans with PTSD and insomnia: STOP-BANG does not sufficiently detect risk. *J Clin Sleep Med* 2022;18:67-73.

64.   Fehr BS, Katz WF, Van Enkevort EA, Khawaja IS. Obstructive Sleep Apnea in Posttraumatic Stress Disorder Comorbid With Mood

Disorder: Significantly Higher Incidence Than in Either Diagnosis Alone. *Prim Care Companion CNS Disord* 2018;20.

65. El-Solh AA, Adamo D, Kufel T. Comorbid insomnia and sleep apnea in Veterans with post-traumatic stress disorder. *Sleep Breath* 2018;22:23-31.

66. Zhang Y, Weed JG, Ren R, Tang X, Zhang W. Prevalence of obstructive sleep apnea in patients with posttraumatic stress disorder and its impact on adherence to continuous positive airway pressure therapy: a meta-analysis. *Sleep Med* 2017;36:125-132.

67. Lee HJ, Lee DA, Shin KJ, Park KM. Glymphatic system dysfunction in obstructive sleep apnea evidenced by DTI-ALPS. *Sleep Med* 2022;89:176-181.

68. Ju YE, Finn MB, Sutphen CL et al. Obstructive sleep apnea decreases central nervous system-derived proteins in the cerebrospinal fluid. *Ann Neurol* 2016;80:154-159.

69. Wassing R, Lakbila-Kamal O, Ramautar JR, Stoffers D, Schalkwijk F, Van Someren EJW. Restless REM Sleep Impedes Overnight Amygdala Adaptation. *Curr Biol* 2019;29:2351-2358.

70. Memon J, Manganaro SN. Obstructive Sleep-disordered Breathing. *StatPearls Publishing.* 2022.

71. Goldstein AN, Walker MP. The role of sleep in emotional brain function. *Annu Rev Clin Psychol* 2022;10:679-709.

72. Labarca G, Gower J, Lamperti L, Dreyse J, Jorquera J. Chronic intermittent hypoxia in obstructive sleep apnea: a narrative review from pathophysiological pathways to a precision clinical approach. *Sleep Breath* 2020;24:751-760.

73. Orru G, Storari M, Scano A, Piras V, Taibi R, Viscuso D. Obstructive Sleep Apnea, oxidative stress, inflammation and endothelial dysfunction- An overview of predictive laboratory biomarkers. *Eur Rev Med Pharmacol Sci* 2020;24:6939-6948.

74. Wang J, Yu W, Gao M et al. Impact of Obstructive Sleep Apnea Syndrome on Endothelial Function, Arterial Stiffening, and Serum Inflammatory Markers: An Updated Meta-analysis and Metaregression

of 18 Studies. *J Am Heart Assoc* 2015;4.

75. Gupta MA, Jarosz P. Obstructive Sleep Apnea Severity is Directly Related to Suicidal Ideation in Posttraumatic Stress Disorder. *J Clin Sleep Med* 2018;14:427-435.

76. Corfield EC, Martin NG, Nyholt DR. Co-occurrence and symptomatology of fatigue and depression. *Compr Psychiatry* 2016;71:1-10.

77. Krieger J, Laks L, Wilcox I et al. Atrial natriuretic peptide release during sleep in patients with obstructive sleep apnoea before and during treatment with nasal continuous positive airway pressure. *Clin Sci (Lond)* 1989;77:407-411.

78. Guilleminault C, Stoohs R, Kim YD, Chervin R, Black J, Clerk A. Upper airway sleep-disordered breathing in women. *Ann Intern Med* 1995;122:493-501.

79. Guilleminault C, Lin CM, Goncalves MA, Ramos E. A prospective study of nocturia and the quality of life of elderly patients with obstructive sleep apnea or sleep onset insomnia. *J Psychosom Res* 2004;56:511-515.

80. Weiss JP, Everaert K. Management of Nocturia and Nocturnal Polyuria. *Urology* 2019;133S:24-33.

81. Romero E, Krakow B, Haynes P, Ulibarri V. Nocturia and snoring: predictive symptoms for obstructive sleep apnea. *Sleep Breath* 2010;14:337-343.

82. Spalka J, Kedzia K, Kuczynski W et al. Morning Headache as an Obstructive Sleep Apnea-Related Symptom among Sleep Clinic Patients-A Cross-Section Analysis. *Brain Sci* 2020;10.

83. Ruzicka M, Knoll G, Leenen FHH, Leech J, Aaron SD, Hiremath S. Effects of CPAP on Blood Pressure and Sympathetic Activity in Patients With Diabetes Mellitus, Chronic Kidney Disease, and Resistant Hypertension. *CJC Open* 2020;2:258-264.

84. Guilleminault C, Faul JL, Stoohs R. Sleep-disordered breathing and hypotension. *Am J Respir Crit Care Med* 2001;164:1242-1247.

85. Marin JM, Carrizo SJ, Vicente E, Agusti AG. Long-term cardiovascular outcomes in men with obstructive sleep apnoea-hypopnoea with

or without treatment with continuous positive airway pressure: an observational study. *Lancet* 2005;365:1046-1053.

86. Qaseem A, Holty JE, Owens DK, Dallas P, Starkey M, Shekelle P. Management of Obstructive Sleep Apnea in Adults: A Clinical Practice Guideline From the American College of Physicians. *Ann Intern Med* 2013.

87. Lin CH, Lurie RC, Lyons OD. Sleep Apnea and Chronic Kidney Disease: A State-of-the-Art Review. *Chest* 2020;157:673-685.

88. Gold AR, Dipalo F, Gold MS, Broderick J. Inspiratory airflow dynamics during sleep in women with fibromyalgia. *Sleep* 2004;27:459-466.

89. Sabil A, Bignard R, Gerves-Pinquie C et al. Risk Factors for Sleepiness at the Wheel and Sleep-Related Car Accidents Among Patients with Obstructive Sleep Apnea: Data from the French Pays de la Loire Sleep Cohort. *Nat Sci Sleep* 2021;13:1737-1746.

90. Sharafkhaneh A, Giray N, Richardson P, Young T, Hirshkowitz M. Association of psychiatric disorders and sleep apnea in a large cohort. *Sleep* 2005;28:1405-1411.

91. Oksenberg A, Froom P, Melamed S. Dry mouth upon awakening in obstructive sleep apnea. *J Sleep Res* 2006;15:317-320.

92. Tamanna S, Campbell D, Warren R, Ullah MI. Effect of CPAP Therapy on Symptoms of Nocturnal Gastroesophageal Reflux among Patients with Obstructive Sleep Apnea. *J Clin Sleep Med* 2016;12:1257-1261.

93. Mun JK, Choi SJ, Kang MR, Hong SB, Joo EY. Sleep and libido in men with obstructive sleep apnea syndrome. *Sleep Med* 2018;52:158-162.

94. Pascual M, de BJ, Barbe F et al. Erectile dysfunction in obstructive sleep apnea patients: A randomized trial on the effects of Continuous Positive Airway Pressure (CPAP). *PLoS One* 2018;13:e0201930.

95. Mariman A, Delesie L, Tobback E et al. Undiagnosed and comorbid disorders in patients with presumed chronic fatigue syndrome. *J Psychosom Res* 2013;75:491-496.

96. Pan T, Liu S, Ke S, Wang E, Jiang Y, Wang S. Association of obstructive sleep apnea with cognitive decline and age among non-demented older adults. *Neurosci Lett* 2021;756:135955.

97. Seda G, Matwiyoff G, Parrish JS. Effects of Obstructive Sleep Apnea and CPAP on Cognitive Function. *Curr Neurol Neurosci Rep* 2021;21:32.

98. Lusic KL, Pavlinac D, I, Pecotic R, Valic M, Dogas Z. Psychomotor Performance in Patients with Obstructive Sleep Apnea Syndrome. *Nat Sci Sleep* 2020;12:183-195.

99. Slowik JM, Collen JF. Obstructive Sleep Apnea. *StatPearls Publishing*, 2022.

100. Berry RB, Sriram P. Auto-adjusting positive airway pressure treatment for sleep apnea diagnosed by home sleep testing. *J Clin Sleep Med* 2014;10:1269-1275.

101. Johnson PL, Edwards N, Burgess KR, Sullivan CE. Detection of increased upper airway resistance during overnight polysomnography. *Sleep* 2005;28:85-90.

102. Pevernagie DA, Gnidovec-Strazisar B, Grote L et al. On the rise and fall of the apnea-hypopnea index: A historical review and critical appraisal. *J Sleep Res* 2020;29:e13066.

103. Galbiati A, Sforza M, Fasiello E et al. The association between emotional dysregulation and REM sleep features in insomnia disorder. *Brain Cogn* 2020;146:105642.

104. Guilleminault C, Winkle R, Korobkin R, Simmons B. Children and nocturnal snoring: evaluation of the effects of sleep related respiratory resistive load and daytime functioning. *Eur J Pediatr* 1982;139:165-171.

105. Guilleminault C, Stoohs R, Clerk A, Cetel M, Maistros P. A cause of excessive daytime sleepiness. The upper airway resistance syndrome. *Chest* 1993;104:781-787.

106. Ruehland WR, Rochford PD, O'Donoghue FJ, Pierce RJ, Singh P, Thornton AT. The new AASM criteria for scoring hypopneas: impact on the apnea hypopnea index. *Sleep* 2009;32:150-157.

107. Younes M, Azarbarzin A, Reid M, Mazzotti DR, Redline S. Characteristics and reproducibility of novel sleep EEG biomarkers and their variation with sleep apnea and insomnia in a large community-based cohort. *Sleep* 2021;44.

108. Younes M, Schweitzer PK, Griffin KS, Balshaw R, Walsh JK. Comparing two measures of sleep depth/intensity. *Sleep* 2020;43.

109. Zeineddine S, Rowley JA, Chowdhuri S. Oxygen Therapy in Sleep-Disordered Breathing. *Chest* 2021;160:701-717.

110. Gozal E, Sachleben LR, Jr., Rane MJ, Vega C, Gozal D. Mild sustained and intermittent hypoxia induce apoptosis in PC-12 cells via different mechanisms. *Am J Physiol Cell Physiol* 2005;288:C535-C542.

111. Sanders MH, Kern N. Obstructive sleep apnea treated by independently adjusted inspiratory and expiratory positive airway pressures via nasal mask. Physiologic and clinical implications. *Chest* 1990;98:317-324.

112. Krakow B, Ulibarri V, Melendrez D, Kikta S, Togami L, Haynes P. A daytime, abbreviated cardio-respiratory sleep study (CPT 95807-52) to acclimate insomnia patients with sleep disordered breathing to positive airway pressure (PAP-NAP). *J Clin Sleep Med* 2008;4:212-222.

113. Ulibarri VA, Krakow B, McIver ND. The PAP-NAP one decade later: patient risk factors, indications, and clinically relevant emotional and motivational influences on PAP use. *Sleep Breath* 2020;24:1427-1440.

114. Krakow B, Foley-Shea M, Ulibarri VA, McIver ND, Honsinger R. Prevalence of potential nonallergic rhinitis at a community-based sleep medical center. *Sleep Breath* 2016;20:987-993.

115. Koufman JA. Laryngopharyngeal reflux is different from classic gastroesophageal reflux disease. *Ear Nose Throat J* 2002;81:7-9.

116. Dicus Brookes CC, Boyd SB. Controversies in Obstructive Sleep Apnea Surgery. *Oral Maxillofac Surg Clin North Am* 2017;29:503-513.

117. Georgalas C. The role of the nose in snoring and obstructive sleep apnoea: an update. *Eur Arch Otorhinolaryngol* 2011;268:1365-1373.

118. Uwiera TC. Considerations in Surgical Management of Pediatric Obstructive Sleep Apnea: Tonsillectomy and Beyond. *Children (Basel)* 2021;8.

119. Friedman JJ, Salapatas AM, Bonzelaar LB, Hwang MS, Friedman M. Changing Rates of Morbidity and Mortality in Obstructive Sleep Apnea Surgery. *Otolaryngol Head Neck Surg* 2017;157:123-127.

120. Kent D, Stanley J, Aurora RN et al. Referral of adults with obstructive sleep apnea for surgical consultation: an American Academy of Sleep Medicine systematic review, meta-analysis, and GRADE assessment. *J Clin Sleep Med* 2021;17:2507-2531.

121. Li K, Quo S, Guilleminault C. Endoscopically-assisted surgical expansion (EASE) for the treatment of obstructive sleep apnea. *Sleep Med* 2019;60:53-59.

122. Chesler BE. Emotional eating: a virtually untreated risk factor for outcome following bariatric surgery. *ScientificWorldJournal* 2012;2012:365961.

123. Ming X, Yang M, Chen X. Metabolic bariatric surgery as a treatment for obstructive sleep apnea hypopnea syndrome: review of the literature and potential mechanisms. *Surg Obes Relat Dis* 2021;17:215-220.

124. Wang D, Modik O, Sturm JJ et al. Neurophysiological profiles of responders and non-responders to hypoglossal nerve stimulation: a single institution study. *J Clin Sleep Med* 2021.

125. Morse E, Han C, Suurna M. Hypoglossal Nerve Stimulator Implantation in an Ambulatory Surgery Center Versus Hospital. *Laryngoscope* 2022;132:706-710.

126. Javaheri S, Javaheri S. Update on Persistent Excessive Daytime Sleepiness in OSA. *Chest* 2020;158:776-786.

127. Nineb A, Rosso C, Dumurgier J, Nordine T, Lefaucheur JP, Creange A. Restless legs syndrome is frequently overlooked in patients being evaluated for polyneuropathies. *Eur J Neurol* 2007;14:788-792.

128. Chenini S, Barateau L, Guiraud L et al. Depressive Symptoms and Suicidal Thoughts in Restless Legs Syndrome. *Mov Disord* 2022.

129. Para KS, Chow CA, Nalamada K et al. Suicidal thought and behavior in individuals with restless legs syndrome. *Sleep Med* 2019;54:1-7.

130. Roux FJ. Restless legs syndrome: impact on sleep-related breathing disorders. *Respirology* 2013;18:238-245.

131. Exar EN, Collop NA. The association of upper airway resistance with periodic limb movements. *Sleep* 2001;24:188-192.

132. Heim B, Ellmerer P, Stefani A et al. Factors associated with

augmentation in patients with restless legs syndrome. *Eur J Neurol* 2022;29:1227-1231.

133. Bayard S, Langenier MC, Dauvilliers Y. Decision-making, reward-seeking behaviors and dopamine agonist therapy in restless legs syndrome. *Sleep* 2013;36:1501-1507.

134. Elena H, Leslie B, Skeba P, Wang A, Earley CJ, Allen RP. Effects of new PLM scoring rules on PLM rate in relation to sleep and resting wake for RLS and healthy controls. *Sleep Breath* 2021;25:381-386.

135. Winkelman JW. The evoked heart rate response to periodic leg movements of sleep. *Sleep* 1999;22:575-580.

136. Allen RP, Picchietti DL, Auerbach M et al. Evidence-based and consensus clinical practice guidelines for the iron treatment of restless legs syndrome/Willis-Ekbom disease in adults and children: an IRLSSG task force report. *Sleep Med* 2018;41:27-44.

137. Hornyak M, Voderholzer U, Hohagen F, Berger M, Riemann D. Magnesium therapy for periodic leg movements-related insomnia and restless legs syndrome: an open pilot study. *Sleep* 1998;21:501-505.

138. Marshall NS, Serinel Y, Killick R et al. Magnesium supplementation for the treatment of restless legs syndrome and periodic limb movement disorder: A systematic review. *Sleep Med Rev* 2019;48:101218.

139. Liu HM, Chu M, Liu CF, Zhang T, Gu P. Analysis of Serum Vitamin D Level and Related Factors in Patients With Restless Legs Syndrome. *Front Neurol* 2021;12:782565.

140. Kolla BP, Mansukhani MP, Bostwick JM. The influence of antidepressants on restless legs syndrome and periodic limb movements: A systematic review. *Sleep Med Rev* 2018;38:131-140.

141. Guilleminault C, Palombini L, Pelayo R, Chervin RD. Sleepwalking and sleep terrors in prepubertal children: what triggers them? *Pediatrics* 2003;111:e17-e25.

142. Guilleminault C, Kirisoglu C, Bao G, Arias V, Chan A, Li KK. Adult chronic sleepwalking and its treatment based on polysomnography. *Brain* 2005;128:1062-1069.

143. Kales JC, Cadieux RJ, Soldatos CR, Kales A. Psychotherapy with

night-terror patients. *Am J Psychother* 1982;36:399-407.

144. Ntafouli M, Galbiati A, Gazea M, Bassetti CLA, Bargiotas P. Update on nonpharmacological interventions in parasomnias. *Postgrad Med* 2020;132:72-79.

145. Schenck CH, Bundlie SR, Ettinger MG, Mahowald MW. Chronic behavioral disorders of human REM sleep: a new category of parasomnia. *Sleep* 1986;9:293-308.

146. Buskova J, Kemlink D, Ibarburu V, Nevsimalova S, Sonka K. Antidepressants substantially affect basic REM sleep characteristics in narcolepsy-cataplexy patients. *Neuro Endocrinol Lett* 2015; 36:430-433.

147. Malhotra R, Avidan AY. Neurodegenerative Disease and REM Behavior Disorder. *Curr Treat Options Neurol* 2012;14:474-492.

148. Brock MS, Powell TA, Creamer JL, Moore BA, Mysliwiec V. Trauma Associated Sleep Disorder: Clinical Developments 5 Years After Discovery. *Curr Psychiatry Rep* 2019;21:80.

149. Webster JB, Bell KR, Hussey JD, Natale TK, Lakshminarayan S. Sleep apnea in adults with traumatic brain injury: a preliminary investigation. *Arch Phys Med Rehabil* 2001;82:316-321.

150. Walters AS, Wagner ML, Hening WA et al. Successful treatment of the idiopathic restless legs syndrome in a randomized double-blind trial of oxycodone versus placebo. *Sleep* 1993;16:327-332.

151. Bodizs R, Sverteczki M, Meszaros E. Wakefulness-sleep transition: emerging electroencephalographic similarities with the rapid eye movement phase. *Brain Res Bull* 2008;76:85-89.

152. McKellar P, Simpson L. Between wakefulness and sleep: hypnagogic imagery. *Br J Psychol* 1954;45:266-276.

153. Pearson J. The human imagination: the cognitive neuroscience of visual mental imagery. *Nat Rev Neurosci* 2019;20:624-634.

154. Becker CB, Zayfert C, Anderson E. A survey of psychologists' attitudes towards and utilization of exposure therapy for PTSD. *Behav Res Ther* 2004;42:277-292.

155. Brom D, Stokar Y, Lawi C et al. Somatic Experiencing for Posttraumatic

Stress Disorder: A Randomized Controlled Outcome Study. *J Trauma Stress* 2017;30:304-312.

156. McPartland J, Miller B. Bodywork therapy systems. *Phys Med Rehabil Clin N Am* 1999;10:583-602, viii.

157. Timulak L, McElvaney J, Keogh D et al. Emotion-focused therapy for generalized anxiety disorder: An exploratory study. *Psychotherapy (Chic)* 2017;54:361-366.

158. Herrmann IR, Greenberg LS, Auszra L. Emotion categories and patterns of change in experiential therapy for depression. *Psychother Res* 2016;26:178-195.

159. Greenberg LS. Emotions, the great captains of our lives: their role in the process of change in psychotherapy. *Am Psychol* 2012;67:697-707.

160. Greenberg LS, Pascual-Leone A. Emotion in psychotherapy: a practice-friendly research review. *J Clin Psychol* 2006;62:611-630.

161. Greenberg LS, Malcolm W. Resolving unfinished business: relating process to outcome. *J Consult Clin Psychol* 2002;70:406-416.

162. Greenberg LS, Bolger E. An emotion-focused approach to the overregulation of emotion and emotional pain. *J Clin Psychol* 2001;57:197-211.

163. Greenberg LS. Ideal psychotherapy research: a study of significant change processes. *J Clin Psychol* 1999;55:1467-1480.

164. Krakow B, Krakow J, Ulibarri VA, Krakow J. Nocturnal time monitoring behavior ("clock-watching") in patients presenting to a sleep medical center with insomnia and posttraumatic stress symptoms. *J Nerv Ment Dis* 2012;200:821-825.

165. Churchill R, Moore TH, Furukawa TA et al. 'Third wave' cognitive and behavioural therapies versus treatment as usual for depression. *Cochrane Database Syst Rev* 2013;CD008705.

166. Whittall H, Pillion M, Gradisar M. Daytime sleepiness, driving performance, reaction time and inhibitory control during sleep restriction therapy for Chronic Insomnia Disorder. *Sleep Med* 2018;45:44-48.

167. Kyle SD, Miller CB, Rogers Z, Siriwardena AN, Macmahon KM, Espie CA. Sleep restriction therapy for insomnia is associated with

reduced objective total sleep time, increased daytime somnolence, and objectively impaired vigilance: implications for the clinical management of insomnia disorder. *Sleep* 2014;37:229-237.

168. McEntire DM, Kirkpatrick DR, Kerfeld MJ et al. Effect of sedative-hypnotics, anesthetics and analgesics on sleep architecture in obstructive sleep apnea. *Expert Rev Clin Pharmacol* 2014;7:787-806.

169. Seda G, Sanchez-Ortuno MM, Welsh CH, Halbower AC, Edinger JD. Comparative meta-analysis of prazosin and imagery rehearsal therapy for nightmare frequency, sleep quality, and posttraumatic stress. *J Clin Sleep Med* 2015;11:11-22.

170. Wile IS. Auto-suggested dreams as a factor in therapy. *American Journal of Orthopsychiatry* 1934;4:449-463.

171. Barrett D. The "Royal Road" Becomes a Shrewd Shortcut: The Use of Dreams in Focused Treatment. *Journal of Cognitive Psychotherapy* 2002;16.

172. BaHammam AS, Almeneessier AS. Dreams and Nightmares in Patients With Obstructive Sleep Apnea: A Review. *Front Neurol* 2019;10:1127.

173. Tamanna S, Parker JD, Lyons J, Ullah MI. The effect of continuous positive air pressure (CPAP) on nightmares in patients with posttraumatic stress disorder (PTSD) and obstructive sleep apnea (OSA). *J Clin Sleep Med* 2014;10:631-636.

174. Ter Heege FM, Mijnster T, van Veen MM et al. The clinical relevance of early identification and treatment of sleep disorders in mental health care: protocol of a randomized control trial. *BMC Psychiatry* 2020;20:331.

175. Lopez R, Barateau L, Evangelista E, Dauvilliers, Y. Depression and Hypersomnia: A Complex Association. 2017 Sep;12(3):395-405. *Sleep Med Clin* 2017;12:395-405.

176. McCall WV, Benca RM, Rosenquist PB et al. Reducing Suicidal Ideation Through Insomnia Treatment (REST-IT): A Randomized Clinical Trial. *Am J Psychiatry* 2019;176:957-965.

177. Drapeau CW, Nadorff MR. Suicidality in sleep disorders: prevalence, impact, and management strategies. *Nat Sci Sleep* 2017;9:213-226.

178. Rabbi Yaakov Culi. Shemot/Parasht Yitro. *Meam Loez*. 1730;17.

179. Frankl VE. Basic concepts of logotherapy. *Confin Psychiatr* 1961;4:99-109.

180. Moshe Rabbeinu. Deuteronomy 30:19. *Chumash*. 1312.

181. Krakow B, Ulibarri VA, Foley-Shea MR, Tidler A, McIver ND. Adherence and Subthreshold Adherence in Sleep Apnea Subjects Receiving Positive Airway Pressure Therapy: A Retrospective Study Evaluating Differences in Adherence Versus Use. *Respir Care* 2016;61:1023-1032.

182. Bao G, Guilleminault C. Upper airway resistance syndrome--one decade later. *Curr Opin Pulm Med* 2004;10:461-467.

INDEX

A

ABPAP (auto-adjusting bilevel) therapy, 72–74, 78, 80, 301, 321-323

acceptance and commitment therapy, 264

adaptive servo-ventilation (ASV), 72–74, 94, 320–21, 322, 323

Adderall, 274

aerophagia, 94, 134, 337–40

Afrin nasal spray, 98

AIRMAX nasal dilator, 102, 277

airway collapse, in sleep-disordered breathing, 18
    graphics, 66, 67

allergic rhinitis (AR), 97–101, 340, 355-356

Ambien, 132, 364

American Academy of Dental Sleep Medicine, 105

American Academy of Sleep Medicine, 30, 57

American Psychiatric Association, xxiii

anger, processing, 186–87, 194

antidepressants
    emotional processing, 190
    hypersomnia, 273
    leg movement disorders, 137–39, 269
    PLMD, 124, 126, 137–39
    REM suppression, 41, 118
    sleep, 40, 141, 272

APAP (auto-CPAP), 307, 320

apnea, sleep, 17–18, 19–20, 26–27, 325
    missing the diagnosis, 300-31
    treating nightmares, 255–56

apnea-hypopnea index (AHI), 38, 42–43, 49, 56–57, 62, 73,
    SDB severity, 34–35

arousals,
    breathing events, 34, 49, 328
    fragmented sleep, 53–55
    leg movement disorders, 126, 133
    spontaneous, 55

Astelin nasal spray, 100, 340

Astepro nasal spray, 100, 340

atrial natriuretic peptide (ANP), 25–26

Atrovent nasal spray, 100, 340

attitude, in coping with sleep disorders, 281–82

augmentation, in leg movement disorders, 128-129, 132, 136, 270, 358

aural imagery, for insomnia, 239

auto-adjusting pressures, See PAP Therapy, ABPAP, ASV

avoidance behavior, 163, 173
    mental health, 179–80
    PTSD, 180, 217–18

awakenings, in fragmented sleep, 52–53
    alertness following, 29
    middle of night, 228, 236
    PAP therapy decreases, 68, 74, 333
    sleeping pills, 268

special categories of, 54–55

use of imagery after, 210

B

bad/broken sleep, effect on the mind, xxiii, 1–8

graphic, 63, *64*

Beck, Aaron, 222

Berlin, Irving, 299

Bleep Basic PAP mask, 86, 88, 309

"brain-washing," 1, 5, 18, 38, 276, 279, 304–5

breathing, complexity in SDB, 24–31

breathing, influence on sleep disorders, 16–23

breathing exercises, for insomnia, 239

Breeze PAP mask, 309

bruxism, sleep, 145

Buteyko breathing, 239

C

caffeine, for hypersomnia, 119, 274, 278

excess signals sleep disorder, 21

carbon dioxide (CO_2), in PAP therapy, 312

case studies

Albert, insomnia, 195–200, 208–9

C-Flex patient, 77–78

Claire, fatigue and sleepiness, 62–63

Esmeralda, insomnia, 146–47

female sexual assault survivors, 30–31

imagery rehearsal therapy, 166–67

Janet, insomnia and nightmares, 201–6, 208–9, 211–12, 215–18

leg jerks and oral appliance therapy, 138

PAP-NAP therapy for EPI, 93–95

PTSD patients with OSA or UARS, 23

trauma survivors versus average sleep center patients, 31

Vietnam veteran, PTSD and nightmares, 14–15

cataplexy, 271–72

catharsis, 221–22

central sleep apnea (CSA), 17–18, 50-51, 73

clock-watching, in insomnia, 234–36

Clonazepam, 132, 142

cognitive-behavioral therapy (CBT), 222–23

for insomnia (CBT-I), 218, 224–41, 302, 360–61

Colorku, 238–39

complex insomnia, 23

CPAP (continuous positive air pressure) therapy

auto-, 71, 77, 81, 307

failures, 68–70, 76

pressure intolerance in, 71–72

treat OSA/UARS, 65–66, 71–73, 320–21

creative destruction, and change, 32

Crosby, Bing, 299

D

daily activities, in coping with sleep disorders, 287–89

Damon, Matt, 297

daytime sleepiness, stimulants for, 119–20

delta sleep, 35–37, 331

   definition, 5-7

   graphics, measurement of, 44, *58, 59*

   normalizing levels, 148, 265, 279

   pharmaceutical drugs, 41,266-267

   response to PAP, 61, 301

   sleep-disordered breathing, 18, 20, 23, 38

   sleep fragmentation, 10-11, 53

depression, with hypersomnia, 273–74

depth of sleep, *58,* 59, 140

Diagnostic and Statistical Manual of Mental

   Disorders, Version 5, sleep disorders

     under, xxiii–xxiv

dialectical behavioral therapy, 264

diaphragmatic breathing, for insomnia, 239

disordered sleep, effect on the mind and

   body, 1–8, 28-29

dopamine derivatives, for leg movement

   disorders, 128–30, 134

dream therapy, 250–53

durable medical equipment (DME)

   companies, 81–84, 310, 311, 340–44

E

Eclipse DreamPort PAP mask, 86

electroencephalography (EEG), in sleep

   diagnosis, 3, 44, 51-54, 126

Ellis, Albert, 222

emotional intel, 195, 199

   connecting to real-time emotions, 187–89

emotional processing

   artichoke analogy, 214–15

   cascading emotions in, 212–14

   correct method, 183–85

   PAP therapy, 219–20

   self-contained, 195–200

emotion-focused therapy (EFT), 168–81,

   190–91

   insomnia, 169–81, 361–63

   sleep-related, 182–91

     applying in insomnia, 192–223

   three steps, 170-174, 179, 184, 196, 198

   weight loss, 113

emotions

   connecting emotional intel, 187–89

   feeling negative, 177–78

   primary vs secondary, 171, 190, 199

   purpose of, 192–93

endoscopic-assisted surgical expansion

   (EASE), 109–10

esophageal manometry, 42

Excite OSA tongue-retaining device, 121

expiratory pressure intolerance (EPI),

   71–78, 93, 325–27

expiratory pressure relief, in PAP therapy,

   320

eye movement desensitization and

   reprocessing (EMDR), 257, 292

F

fear, processing, 194–95

feeling, vs thinking about feeling, 172–73,

   177–78, 185, 220–21

feelings, location of, 173–77, 182

flow limitation event (FLE), 34, 42, 49,

   50-54, 62, 65

graphic, 66, *67*

pressurized air, 69, 73, 77–78, 320, 325, 330

surgical failure, 109

See also RERA, UARS

forgiveness, in coping with sleep disorders, 295–96, 298–99

4-7-8 breathing, for insomnia, 239

Fragmentation, *See* sleep fragmentation

Frankl, Viktor, 291

Freud, Sigmund, 221, 222

full face mask (FFM), 85, 309–10, 313, 316, 349–50

   advantages of, 316–17

G

GABA derivatives, for leg movement disorders, 131–32

gastroesophageal reflux disease (GERD), 94

Gehrig, Lou, 294

GGZ Drenthe Mental Health Institute, 271

glymphatic system, 279, 304–6

Good Will Hunting, 297

Gozal, David, 61

graphics

   airway collapse, 66, *67*

   sleep, 44–46

   sleep breathing, 47–51

   sleep fragmentation, 51–54

gratitude, in coping with sleep disorders, 293–95

Greenberg, Leslie, 190, 363

Guilleminault, Christian, 42, 49, 141

guilt, and shame, in trauma survivors, 295–97

H

headaches

   morning, OSA/SDB, 27–28, 146

   tension, 184

Hickman, Lynne, 93

Hollifield, Michael, 244, 247

home medical equipment (HME)

   companies, 81–84, 340–44

home sleep test (HST), 33–34, 84

Horizant, 131

humidifiers, in PAP therapy, 335–37

humor, in coping with sleep disorders, 282–85

HVNSleep Pod, 121

hydrocodone, 130

hypersomnia

   depression, 273–74

   medications for, 271–73, 274–75

hypnagogic imagery, 162

hypoglossal nerve stimulator (HGNS), 115–17

hypoxia, 61, 111

I

I Love Lucy, 283

identity formation, through work, 285–86

idiopathic hypersomnia (IHS), 272, 277

imagery rehearsal therapy (IRT), for nightmares, 246–48, 257–58, 259–60, 365

   and dream therapy, 251–53

tips on use, 248–49

imagery distraction (mind's eye), 150–51,
    156–67
    daytime practice of, 159–61
    for insomnia, 156–57, 237–39, 359–60
    for nightmares, 163–64
    other uses of, 166–67
    in PAP therapy, 80–81
    and time monitoring behavior
        (TMB), 210–11
    unpleasant imagery in, dealing with,
        162–64

insomnia, 11–13, 13–14, 16–17, 148–51
    alternative medical treatments for,
        363–64
    aural imagery for, 239
    breathing exercises for, 239
    case studies
        Albert, 195–200, 208–9
        Esmeralda, 146–47
        Janet, with nightmares, 201–6, 208–9,
            211–12, 215–18
    CBT-I for, 360–61
    clock-watching in, 234–36
    cognitive behavioral therapy (CBT) for,
        224–41
    complex, 23
    diaphragmatic breathing for, 239
    EFT, 169–81, 361–63
    imagery distraction and, 156–57, 237–39
    medications and, 178–79, 241
    nonlinear thinking for, 236–39
    post-awakening routines, 228–29, 230–32

SDB, 29, 224
    sleep restriction therapy (SRT) for,
        226–28, 240–41
    stimulus control in, 229–30
    TFI system and, 151–54
    time monitoring behavior (TMB) in,
        209–10, 234–36
    tracking PAP progress through, 331–33

Insomnia Cures, 232

insurance companies, coverage of sleep
    disorders, 57, 65, 280

iron (serum ferritin), in treatment of leg
    movement disorders, 134–35, 270

L

lab titration testing, 69

leg movement disorders, 124–27, 133, 331,
    357–59
    aerophagia, 338
    antidepressants and, 126, 137–39, 358
    arousals, 133
    iron (serum ferritin) in treatment of,
        134–35, 358
    L-tyrosine, in treatment of, 136
    magnesium, in treatment of, 135
    medications for, 128–32, 358
    melatonin, in treatment of, 136–37
    mental health patients, 124–25, 139,
        357–58
    natural treatments for, 133–37, 358
    opiates, in treatment of, 130, 147
    oxycodone, for treatment of, 130, 147
    parasomnias and, 140, 141

SDB, 126–27

suicidal ideation in, 124, 128, 138, 139

vitamins, in treatment of, 135

Levine, Peter A., 363

Li, Kasey, 110

logotherapy, 291

losing sleep over losing sleep (LSOLS),
208–9, 232–34

L-tyrosine, in treatment of leg movement
disorders, 136, 270

Lunesta, 364

Lyrica, 131

M

magnesium, in treatment of leg movement
disorders, 135

Maimonides Sleep Arts & Sciences, 62

maladaptive emotional processing, 186

mandibular advancement devices (MAD),
103; *See* oral appliance therapy

mandibular distraction osteogenesis
(MDO), 109–110

Man's Search for Meaning, 291

mask liners, PAP, 85–86

masks, PAP, *See* PAP masks

maxillomandibular advancement (MMA),
109–10

meaning, search for, in coping with sleep
disorders, 290–92

medical system, dealing with frustrations
of, 80–95

Medicare, 57, 327, 331, 341-343

medications

failure to resolve sleep disorders, 6–7

insomnia, 178–79

PLMD, 128–32

REM-suppressant, 118–19

restless legs syndrome, 128–32

sleep disorders, 117–20, 261–71

considerations with, 268–71

efficacy of, 266–68

sleep testing, 40

melatonin, in treatment of leg movement
disorders, 136–37

Melendrez, Dominic, 63, 66

mental health patients

avoidance behavior in, 179–80

humor, as coping mechanism in, 284–85

leg movement disorders in, 124–25, 139

nightmares in, 364–65

OSA in, 30–31, 122

SDB in, 30–31, 122

sleep disorders in, 279–80

sleep fixation pathways in, 206–8

sleep medications and, 266–67

UARS in, 30–31, 122

methadone, 130

micro-CPAP devices, 121

mind's eye imagery, *See* imagery distraction

Mirapex, 128, 146

mouth breathing, in PAP therapy, 97,
309–10, 315–16, 330

mouth taping, in PAP therapy, 319–20, 330

N

napping, 275–78, 303

OSA, 276–77

narcissistic personality disorder, 282–83

narcolepsy, 271–72

nasal cannula pressure transducer (NCPT), 33, 42

nasal dilator strip (NDS) therapy, 101–2, 356

nasal dilators, 102, 277

nasal hygiene, 96–97, 355–56

nasal pillows, 85, 309, 314, 316, 317, 339

Nasalcrom nasal spray, 98

Neidhardt, Joseph, 164, 248

Neupro, 128–29

Neurontin, 131, 146–47

Night Balance, positional therapy device, 114

night terrors, 140–42

Nightmare Treatment Summit (2016), 247

nightmares, 11–13, 13–14, 16–17, 148–51

    case studies,

        Janet, 201–6, 208–9, 211–12, 215–18

        Vietnam veteran, with PTSD, 14–15

    imagery distraction for, 163–64

    imagery rehearsal therapy (IRT) for, 246–48, 257–58, 259–60, 365

        dream therapy, 251–53

        tips on use of, 248–49

    learned behavior theory of, 245–46, 249–51

    mental health patients, 364–65

    psychotherapies for, 257

    PTSD, 243–45, 247, 253–54

    REM behavior disorder and treatment of, 258

REM sleep and, 255–56

sleep apnea and, 255–56

treatments for, 242–60, 253–55, 364–65

Noah, William, 121

nocturia, due to SDB, 24–27

nocturnal eating disorders, 144

nonallergic rhinitis (NAR), 97–101, 336, 339–40, 355-356

nonlinear thinking, for insomnia, 236–39

noradrenergic activity, 254

The Nose Knows, video series, 355

NREM (non-REM) sleep

    graphics, 44–46

    measurement of, 58–59

    See also delta sleep

Nuvigil, 274

O

obstructive sleep apnea (OSA), 17–18, 19–20; *See* also PAP therapy

    diagnosing, 32-43

    morning headaches, 28

    napping, 276–77

    nocturia, 24–27

    PTSD patients, 23

    symptoms of, 28–29

opiates, for leg movement disorders, 130, 147

oral appliance therapy (OAT), 103–5

OSCAR software, for PAP, 90, 333, 348

Overeaters Anonymous (OA), 112–13

oxycodone, for leg movement disorders, 130, 147

oxygen, breathing disorders, 60–61

oxygen desaturation, 19, 60–61

oxygen fluctuation (fragmentation), 19, 60–61

P

Pad a Check mask liners, 85, 314

PAP (positive air pressure), 65–79

  adapting to, 307–9

    myths about, 310–11

  adjusting pressure settings, 89–91

  alternatives to, 96–122

  auto-adjusting devices, 321–28

  business side of, 81–82

  CPAP, 65–66, 71–73, 320–21

  emotional processing and, 219–20

  expiratory pressure intolerance (EPI), 71–78, 93, 325–27

  fine-tuning equipment, 86–87

  humidifier in, 335–37

  imagery distraction in, 80–81

  mode, 320–21

  mouth breathing in, 97, 309–10, 315–16, 330

  mouth taping in, 319–20, 330

  nightmare treatment, 255–56

  pointers for users, 79, 87–93

  positioning during, 349–51

  pressure setting changes in, 347–49

  sleep-disordered breathing (SDB), 65–79

  troubleshooting guide (PAP Pearls, Appendix A), 307–51

  tube placement in, 334–35

PAP mask liners, 85–86

PAP masks, 83–84, 329–30

  aerophagia, 338–39

  air blasts due to, 318–19

  fitting issues, 84–86, 309–10

  leak and seal, 311–14

  liners, 314–15

  mouth leak, 318

PAP-NAP procedure, 93–95, 330–31

parasomnias, and leg movement disorders, 140, 141

parsimony, in medical research, 304

Patanase nasal spray, 100

Paxil, 118

periodic limb movement disorder (PLMD), 124–27

  aerophagia, 338

  antidepressants and, 126, 137–39

  medications for, 128–32

  natural treatments for, 133–37

  SDB, 126–27

  sleep medications, 269–70

Perlis, Michael, 275

polysomnogram (PSG) test, 34

positional OSA, 115

positional therapy, 114–15

posttraumatic stress disorder (PTSD), 11, 14–15, 142, 143–44

  avoidance behavior in, 180, 217–18

  imagery distraction and, 162–64

  nightmares in, 243–45, 247, 253–54, 259–60

  OSA and, 23

therapy in, 292

UARS and, 23

Prazosin, 245, 253–55

prescription drugs, *See* medications

pressure intolerance, in CPAP, 71–72, *See*
also EPI

Provigil, 274, 275

Prozac, 118

psychosomatic reaction, 183–84, 189–90

responding to, 185–87

psychotropic medications, for sleep
disorders, 261–71

R

racing thoughts, 148–55, 230–31

emotion driven, 169-170, 173, 178, 362

imagery to reduce, 158, 162

insomnia, 224-225, 236-237

thwarts sleepiness, 219

See Respiratory threat matrix model of
chronic insomnia

religion, in coping with sleep disorders,
289–90, 291–92, 296

REM (rapid eye movement) sleep, 35–37, 331

definition, 5, 36

fragmentation vs consolidation, 11, 18,
20, 28, 38, 53, 61, 77, 118

graphics, 46, *47*

hypoxia, 60, 111

medications, in sleep testing, 40–41

nightmares, 255–56

PAP therapy, 68-69, 74, 301, 331, 348

REM-dependent OSA, 119

quality of sleep, 6, 10, 23, 46, 61, 279

symptoms when insufficient, 11, 17, 20,
28-29, 40-41, 118, 265

REM behavior disorder (RBD), 142–43

anti-depressants, 142

Clonazepam, 142

treatment of nightmares, 258

Remeron, 118

REM-suppressant medications, 118–19

RemZzzs mask liners, 85, 88, 314

Requip, 128

ResMed PAP mask, 86, 88

respiratory disturbance index (RDI), 43,
57, 62, 66, 73, 117

respiratory effort-related arousal (RERA),
34, 328

respiratory threat matrix model of chronic
insomnia, 224

restless legs syndrome (RLS), 124–27,
357–59

antidepressants and, 126, 137–39

medications for, 128–32, 358

natural treatments for, 133–37, 358

SDB, 126–27

sleep medications, 269–70

re-titration (REPAP) testing, 69, 90

reverse polarity, 174–76, 198

rhinitis, 96, 97–101, 339–40, 355–56

Ritalin, 274

S

Safer, Stephen, 170

Schmidt-Nowara, Wolfgang, 52

self-esteem, and work, 286–87

self-talk, in emotional processing, 200

Sensimist nasal spray, 98, 100

septoplasty, 107–8

Seroquel, 266

shame, and guilt, in trauma survivors, 295–97

Sinemet, 128

sinus surgery, 107

sleep

  biological process of, 1–2

  losing, over losing sleep (LSOLS),
    208–9, 232–34

sleep apnea, 17–18, 19–20, 26–27, 325

  treating nightmares, 255–56

  See also PAP Therapy, sleep-disordered
    breathing

sleep breathing disorders, 16–23

  detecting, 20–22, 32-34, 39-43

  effect on the mind, 1–8

  severity, 34-35, 38-39

sleep breathing graphics, 47–51

sleep bruxism, 145

sleep depth, measurement of, 57–59

sleep disorders

  breathing, 16–23

  coping with, 281–300

    difficulty in, 298–99

  diagnosis of, 32–43

  vs. disturbances, 9–10

  DSM-5, xxiii–xxiv

  effect on the mind, 1–8

  four primary, 10–13

  kicking, 123–47

leg movement, 124–27, 133

media coverage of, xxiv

medications for, 117–20, 261–71

  considerations with, 268–71

  efficacy of, 266–68

mental health patients, 279–80

movement, 123–47

physical component, versus psychological,
  2–4, 6

psychotropic medications for, 261–71

screaming, 123–47

seizure, 145–46

types of, 9–15

Sleep Dynamic Therapy, 155, 239

  Quick Start (Appendix B), 352–65

sleep efficiency, 227

sleep fixation pathways, 206–8

sleep fragmentation, 10, 19, 51–54

  graphics, 44, 51–54, 64

  impact on REM and delta sleep, 11, 77,
    256

  leg jerks, 133

  nightmares and SDB, 256

  OSA/UARS, 16, 19, 38, 55, 62, 241

  oxygen therapy, 61

  poor sleep quality, 51, 56

  REM, 118

  spontaneous arousals, 55

sleep graphics, 44–46

sleep movement disorders, 123–47

sleep position, 349–51, 355–56

sleep quality, 301–6

  importance of, 2, 353–55

measurements, problems with, 55–56
necessity of, 4–6
vs. quantity, 2, 7, 301
tracking PAP progress through, 331–33
Sleep Research Pearls
#1, CPAP cures PTSD, 14–15
#2, high rates OSA/UARS in PTSD, 22–23
#3, hidden SDB in PTSD, 30–31
#4, Dr. Guilleminault and UARS, 42–43
#5, Claire's subtle UARS, 61–63
#6, discovering EPI and dual pressure therapy, 77–79
#7, development of PAP-NAP, 93–95
#8, delays in diagnosing physical sleep disorders, 121–22
#9, Esmeralda's leg movements, 146–47
#10, old vs. new approach to sleep in mental health, 154–55
#11, potent, practical use of mind's eye, 166–67
#12, avoidance behavior and mental health problems, 179–81
#13, knowing and applying psychosomatic concepts, 189–91
#14, very brief history of psychiatry and psychology, 221–23
#15, sleep restriction therapy controversy, 240–41
#16, IRT enters the healthcare scene, 259–60
#17, professional sleep and mental health collaborations, 279–80
#18, intro to Epilogue, 300
Pearl of All Pearls, 80–81
sleep restriction therapy (SRT), for insomnia, 218, 226–28, 230, 240–41
sleepiness controversy, 240-241
sleep seizure disorder, 145–46
sleep technician, 329
finding competent, 82–83
with limited experience, obstacles due to, 344–47
sleep terrors, 140–42
sleep testing
finding the best facility, 75–77
making the most of, 73–75
sleep laboratory, 39–42
titration study, tips for successful, 328–31
sleepiness
daytime, 271–73
emotional processing, 219
vs. tiredness, 174, 225–26
sleep-disordered breathing (SDB), 16–22, 355–57
breathing complexity of, 24–31
mental health patients, 30–31, 122
markers of, reliable, 22
nocturia due to, 24–27
PAP therapy for, 65–79
PLMD, 126–27
severity of, 34–35, 38–39
gauging, 44–63
symptoms of, 20–22
SleepMapper software, 333
sleep-related eating disorder (SRED), 144

sleep-related emotion-focused therapy,
182–91

sleep terrors, 140-142

sleepwalking, 123

SOLO (stop, observe, let, observe)
technique, 187

somatic reexperiencing, 363

Sound Sleep, Sound Mind, 154–55

spontaneous arousals, 55

spirituality, in coping with sleep disorders,
289–90, 251–52

Stark Law, 82

stimulants, for hypersomnia, 119–20,
274–75

stimulus control, in insomnia, 229–30, 232

Strattera, 274

stress, as code word, 171–72

suicidal ideation,
leg movement disorders, 124, 128, 132,
138, 139

losing sleep over losing sleep, 233

professional attention, 220-221, 264

REM and depression, 40

sleep fixations, 207

sleep impairment effect, 4-7, 9-10, 12, 18

sleep-disordered breathing, 20, 22, 35, 59

treating sleep disorders, 279, 352, 364-365

super sleep, 301-306

surgery for sleep apnea
jaw and dental, 109–10

nasal, throat, and sinus, 105–9

talk therapy (talking cure), 185, 222, 262,
263, 362–63

TFI (thoughts, feelings, images) system,
150–51
and insomnia, 151–54, 156–67, 224,
237

therapy, in coping with sleep disorders,
292–93

thinking, versus feeling, 172–73, 177–78,
185, 220–21

time monitoring behavior (TMB), in
insomnia, 209–10, 234–36
imagery distraction, 210–11

tiredness, versus sleepiness, 21-22, 151,
174, 225- 226, 240

tongue-retaining devices (TFDs), 104–5

tonsillectomy, 108

trauma survivors, lingering shame and guilt
in, 295–97

trauma-associated sleep disorder (TASD),
143–44

traumatic brain injury (TBI), 142–45

Trazodone, 266

tube placement, in PAP therapy, 334–35

turbinoplasty, 107–8

Turning Nightmares into Dreams workbook,
249

T

U

Ulibarri, Victor, 95

upper airway resistance syndrome (UARS),
17–18, 19–20, 42–43
home sleep testing, 33–34

morning headaches, 28

napping, 276–77

nocturia, 24–27

PTSD patients, 23

SDB severity, 38

symptoms of, 28–29

See also graphics, Figs 5.4, 5.6, 5.7,
6.1, 6.2

uvulectomy (UV), 106–7

uvulopalatopharyngoplasty (UPPP),
106–7

V

valium, 132

V-Com device, 121

vitamins, in treatment of leg movement
disorders, 135, 270

W

Wakix, 272, 275

weight loss

EFT for, 113

to reduce OSA severity, 111–14

to reduce SDB severity, 356–57

White Christmas, 299

Williams, Robin, 297

Winkelman, John, 133

work, in coping with sleep disorders,
285–87

non-work activities, 287–89

X

xylitol nasal spray, 100–101, 340

Y

Younes, Magdy, 59

ACKNOWLEDGMENTS

M y earliest encounters with physician faculty at the U. of Maryland School of Medicine (Baltimore) in the late summer of 1979 repeatedly invoked the theme: "your patients will prove your greatest library." No truer words were spoken, and I cannot thank enough thousands of patients whom we treated at Maimonides Sleep Arts & Sciences in Albuquerque since 2002. I am immeasurably grateful for the experience and knowledge they provided and was honored to have their sleep care entrusted to me and my fantastic staff.

So many of our staff and sleep technologists contributed to our understanding and our insights about the true complexity of sleep disorders in mental health patients, and they markedly enhanced our clinical and research efforts. These individuals were the driving force to maintain the operations and services of the sleep center during this past decade, and their work was greatly appreciated and indispensable. Special thanks to Brett Cunningham, Esme Dominguez, Ana Dynarski, Michelle Sturgess and Carli Yonemoto.

Similarly, the work of our many research coordinators and investigators stimulated, enlivened, and fortified our capacity to look for answers to the abundant questions the field of sleep medicine persistently raises. Special thanks to my most important research collaborators of the past decade go to Dr. Natalia McIver and Victor Ulibarri as well as contributors Shara Kikta, Dominic Melendrez, and Dr. Edward Romero.

Through this past decade, I have been blessed with so many contacts, conversations and collaborations with friends and colleagues in various sleep research fields as well as in psychiatry and psychology. I will no doubt forget some names for which I apologize in advance. However, here is at least a partial list of those who I wish to thank for their insights, contributions, and to be sure their criticisms, including Richard Allen, Robert Baade, Adam Benjafield, Marietta Bibbs, Rob Brough, Ronald Chervin, Spencer Dawson, Linda Dutcher, Fritz Eberle, Jack Edinger, Ron Escudero, Colin Espie,

Peggy Fancher, Peter Farrell, Annika Gieselmann, Avram Gold, Christian Guilleminault, Michael Hollifield, Richard Honsinger, Jean-Jacques Hosselet, Thomas Joiner, Forouz Jowkar, Leon Lack, Jaap Lancee, William Lanier, David Leech, Kasey Li, Jason Mayfield, Tom Meade, James Metz, Bret Moore, Charles Morin, Vince Mysliwiec, Michael Nadorff, Steven Park, Michael Perlis, Wilfred Pigeon, Maurizio Pompili, David Rapoport, Jena Richter, Wolfgang Schmidt-Nowara, Ron Schrader, Alan Schwartz, Richard Seligman, Roger Smith, Victor Spoormaker, Aly Suh, Robert Thomas, Alyssa Tidler, Scott Webber, Saul Wiesel, John Winkelman, Dmitri and Marianne Zaichkine. To be clear, I am not suggesting all these folks endorsed my work, my research or my book; nonetheless throughout the past decade they have provided me with a great deal of insight and wisdom and occasional sparring from their respective fields of sleep, healthcare, and psychotherapy, helping me to refine my own work.

Among those providing specific editorial assistance, I wish to thank Jerald Gottlieb, Brook Roberts, Matthew Rodgers, Victor Ulibarri, and Leonard Zema. Thanks to my Cover Crew for so much energy, creativity and inspiration in designing the front of the book. Thanks to Fritz Eberle, Penny and Larry Krakow, Reyna and Eli Mamann, Roger Smith, Stephen Safer, Bette Weigert. And a final thank you for publishing assistance from Lindsay Ahl, the team at Cascadia Author Services and Paul Tabili.

Personally, I am indebted to the support and wisdom from my family, including my wife, daughter, son and son-in-law as well as my brothers and sister and numerous cousins, nieces and nephews.

Above all else, I wish to thank our Creator for providing me with the wherewithal and knowledge to complete this book in the hopes it will provide succor to those who have suffered far too long from the misery of unrecognized and untreated sleep disorders.

ABOUT THE AUTHOR

B arry Krakow began napping daily, age 13, and continued napping another 31 years until diagnosed with UARS by Dr. Christian Guilleminault at Stanford U. Sleep Disorders Center in 1993. The trip to Stanford led to board-certification in sleep medicine in 1994. Prior to this career change from internal medicine, Dr. Krakow was providentially taken under wing in 1988 by Dr. Robert Kellner and Dr. Joseph Neidhardt (Psychiatry Department, U. of New Mexico School of Medicine) to assist in research on and development of the revolutionary intervention, "Imagery Rehearsal Therapy" for chronic nightmares.

In 1997, Dr. Krakow attempted his first UARS treatment (nasal septoplasty) and then applied Dr. Tom Meade's original Snore Guard oral appliance and later his Therasnore device. Next, he used Dr. Wayne Halstrom's Silencer device with stunning results. He wrote two books and opened a nonprofit sleep research facility, the Sleep & Human Health Institute, which received the first NIMH grant to study the impact of a disaster on trauma survivors and their sleep. In 2002 he opened a state-of-the-art sleep center, specializing in treatment for mental health patients, Maimonides Sleep Arts & Sciences. During this five year stretch, napping behavior was put to bed.

For the next decade, Dr. Krakow tested every mode of PAP therapy; and, in 2012 entered into a co-dependent relationship with the miraculous, life-saving ResMed ASV device (currently the ASVAuto mode) to gain the highest quality of slumber, energizing further efforts to pioneer treatments for mental health patients suffering from insomnia, nightmares, sleep breathing disorders, and sleep movement disorders.

Since 2017, his TEDx talk, "Why do we wake up at night?" remains one of the most popular insomnia videos posted by a practicing clinical sleep medicine specialist, approaching a million views. His newly penned Substack newsletter can be accessed at https://fastasleep.substack.com. Dr. Krakow is currently Professor of Psychiatry and Behavioral Health at Mercer U. School of Medicine, where he is collaborating in one of the first formal programs to teach sleep disorders assessments and interventions to psychiatry residents.

To learn about his Sleep Health Coaching services, please visit www. barrykrakowmd.com. He lives in Savannah, Georgia with his wife, Jessica, two dogs and a cat, all of whom enjoy a refreshing, life-saving Sabbath nap on Saturday afternoons.

www.ingramcontent.com/pod-product-compliance
Lightning Source LLC
Chambersburg PA
CBHW072059040426
42334CB00041B/1358